Making Physicians

Clio Medica

STUDIES IN THE HISTORY OF MEDICINE AND HEALTH

VOLUME 106

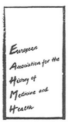

The titles published in this series are listed at *brill.com/clio*

Making Physicians

*Tradition, Teaching, and Trials at
Leiden University, 1575–1639*

VOLUME 1

By

Evan R. Ragland

BRILL

LEIDEN | BOSTON

This publication is made possible in part by support from the Institute for Scholarship in the Liberal Arts, College of Arts and Letters, the University of Notre Dame, USA.

Cover illustration: Idealized portrait of Petrus Paaw dissecting. Engraving by Andries Stock after a drawing by Jacques de Gheyn II, 1615. Credit: CC BY. Wellcome Collection, 24757i. See also Figure 12.

Volume 2: *Experimental Medicine: Anatomy, Chymistry, and Clinical Practice at Leiden University, 1639–1672*, by Evan R. Ragland. CLIO 107. Hardback ISBN: 978-90-04-51573-4; E-book ISBN: 978-90-04-51574-1.

The Library of Congress Cataloging-in-Publication Data is available online at https://catalog.loc.gov
LC record available at https://lccn.loc.gov/2022008092

Typeface for the Latin, Greek, and Cyrillic scripts: "Brill". See and download: brill.com/brill-typeface.

ISSN 0045-7183
ISBN 978-90-04-46511-4 (hardback)
ISBN 978-90-04-51572-7 (e-book)

For Zoe

Contents

Acknowledgments

I cannot begin without thanking Zoe Ragland, who was with me before all this started and is still at my side as it comes to a close. Researching and writing books takes hundreds of long days over many years. She has made every day so much better.

I thank my editor, Frank Huisman, and the staff at Brill for giving their guidance and help. Two anonymous reviewers went far beyond the usual scholarly duties to review the original manuscript, which encompassed what are now two long books. Their attention to the details and views of the larger story helped a great deal as I divided the manuscript, rewrote the introduction and conclusion, and made many changes and corrections. Of course, the remaining errors remain my own.

This book is unusual since it is not the revised version of my dissertation. Instead, it has largely been the work of three semesters on fellowship leave and many evenings, weekends, summers, and "break" periods between semesters. As I began revising my dissertation, I researched and wrote a new chapter about what came before the experimentalism of Leiden University medical education in the 1640s through the 1670s. I wanted to tell more of a story of change over time. The sources only seemed to multiply, and reading steadily through textbooks and then pulling threads here and there quickly unraveled my prior view based on the standard narratives about Galenic medicine. Following the leads of the sources through philosophical theory, making medicines, therapy, anatomy, and clinical practices took me to all sorts of new places. One chapter became three, then six, then seven. I think I have a better account of the "before" part of the story now.

Since this book did not build significantly from research support and advising during the dissertation process, further support played a vital role. A research and travel grant from the Institute for Scholarship in the Liberal Arts at the University of Notre Dame started the intensive research process. A further subvention from the Institute for Scholarship in the Liberal Arts at the University of Notre Dame supported the publication process. A generous fellowship from the American Council of Learned Societies was essential in providing a year on leave to research and write full-time. A later semester's sabbatical gave me time to revise and extend the crucial chapters on medicines and knowing diseases. My initial dissertation research in archives in Europe received support from a National Science Foundation Doctoral Dissertation Research Grant, number 0750694, and a Scaliger Fellowship from the Scaliger Instituut at Leiden University. Some of my dissertation work has appeared in articles, which I cite in this book. That work received superb support from the Chemical Heritage Foundation (now the Science History Institute) and a dissertation fellowship from Indiana University Bloomington. Of course, my education in the excellent History and Philosophy of Science and Medicine department at Indiana remains indebted especially to Nico Bertoloni Meli, Bill Newman, Jutta Schickore, and Sandy Gliboff. Arthur Field introduced me to the historiography of the Renaissance. Nico Bertoloni Meli started me on my research into Leiden medicine, and has provided advice and comments along the way.

Libraries and librarians should never be forgotten. The rare books staff at Leiden University supported my steady survey of hundreds of seventeenth-century medical disputations. Archivists at the Leiden Regionaal Archief and the Stadsarchief Amsterdam helped me to find useful sources. Further research with documents in the Sloane Collection at the British Library still yields rich finds. I always received quick and excellent assistance from the staff of the Rare Books and Special Collections at Notre Dame. I have received quite a few interlibrary loans in very good time from the staff at Notre Dame and lending libraries. The Bayerische StaatsBibliothek has been an invaluable online resource for research and images, especially during the COVID-19 pandemic. The staff of the Museum Boerhaave in Leiden helped me find essential, rare sources.

A number of audiences gave welcome encouragement, questions, and critiques. I thank especially colleagues at Cambridge University, the University of Minnesota, Indiana University Bloomington, Johns Hopkins University, Cedars-Sinai Medical Center, the University of Notre Dame, and the Max-Planck-Institut für Wissenschaftsgeschichte.

Colleagues at the University of Alabama Huntsville provided a beautiful community for my first full-time teaching job. At the University of Notre Dame, where I researched and wrote this book, I thank all the members of the Department of History and the program in the History and Philosophy of Science. Chris Hamlin has been my mentor, conversation partner, sounding board, co-teacher, and reader of drafts of some of the material here. I was a bit starstruck to call him a colleague; I am honored to call him a friend. Robert Goulding's expertise in Renaissance history of science, his excellent leadership, and his good cheer have been a steady help. Paul Ocobock has given much good advice and many pep-talks, usually when he least expected another visit. John Deak made my first years at Notre Dame much more welcoming. Dan Hobbins gave good advice and encouragement. Brad Gregory, as always, gave much to think about. Tawrin Baker and Phil Sloan helped to form a vital community of scholars of early modern medicine and life sciences. My department chairs, Jon Coleman and Elisabeth Köll, provided patient support and firm deadlines. I thank them both from my heart. Chris Hamlin and Bob Sullivan have been steadfast, wise, and humane advisors.

Away from Notre Dame, other scholars have provided vital engagement. I will always remember the late Harm Beukers for his patient advice in our meeting in Leiden years ago. His scholarship is a model of concision and mastery of the details. Dániel Margócsy always offered a warm welcome and excellent scholarship. Hal Cook gave good advice on parts of the second book and opened up the wider world of Dutch medicine. Saskia Klerk gave an excellent introduction to early modern Dutch pharmacology. Marieke Hendriksen showed me the importance of the later Leiden anatomical collections and the aesthetic dimension. Jole Shackelford gave helpful suggestions and pointers to things to read. Larry Principe, as always, was a sharp and warm interlocutor. Peter Distelzweig and Benny Goldberg continue to enrich my understanding of early modern philosophy and medicine. Richard Oosterhoff is an exemplary young historian who shows how to practice scholarship as friendship. Gideon Manning was a fine host and, as always, articulated incisive responses. Joel Klein shared his excellent work on Sennert and German chymistry. Matthew Gaetano is always a ready source of expertise on Aristotelian philosophy and early modern theology. There are many more people to thank for the second book, based on the dissertation. To those I have missed for this book: thank you, and my apologies.

Friends and colleagues have read parts of this book in various drafts. I thank especially R. Allen Shotwell for reading much and his ready, expert replies to email queries. Nico Bertoloni Meli, Matthew Gaetano, Tomàs Valle, and Eric Jorink all read significant amounts of earlier drafts and all gave valuable comments. I thank Tomàs Valle and Matthew Gaetano in particular for their persistence and keen editing. Nuno Castel-Branco shared his excellent work on Steno and gave comments on parts of this book. I also thank Arnaud Zimmern, Britta Eastburg-Friesen, Hannah Stevenson, and Zoe Ragland for reading parts of the final manuscript. I thank Britta and Zoe, especially for their eagle-eyed editing.

I wrote or revised much of this book at home, and quite a bit of it during the ongoing pandemic. Although I think it has some valuable things to say, and helps to keep home and hearth together, it has also tended to keep me from my children. I want to thank each of them—Charlotte, Josiah, Christopher, and Lucy—for their patience and impatience. I also want to mark clearly the joy they bring by existing. I am happy to say to them that the book is finally (nearly) done. The next is well on the way, too. My relatives and friends have provided encouragement and friendly inquiries. Claudia and Kevin Wood have helped the most and the longest. I also thank my mother and father for supporting my earlier education and raising me up.

At the end, as at the beginning, I thank Zoe most of all. Thank you.

Illustrations

Bodies of Knowledge in the Late Renaissance

On June 20th 1624, at two in the morning, the young student Petrus Balen died. The next morning, professors and fellow students at Leiden University quickly gathered to dissect his body. For them, his dead body offered live possibilities for cutting down to the hidden causes of his disease and death. The university's professor of anatomy and surgery, Otto Heurnius, arranged for the post-mortem dissection as soon as possible, just two hours after breakfast. Surrounded by students, the States College regent in charge of the scholarship students, and Balen's grieving widow, Heurnius and a surgeon, Joannes Lambertus, located the cause of death in the cadaver: his body's esophageal muscles and the esophagus itself had constricted tightly closed, compressed by a swelling around a collection of morbid matter in his neck. Heurnius and the other witnesses noted the rotten, blackened color of all the anatomical parts around the matter. This morbid matter, thick like the dregs of olive oil but ashy in color, adhered to all the neighboring parts.[1] As in most other recorded cases, professors and students ascribed Balen's death to faults of local anatomical structure and action, qualitative changes, and the movements of the humors.

Petrus Balen had been a good student, noted as "very modest, pious, and very diligent," who suffered from a meager bodily strength.[2] He had died a good death: "His voice and mind were whole up to the moment he breathed out his soul, his eyes perpetually fixed on the heavens, and with hands extended, with prayer, with ardent vows, calling to be joined with the Savior." Balen likely held one of two city scholarships to study theology at Leiden; like many other theology students he was supported by his home city to learn and then teach orthodox Reformed theology.[3] A bright native of Leiden, Balen had originally matriculated to study law at the young age of thirteen, in June of 1611.[4] Since he was younger than fourteen, his Latin skills must have passed examination.[5]

---

1 Otto Heurnius, *Historiae*, 28.

2 Otto Heurnius, *Historiae*, 28.

3 Otterspeer, *Groepsportret*, 1, 153, 160. Festus Hommius was the States College regent at the time. Throughout, I have tended to use the Latin forms of scholars' names. This follows the practice of the scholarly communities of the time and often matches versions in present-day scholarship. I have departed from this rule, as in the case of Petrus Paaw, when non-Latin forms appeared much more often in the secondary literature.

4 *Album Studiosorum*, col. 102.

5 Otterspeer, *Groepsportret*, 1, 256.

© EVAN R. RAGLAND, 2022 | DOI:10.1163/9789004515727_002

Yet his lack of vigor had prolonged his studies and weakened his resistance to disorders of his body's parts—to disease. Even the demands of bookish studies required students to train their bodies through hard study, careful listening, and disputation. This was true of medical students as well, who also practiced sensory engagement with medicinal plants and dissected cadavers, and learned diagnosis, therapy, and prognosis at patients' bedsides, either in private homes or the city hospital. Pedagogical practices lived and developed as embodied practices, as the curricula shaped students into the physicians, lawyers, pastors, or clerks of their professional lives.

Balen's case history gives us a view of academic bedside practice. Preparing his body against the harsh cold, Balen had "wanted to make his head tough against winter injury, studying in the museum with an uncovered head and open windows."[6] The coldness penetrated his anatomy, constricting parts and congealing humors. The medical people at Leiden thought that this corruption in his neck, like many other collections of morbid matter, resulted from a standard Galenic process of defective concoction or cooking of the local humors. The structure of Balen's neck anatomy mattered, too, since the natural tightness of his throat increased the chances that thick, sticky humors could get caught in the vessels there. Tragically, Balen's bold attempt to harden his head to the winter cold caused his neck to swell as the thickened local humors built up into an abscess. His neck became rigid like stone, and he could not swallow. His physicians and surgeons tried softening agents and even inserted surgical instruments into the esophagus to attempt to clear it, which caused great pain. Finally, the abscess ruptured, letting out a "huge amount" of matter. But then the flow of this corrupt humor into his chest generated a new disease as it disturbed new body parts, and he fell stricken with a fever. Then the swelling in his neck began again, fatally.

The unpleasant details of this student's disease and tragic death should be important to us now, since they were vital for the professors and students then. The story of Balen's illness and death, and the close description of his post-mortem dissection, come from the medical diary of Otto Heurnius. They raise pressing historical questions as they arrest our attention. Why would a Galenic medical professor such as Otto Heurnius show so much interest in tracking hidden anatomical changes in a patient, and then detailing the grisly morbid appearances in his dissected dead body? To be more specific: in what medical, pedagogical culture did such practices make sense, and even appear as excellent, attractive opportunities for learning? Finally, how did professors

---

6   Otto Heurnius, *Historiae*, 28.

and students come to establish their traditions and make new knowledge, especially from experience and even activities that look like experiments? To answer these questions, we must learn to think like late-Renaissance academic physicians, and describe how students learned to think that way.

Over the next seven chapters, we will take a detailed tour of the Leiden medical school over its first six decades. This was a humanist, collaborative medical culture which embraced the best of the old and aimed for new knowledge through scholarly research; a culture that fulfilled the promise of ancient medical traditions *and* cultivated practical skills. Professors and students trained their minds together with their senses to perceive and understand the causes of health and disease in human bodies. Balen's case narrative and post-mortem investigation give us a snapshot of Leiden's communal practices of knowing bodies and diseases through discursive study as well as sensory and manual engagement with particulars.[7]

This book offers a crash course in early modern Galenic medicine. This means that we will have to hit the books, in this case with early modern textbooks, study guides, student disputations, and their ancient sources. We will also engage, verbally and vicariously, with the material objects they encountered in the university garden, the hospital, anatomy theater, and dissecting rooms. This requires embracing Galenic medicine in its programmatic combination of reason and experience. Throughout, the integration of embodied, shared practices and discursive frameworks and ideas blends more traditional intellectual history with the history of practice. In the end, I draw on evidence from ancient sources and across Renaissance Europe to present a more complete and explicitly revisionist portrait of Galenic medicine.

This portrait may initially appear a bit strange. It certainly did to me, at first. As I read the textbooks and disputations of the medical professors and students, I kept finding discussions of diseases in terms of impaired organ functions, and recipes for remedies to help restore organs' healthy material conditions. This ran against the most common stories of humoral medicine, in which organs and solid parts take a distant back seat to the changes of the humors. But the centrality of the material compositions, structures, actions, and functions of the parts of the body runs throughout Galen's medicine. In the Renaissance revival of healthy and pathological anatomy, it became even

---

7   In using the term "discursive" I am not at all appealing to a Foucauldian notion of "discourse," or another technical understanding, but to the set of written, spoken, and printed texts and speech that made up the verbal, more "bookish" parts of medical education, from lectures to note-taking to printed textbooks and disputations.

more important and tangible for physicians' physiological, pathological, and therapeutic practices.

Throughout the book, I combine close readings of ancient works, especially those of Galen, with studies of early modern texts and the pedagogical practices of university medical education. I retell the normative histories and ideals professors wove from ancient models, the practices of disputation, the recommended book lists, and major philosophical principles and ways of thinking. Temperament theory, drawn from Galenic theory, formed the foundation of their medical ontology and unified their ideas and practices of diagnosis, pathology, and therapy. Like Galen, they held that the primary qualities of hot, cold, wet, and dry mixed to form the matter of organs, drugs, humors, and other materials, and these mixtures, usually called "temperaments" or "complexions," generated the powers or "faculties" of things. They put these frameworks and vocabularies of qualities and faculties to work in their embodied study of medicinal ingredients, living patients' bodies, and dissected cadavers.

Next, I investigate how students learned to make medicines in that framework of theory and rational practice, but also in their direct, sensory engagement with the things they used to make the medicines. I detail the surprising and previously-unknown early adoption of chymical lectures at Leiden, and I provide a new look at the ancient models for knowing drug ingredients, as well as the notetaking practices and bodily, sensory engagement of students with plants in and around the university garden. Drawing the threads together, I then work from Galen's texts to the textbooks of early modern Galenic physicians from Padua, Paris, and especially Leiden to present a revisionist account of Galenic diagnosis, pathology, and therapy. Medical education at Leiden culminated in bedside clinical teaching and post-mortem dissections of patients' cadavers. Contrary to a widespread and persistent narrative of Galenic medicine, for physicians at Leiden and early modern physicians in general, humors and their changed motions, qualities, and quantities often *caused* diseases, but they rarely *constituted* diseases. Instead, early modern Galenists followed Galen in defining and perceiving most diseases as local impairments of organs and simple parts. The "imbalances" of Galenic medicine were not disproportions of the humors in general, but almost always injurious alterations to the healthy temperaments and structures of the organs and parts. These temperaments, in turn, were constituted by mixtures of the hot, cold, wet, and dry qualities and generated the faculties or powers of things. The temperaments and structures of the organs and simple parts (bone, cartilage, sinew, etc.) determined their powers for action or "faculties." When qualitative or structural changes impaired the functions of organs or simple parts in such a way as to cause notable malfunction, pain, or distress, physicians diagnosed diseases. They learned to diagnose these "sick parts" and treat them with targeted remedies.

Across all of these practices—from bookish disputations largely based on ancient texts from the Hippocratic corpus and Galen to post-mortem dissections of patients' cadavers in the hospital dissecting room—professors taught students to combine discursive knowledge and norms with the sensed materiality of particular objects. Ancient models and maxims emphasized the marriage of reason and experience, which mutually reinforced the common Aristotelian-Galenic philosophical epistemology. Knowledge began with the senses, and the fundamental qualities of material things were in theory perceptible: hotness, coldness, wetness, and dryness. To know the faculties or powers of things such as drugs or even body parts, one had to learn from Galen and other authorities, as well as follow the regular actions of organs, or the perceptible effects of drugs and food on human bodies. Even these seemingly mysterious "faculties," then, came into knowledge first of all from perceiving the effects of sensible things in the world, and in principle could be explained in terms of the fundamental stuff of the natural world. To know plants rightly, students needed to hear their professors lecture on ancient sources such as Dioscorides' compendium of *materia medica*, or Galen's *On the Faculties and Mixtures of Simple Drugs*. To see and diagnose patients correctly, students learned to diagnose the changes to the temperaments and structures of different organs or parts through perceptible signs and symptoms. These changes of organs and simple parts generated the impaired functions which constituted diseases. In the bodies of patients who died from their diseases, like Petrus Balen, students and professors could observe and correlate the hidden morbid appearances in cadavers, appearances revealed through careful dissections with surgeons.

Rather than opposing more empirical ways of knowing, humanist, bookish scholarship supported, directed, and energized sensory, bodily engagement with things. The language, models, guiding principles, anecdotes, and even stanzas from ancient texts trained students through lectures, reading, disputation, and note-taking. In his detailed description of the post-mortem dissection of another hospital patient, professor Otto Heurnius naturally added a four-line Latin quotation from the ancient Roman poet Ovid's *Metamorphoses*. But his humanist attention to the descriptive details of things also allowed him to connect new morbid phenomena across dissected patients' cadavers, such as a yolk-like, slippery substance in the hearts of two women who died suddenly, or the "droplets," abscesses, ulcers and "tiny tubercles" dotting the dissected lungs of the bodies of patients suffering from "phthisis" or consumption.[8] Even in these small pathological innovations, ancient

---

8 Otto Heurnius, *Historiae*, 22. The presence of tubercles identified in the post-mortem dissections, along with the symptoms of the patients, strongly suggests that we would identify many of these as cases of tuberculosis.

texts informed their practices. After all, from Galen on, physicians had been taught to think of ulcers and ulceration of the lungs as the definitive cause of phthisis. Otto's father, Johannes, stuffed his lectures and textbooks with references to ancient sources—Galen, Hippocrates, Celsus, Aretaeus—and used his erudite commentary on the Hippocratic *Aphorisms* to reflect on medical practice. Early modern histories of the discipline of medicine, and of chymistry, picked from a vast humanist field of ancient poets and writers, advertised their expertise in reason and experience, and shaped their identities and goals. Being a physician and practicing Galenic medicine always involved the mutual interrelation of discursive practices *and* sense-based engagement with things.

Although ancient texts indeed had the authority of expertise and long, apparently successful use in practice, they helped to direct rather than block innovation. Building pedagogical cultures with these practices and ideas, professors gradually added new knowledge of plants from local and global networks, chymical remedies and operations, and even the hidden changes of organs in disease and death. This volume demonstrates that early modern medical professors and students *before* the rise of experimentalism already developed robust practices—shared ways of acting, thinking, sensing, writing, and interacting toward communal goals—that gradually came to look like experimental trials and at times even generated new knowledge. A second, forthcoming volume details the rise of the new experimental*ist* university medical culture, in which students and professors performed systematic experimental investigations on a range of subjects in anatomy, chymistry, and clinical practice, and aimed to develop not only new pieces of knowledge but new theories and grand systems.[9] For them, experimentation was the essential activity for properly practicing anatomy, chymistry, and medicine. Experiments acted as the ground and test of knowledge claims. Even before this shift, though, early modern universities such as Leiden were productive training grounds for combining reason and experience, and even experimental trials, to make new practices and knowledge, and, later, labor in the construction of the new sciences.

---

9 This book, tentatively titled *Experimental Medicine: Experimentalist Anatomy, Chymistry, and Clinical Practice at Leiden University, 1639–1672 and Beyond*, is complete and documents in detail the rise of experimentalist medical culture from the late 1630s through the 1670s, and its surprising legacy into new experimental physiology and medicine of the 1800s. I have also made preliminary studies: Ragland, "Experimenting." Ragland, "Mechanism." Ragland, "Chymistry." Ragland, "Experimental Clinical Medicine."

1   Following Galen to Find the Seats and Causes of Disease

Everyone knows that premodern physicians generally practiced Galenic medicine, but what was Galenic medicine? The widespread, established view among most historians of medicine is that Galenic medicine mostly ignored the solid parts of the body, that general humoral imbalances constituted most diseases, that anatomy did not matter for therapy, and that physicians before the eighteenth century showed little interest in pathological anatomy founded in post-mortem dissections.[10] As I demonstrate in this book, all of these characterizations are false.

In this traditional view, the famed Renaissance rise in status and spread of anatomical teaching and research had little-to-nothing to do with medical practice or treating disease.[11] Early modern post-mortem dissections for understanding disease and death were rare and marginal to medical practice, and concentrated on rarities and wonders rather than common disease phenomena.[12] Instead, even Galen's medicine, for all of its anatomical sophistication, relied on humoralism for "explaining disease," and only later Paris medicine around 1800 broke away, newly "situating disease in the organs rather than the humors."[13] In this common story, specific organs and especially pathological dissections were not at all important for "humoral" medicine, which attended primarily to the whole body and the general balance or imbalance of the four humors (blood, yellow bile, black bile, and phlegm).[14] Finally, this story ends by celebrating the supposed rise of post-mortem dissections in Paris hospitals

---

10   For the claim that Hippocratic and Galenic physicians "often ignored the solid parts of the body" and that only later eighteenth-century physicians included anatomical seats of disease and local lesions, see Maulitz, "The Pathological Tradition," 169–170, and compare Maulitz, "Pathology." For the claim that thinking in terms of anatomical seats of diseases "directly opposed" humoral thinking, see Reiser, "The Science of Diagnosis," 827. For claims about the uselessness of anatomy for medical practice and therapy, see Cook, *Matters of Exchange*, 37, 393–394 and Cunningham, *Anatomist Anatomis'd*, 198. For claims about balance and imbalance conceived in terms of the whole-body or general proportions and mixtures of humors, see Lindemann, *Medicine*, 18, 13.

11   Pace, e.g., French, *Dissection and Vivisection*, 1–2; Cunningham, *Anatomist Anatomis'd*, 197; Cook, *Matters of Exchange*, 37. For a more nuanced view, see Bertoloni Meli, *Mechanism, Experiment, Disease*, 14–15.

12   This view continues from Long, *A History of Pathology*, 31, 43, 47.

13   Bynum, *History of Medicine*, 15, 55. E.g., Duffin, *History of Medicine*, 71–73, 76, 78, notes that Galen associated some pathological explanations with anatomy, but retains most of the standard narrative.

14   E.g, Lindemann, *Medicine and Society*, 13, 17–18, 100. Maulitz, "The Pathological Tradition," 169–170. Reiser, "The Science of Diagnosis," 827. Maulitz, "Pathology." Against this standard view, see the chapters in De Renzi, et al., *Pathology in Practice*, especially Stolberg,

around 1800, and claims that medical teaching before then did not significantly rely on clinical, bedside instruction. In the rare cases when it did, professors used hospital teaching only to demonstrate or perform static knowledge, rather than generate new knowledge.[15] The evidence from Leiden teaching, select Italian universities, and Galen's own works refutes each one of the interlocking claims in this mythic narrative.

Very recent work has called this widespread view into question, especially with examples from Italian, notably Paduan, medical practices from the mid-1500s and later.[16] These scholars have also emphasized the need for fresh narratives to replace the idea of a discrete break with the development of the organ-based anatomical-clinical medicine of the Paris hospital school at the end of the 1700s.[17] But we have yet to construct a replacement history, especially one that integrates all the core medical practices—diagnosis, prognosis, making and administering medicines, thinking anatomically and pathologically, and performing and witnessing dissections—*within* the pedagogical context of making new physicians *and* new knowledge.

In this book, I use Leiden university teaching and learning as a focus to recover just such a comprehensive view. I begin with the founding of Leiden University in 1575. A symbol of Dutch resistance and aspirations after Spanish destruction, the university remained a place of eclectic learning, research, relative religious toleration, heavy drinking, and student agency. In Anthony Grafton's estimation, Leiden was also "the most innovative university in Europe," and his expert call for more learning about it still merits scholarly enthusiasm and erudition.[18] Comprehensive histories of medical teaching and practice there have been a major desideratum.

"Post-mortems," some remarks from Stolberg, *Experiencing Illness*, 71–74, and chapters five, six, and seven below.

15   Lindemann, *Medicine and Society*, 144–148 and 157–165.

16   Regular private post-mortem dissections began much earlier, around 1300 in Italy. Park, *Secrets of Women*. Park, "The Criminal and the Saintly Body," 1–33. For sources undermining the old narrative of medicine shifting from diseases as general humoral imbalances to organ- or part-based diagnosis and pathology with the Paris hospital medicine, see the following: Bylebyl, "Commentary." Bylebyl, "The Manifest and the Hidden." Stolberg, *Experiencing Illness*. De Renzi, Bresadola, and Conforti, "Pathological Dissections in Early Modern Europe." Stolberg, "Post-mortems." De Renzi, "Seats and Series." Donato, *Sudden Death*. Shotwell, "The Great Pox." Skaarup, *Anatomy and Anatomists in Early Modern Spain*. Bertoloni Meli, *Visualizing Disease*. Keel, *L'avenement de la medicine clinique*. Wear, *Knowledge & Practice*, 116–126, 146–148. Bouley, *Pious Postmortems*.

17   De Renzi, Bresadola, and Conforti, "Pathological Dissections."

18   Grafton, "Libraries and Lecture Halls," 241. Grafton, *Joseph Scaliger*. For excellent topical articles, see Lunsingh Scheurleer and Posthumus Meyjes, ed., *Leiden University in the*

Sketched line by line from close readings of unstudied primary sources, this book paints an integrated picture of medical pedagogy, disciplinary history, philosophical theory, rational practice, training with medicinal simples, anatomical practices, and bedside and clinical teaching. As I show, in early modern Galenic medicine, and Galen's own ancient medicine, humors often *caused* disease states by impairing the functions of organs, but humoral changes rarely *constituted* diseases on their own. In treating patients, anatomical knowledge enabled the physician to locate the precise "seat" (*sedes*) of the disease that hindered the proper functioning of the diseased organ.[19] Physicians and students localized disease to specific organs or body parts, or specific regions of organs and parts. Phlegmy buildup in the lungs could cause consumption or phthisis, but only the impaired lungs resulted in the overheated liver, poor nutrition, wasting, and coughing up pus and blood characteristic of the disease.

Building on earlier scholarship, I show that Leiden professors borrowed from the models of their own university training, especially from the University of Padua, to establish a strong *tradition* of anatomical-clinical medical teaching and research, one that increasingly aimed to generate new knowledge of diseases and treatments, and sometimes succeeded. Professors gained new knowledge of new parasites from the Dutch colonies, and investigated indigenous remedies for them. They tried chymical medicines and explained chymical practices and substances to students in lectures. Through anatomies, they claimed to identify new anatomical structures, such as tiny bones in the human ear, as well as pathological changes and substances, especially morbid structures in the lungs of patients suffering from phthisis or consumption. At least by 1598, students attended the private post-mortem dissections of the professor of anatomy, Petrus Paaw, to see the hidden seats and proximate causes of

---

Seventeenth Century. For a beautiful portrait of the university that touches on multiple themes, see Otterspeer, *Groepsportret met Dame I* and Otterspeer, *Groepsportret met Dame II.* For Leiden physics, see especially Ruestow, *Physics at Seventeenth and Eighteenth-Century Leiden* and Wiesenfeldt, *Leerer Raum in Minervas Haus.* For studies of Leiden anatomy, the best is Huisman, *The Finger of God.* See also Lunsingh Scheurleer, "Un Amphithéâtre d'Anatomie Moralisée." For the eighteenth-century anatomical collections, see especially Hendriksen, *Elegant Anatomy.* For the broader history of science and medicine, see, e.g.: Van Berkel, Van Helden, and Palm, *A History of Science in the Netherlands.* Cook, *Matters of Exchange.* Cook, "The New Philosophy in the Low Countries."

19   Galen's *De locis affectis* (*On the affected places*), as the title suggests, was particularly important in this tradition, but this approach is found across his works, from his influential late summary *The Art of Medicine* (*Tegni, Ars medica*) to his works on diseases, symptoms, and drugs. For historians' remarks on disease localization in pre-modern medicine, see the following: Wilson, "On the History of Disease-Concepts"; Wear, *Knowledge & Practice*, 117–119; Stolberg, "Post-mortems."

diseases. By the later 1630s, students and professors eagerly combined regular bedside instruction in the city hospital with routine post-mortem dissections to identify the causes of disease and death. By the 1660s, this tradition, now inflected by experimentalist anatomy and chymistry, flourished, producing new and influential clinical-anatomical theories, notably a theory of phthisis based on the development of tubercles in the lungs.

What is even more important, recovering a more complete view of medical culture shows that these burgeoning practices of anatomical localization were far from peripheral to academic Galenic medicine—they were *central* to it. I demonstrate the widespread Galenic foundations of these practices by putting close readings of common sources, especially Galen's writings, in conversation with texts from Leiden professors and other academic physicians across Europe.[20] In later chapters, I reconstruct anatomical and clinical practice over several more decades, recovering important continuities in the localization of disease in clinical teaching at the city hospital, and the official search for the causes of diseases through post-mortem dissections, from at least 1636 into the 1660s.

Contrary to common historiographic claims, early modern Galenic physicians did not at all conceive of the human body as "a seething mass of fluids rather than the assemblage of discrete organs and systems."[21] This claim directly contradicts Galen's works, which always emphasized the imbalance of the *qualities* of patient's organs, simple parts, and bodies, and defined diseases at specific anatomical sites from head to toe according to the impaired functions of organs and simple parts. As Galen put it in his influential *On the Affected Places* (*De locis affectis*), "Therefore one must always begin from the organ of the injured action, and then seek what is the manner of the injury."[22] As detailed in chapter five, his other works deployed similar definitions and categories, mapping the geography of disease across the organs and simple parts. Early modern medical professors embraced thinking in terms of parts and organs as the seats for diseases. Johannes Heurnius, the leading teaching professor at Leiden around 1600, taught his students a similar organ- and

---

20   Galen, *De Symptomatum Differentiis* in Galen, *De Morborum et Symptomatum Differentiis et Causis*, 39. Cf. Galen, *De Morborum Differentiis*, in the same work, 3: "a disease is a fault either of an action or a constitution." Galen, *De Affectorum Locorum Notitia*, 3r.

21   Lindemann, *Medicine and Society*, 17–18. Cf. Maulitz, "Pathological Tradition," 169–170. Maulitz, "Pathology." Against this standard view, see some remarks from Stolberg, *Experiencing Illness*, 71–74 and Stolberg, "Post-mortems," as well as Wilson, "On the History of Disease-Concepts." For a longer treatment, see chapters five, six, and seven below. Reiser, "Science of Diagnosis," 827.

22   Galen, *De Affectorum Locorum Notitia*, 6r.

part-based pathology, diagnosis, and therapy: "Diseases, as we said, dwell in the parts. However many ways therefore those become faulty, there are just so many diseases."[23]

Humors changed and flowed, affected by the changes of the seasons, food, drink, the air, exercise and rest, excretion and retention, contagions, miasmas, and effluvia. But then what? They altered the qualitative mixtures and anatomical structures of the simple parts and organs or built up where they should not be, blocking vessels and impairing the functions of organs and simple parts. When humors erred from their natural healthy states and became "peccant," they made organs and parts too hot, cold, wet, or dry, changing their temperaments and the faculties or actions generated by these temperaments. As in Petrus Balen's case, they also damaged or blocked vessels and became corrupt, growing local and deadly corruption in specific anatomical structures and sites. Michael Stolberg's very recent and important summary of localized humoral pathology, as found in post-mortem dissections, reveals a range of processes: the local accumulation of a humor in a cavity, organ, or vessel; the rupture of humors from vessels; the buildup or accretion of humors in smaller spots on organs or parts, as in the formation of abscesses or harder steatomata; the obstruction of vessels and cavities, as in epilepsy supposedly due to obstruction of parts of the brain; the formation of stones and tumors; the formation of cancers; the erosion of parts through ulcers; and the spread of corruption or rot, turning organs and parts into pus and putrefied fluids and matter.[24]

While post-mortem dissections were a late-medieval and early modern practice, and widespread only by the second half of the 1500s, this localization of diseases and humors was not. Even the humoral cornerstone text, the Hippocratic work *Nature of Man*, which laid out a theory of four humors and connected those to the four qualities, seasons, ages of life, etc., moved from humoral changes to *local* bodily disease states: "For when an element is isolated and stands by itself, not only must the place which it left become diseased, but the *place where* it stands in a flood must, because of the excess, cause pain and distress."[25] The rest of the Hippocratic corpus, as Helen King shows, very rarely mentions four humors, concentrating instead on other fluids and bodily locations.[26]

---

23   Johannes Heurnius, *Institutiones Medicinae*, 516.

24   Stolberg, "Post-mortems," 75–78.

25   Hippocrates, *Nature of Man*, I.IV, 11–13. Italics added.

26   King, "Female Fluids."

Galen certainly elevated the *Nature of Man* as a foundational text for medicine, but his works overwhelmingly emphasized healthy balance and morbid
imbalance in terms of the four primary *qualities* (hot, cold, wet, and dry) and
often barely mention humors. As Per-Gunnar Ottoson, Joel Kaye, Nancy Siraisi,
and, at times, Owsei Temkin have pointed out briefly, Galen and his medieval
and early modern followers thought and wrote of balance and imbalance in
health and disease, but of the four *qualities* that made up the mixture of bodily
organs and parts, not of the four humors.[27] As befitting a self-conscious expert
anatomist, Galen always attempted to localize disease states to qualitative or
structural changes of organs and parts. His most widespread and influential
teaching text, his mature summary *The Art of Medicine* (also called the *Tegni*,
Techne iatrike, *Ars parva*, or *Ars medica*), gave the lion's share of attention to the
qualitative temperaments of organs and other solid parts.[28] Galen worked
through the various possible hot, cold, wet, and dry variations of the principal organs—the brain, heart, liver, and testes—and other body parts, and
described how to use signs, symptoms, and anatomy to diagnose the impaired
functions or actions and so the diseased organ, part, or system. The actions
and functions of parts followed from their qualitative mixtures (or temperaments) and their structures, but were not reducible to them. Remedies then
targeted the qualitatively or structurally impaired part with opposing qualities
or purgation of local morbid matter. Humors, of course, change qualitatively,
too, and were important vehicles for bringing qualitative changes to body parts.

Across his works, especially his treatises on diseases and symptoms, Galen
extended and applied this emphasis on qualitative and structural impairments of organs and body parts and their localized treatments.[29] Humors
were plainly not nearly as important to Galen's medicine as the qualitative
temperaments and functions of organs, and the humors appear mostly as local
"fluxes," bringing qualitative changes to local organs, blocking channels, or
putrefying. Patients' letters and records articulate similar views, though with a
far less systematic approach to the qualitative variations of organs and much
less anatomical specificity for humoral and disease localizations, as Michael
Stolberg has shown in his analysis of patient writings from across the sixteenth,
seventeenth, and eighteenth centuries.[30]

---

27   Kaye, *A History of Balance*, 168. Ottoson, *Scholastic Medicine*, 130–132. Temkin, *Galenism*,
      13, 17–18, 138 n. 10. Siraisi, *Avicenna in the Renaissance*, 296–315. Pace, e.g., Maclean, *Logic,
      Signs, and Nature*, 241; and Wear, *Knowledge & Practice*, 37–38; and Lindemann, *Medicine
      and Society*, 13, 17–18.
28   Galen, *The Art of Medicine*, esp. pp. 351–364.
29   Johnston, ed. and trans., *Galen: On Diseases and Symptoms*.
30   Stolberg, *Experiencing Illness*, esp. Part II.

Influential centers for medical education from Padua to Leiden put this Galenic approach to work, cultivating attention to anatomical localization in their medical students through localized treatment systems, basic anatomy, and post-mortem dissections. As Jerome Bylebyl showed decades ago, and Michael Stolberg has recently confirmed and extended, Paduan professors combined the regular search for the anatomical seats of diseases through clinical teaching with some, apparently irregular, post-mortem dissections.[31] In a very recent article, Stolberg briefly and brilliantly has indicated the widespread use of evidence from post-mortem dissections to frame humoral explanations for diseases, mostly in the second half of the 1500s.[32] As A. M. Luyendick-Elshout and Harm Beukers have noted, nearly all of the Leiden medical professors studied at Padua and they established similar pedagogical practices at Leiden.[33] For instance, at Leiden Johannes Heurnius' popular theory textbook, the *Institutes of Medicine* (*Institutiones medicinae*, editions 1592–1666) and his *practica* text, *New Method of the Practice of Medicine* (*Praxis medicinae nova ratio*, editions 1587–1650) both emphasized the localization of diseases in specific body parts as the key to bridging the rational, qualitative schemes of the proper method of healing (*methodus medendi*) and the pragmatic head-to-toe approach of treatment manuals.[34]

Official pedagogical structures put human bodies, philosophical and tangible, living and dead, at the center of students' learning. As at some Italian and Spanish universities such as Padua, Pisa, Rome, Bologna, Valencia, Valladolid, Salamanca, Alcalá de Henares, and others, at Leiden the official courses of study cultivated practical knowledge through direct engagement with a range of things and objects, including human bodies living and dead, plants, chymical medicines and procedures, and animal bodies, as well as ancient and early modern texts.[35] Professors dissected and diagnosed to identify the anatomical

---

31   Bylebyl, "Commentary." Bylebyl, "The Manifest and the Hidden." Stolberg, "Post-mortems."
      Stolberg, "Bedside." Stolberg, "Empiricism." Klestinec, *Theaters of Anatomy*, 67–68.

32   Stolberg, "Post-mortems."

33   Luyendijk-Elshout, "Der Einfluss der italienischen Universitäten auf die medizinische
      Facultät Leiden." Beukers, "Clinical Teaching."

34   Heurnius, *Institutiones.* Johannes Heurnius, *Praxis Medicinae Nova Ratio* (1587). For ease
      of citation, unless otherwise indicated I have used the 1650 edition, which appears to
      present the same text of the corrected 1590 edition but in a single-column format and
      larger typeface: Johannes Heurnius, *Praxis Medicinae Nova Ratio* (1650). For the tensions
      between Galen's model of rational *methodus medendi* and common practice, see Bylebyl,
      "Teaching *Methodus Medendi* in the Renaissance"; Wear, "Explorations in Renaissance
      Writings."

35   Skaarup, *Anatomy and Anatomists in Early Modern Spain*, documents the anatomical
      studies begun at Valencia, Salamanca, Valladolid, Alcalá de Henares in the mid-1500s, as

parts at fault in diseases, for instance in Juan Tomás Porcell's use of a sustained series of pathological dissections of five plague victims in 1564 to identify the diseased organ at fault in his diseased patients.[36] In contrast, the Paris Faculty of Medicine emphasized bookish erudition even for its medical practice courses, and the four bodies a year in two annual anatomical dissections performed by surgeons with a professor discoursing above were generally all the anatomy students experienced officially, from the early 1500s into the 1620s.[37] Of course, Vesalius and other Parisian students notoriously robbed graves for bodies to dissect, and the Paris surgeons established regular and more frequent anatomical dissections.[38] Similarly, medical education at Oxford established two annual dissections only in 1623, though surgeons were dissecting there earlier, and few professors had much experience with cadavers before the 1650s.[39] Leiden medical instruction in its first six decades grew as a harvest of Renaissance, especially Italian, developments.[40] But this growth flourished through the humanist scholars' appreciative and critical engagement with ancient texts and their growing expertise in the direct engagement with material things.[41] Detailed knowledge of various human bodies, in healthy and diseased states, as well as comparative studies of animal bodies, most often and most explicitly offered medical students what they wanted above all: tools and methods for success as physicians.

Leiden professors were following Galen in defining and diagnosing diseases in terms of an injury to the function, action, or operation (Galen's term was

---

well as at Barcelona and Zaragoza, often through the imposition of royal power and support, and the spread of anatomical work in Spain and Portugal. Bylebyl, "The School of Padua." Klestinec, *Theaters of Anatomy.* Stolberg, "Bedside Teaching." Ragland, "'Making Trials.'" Findlen, *Possessing Nature.* Palmer, "Medical Botany."

36   Skaarup, *Anatomy and Anatomists in Early Modern Spain,* 170–177. Lopez Piñero and Terrada Ferrandis, "La Obra de Juan Tomas Porcell." For Italy, see, e.g.: Stolberg, "Postmortems."

37   Guerrini, *Courtiers' Anatomists,* 25–26. Iain Lonie argued that at Paris humanist lexical practices were the *primary* way to obtain practical knowledge: Lonie, "The 'Paris Hippocrates.'" For Padua and the others, see Grendler, *The Universities of the Italian Renaissance,* ch. 9.

38   Guerrini, *Courtiers' Anatomists,* 22, 28–30.

39   Frank, "Medicine," 517, 521, 541, 542, 545.

40   E.g., Bylebyl, "The Manifest and the Hidden." Bylebyl, "Commentary." Stolberg, "Postmortems." Stolberg, "Bedside Teaching." Stolberg, "Empiricism." Klestinec, *Theaters of Anatomy.* Findlen, *Possessing Nature.* Luyendijk-Elshout, "Der Einfluss der italienischen Universitäten auf die medizinische Fakultät Leiden." Beukers, "Clinical Teaching."

41   Bylebyl, "The School of Padua." Bylebyl, "Medicine, Philosophy, and Humanism." Joy, *Gassendi the Atomist.* Blair, *The Theater of Nature.* Raphael, *Reading Galileo.* Levitin, *Ancient Wisdom.* Grafton, "A Sketch Map." Ogilvie, *Science of Describing.*

energeia) of a part. And they put their own Italian university training into practice when they tried to follow the northern-Italian or Paduan model of bedside
clinical instruction in the local hospital.[42] As the leading teaching professor of
theoretical and practical medicine, Johannes Heurnius, put it in his textbook
and lectures, "a disease is a constitution beyond nature of the living body, primarily and in itself wounding an action."[43] Here, as in so many other things,
he echoed Galen, who defined a disease as "a constitution beyond nature, or
the cause of a damaged function."[44] Since actions occur in the body often by
individual organs—the instruments that perform actions—diseases tended to
be localized to specific organs. Heurnius' colleague, the professor of anatomy
Petrus Paaw, agreed: "health is defined according to the natural disposition
of the parts completing actions, and disease as an affect contrary to nature
wounding them."[45]

Recovering a more accurate understanding of Galenic thinking about faculties is part of this book's argument about physicians' programmatic reliance
on sensation as the foundation of knowledge. For example, in Galenic theory
body parts acted according to their capacities or "faculties." These were later
derided as refuges of ignorance and mere word-play by upstart philosophers
such as John Locke, and many historians seem to have followed their disdain.[46]
Yet, as in the case of drugs, the faculties of Galenic bodies derived from their
temperaments—their physical mixtures of the principal qualities hot, cold,
wet, and dry—and their structures. Increasingly, physicians followed Galen
yet again to concentrate on the varieties and structures of the basic contractile
"fibers" that made up many organs. Galenic faculties actually bear striking similarities to the views of mechanical philosophers such as Robert Boyle about chymical properties. They are dispositional, relational, and emergent properties.

Following Galen and other Galenic physicians, scholars identified the faculties of body parts, or medicinal simples or compound drugs, by observing
or interacting with them to identify their regular states and effects on different objects. By thinking in terms of qualities and anatomical structures they
could sense, at least in theory, professors, students, and physicians could live
out their epistemological ideal through their close sensory engagement with

42   Stolberg, "Bedside Teaching." Stolberg, "Empiricism."
43   Heurnius, *Institutiones*, 188.
44   Galen, *De Differentiis Morborum*, in Galen, *De Morborum...Differentiis* (1546), 3. Cf. Galen,
      On the Differentiae of Diseases, 134.
45   Petrus Paaw, *Primitiae Anatomicae* (1615), 3–4.
46   Locke, *An Essay concerning Humane Understanding*, 130. Cook, "Medicine," 426. Bertoloni
      Meli, *Mechanism*, 11.

perceptible objects, from plants to live patients' bodily signs and symptoms, to the evidence and causes of diseases revealed in post-mortem dissections.

Medical ways of thinking explicitly directed physicians away from souls and toward materiality. Speaking *philosophically*, pious early modern scholars would also say that the faculties or powers of a living body flowed from the organic soul or *anima* as the first principle of activity. Physicians, though, dealt with tangible bodies and their material temperaments. Speaking *as physicians*, they argued that faculties came about from or just were the qualitative temperaments of organs and parts, capacities enacted in relation to other objects. So when the temperament or structure of a part altered its ability to enact one of its usual faculties, it was diseased. But most internal affections or diseases remained concealed within patients' bodies. How did students learn to know the hidden causes of diseases?

Everything came together in clinical practice, at least in theory. As Dutch historians of medicine such as J. E. Kroon and Harm Beukers have demonstrated, Leiden established decades of regular clinical teaching in the city hospital, from at least 1636.[47] Anatomy, chymistry, and philosophical theory met to guide students' attention to symptoms in living bodies and, increasingly, lesions revealed in post-mortem dissections. In the old St. Caecilia convent, converted to a municipal hospital for two dozen poor men and women, students and professors examined patients, offered diagnoses, prescribed drugs, noted the effects and progress over time, and performed post-mortem dissections.

In diagnosis, professors and students hunted signs of diseases, or perceptible markers of internal changes of vital organs and parts.[48] Pain and swelling often marked the morbid spot. Loss of action or function did, too. Variations in a patient's pulse followed from changes in their vital faculty, seated in the heart. Altered excrement or urine told about impaired concoction or cooking of nutriment; signs of problems with the liver, stomach, and other organs of the belly. Normally, physicians used natural philosophical theory to reason from the surface signs to the hidden causes. Following Galenic tradition, they emphasized the primary qualities of body parts and drugs as the results of material mixture. They did not spend much time thinking in terms of formal

---

47   Kroon, *Bijdragen*, ch. 4. Beukers, "Clinical Teaching," is more cautious about the realiza-
      tion of the 1591 request to establish hospital teaching. Kroon, *Bijdragen*, 46, presents good
      reasons to think earlier clinical instruction was more likely. Paaw included students at
      private or clinical anatomies at least from 1598 to 1602, as show in chapter six below. See
      also Knoeff, "Boerhaave at Leiden."
48   Maclean, *Logic, Signs, and Nature*, ch. 8. See chapters five, six, and seven below.

explanation or the soul as the form of the living body. The form of a part, rather, was the natural structure of a part.

Throughout Galen's works, the structure and material make-up of a part determined its action, and its action or actions determined the use or functions of each part in the functioning of a healthy body.[49] Galenic physicians used the structure-action-use scheme to think through healthy and impaired (diseased) parts. This fit with the best anatomical work of the time, such as that by Hieronymus Fabricius ab Aquapendente (Girolamo Fabrizi) at Padua.[50] These Renaissance anatomists often followed Galen's distinction between the composition or structure of a part (*historia*), its action (*actio, energeia*), and its use or function (*chreia*).[51] The *historia* set out the temperaments of an organ, and the properties following from the temperaments. A part's action was the "active motion" that contributed to the animal's living functions or uses.[52] The functions and uses contributed to the life of the living animal. From the material mixtures and structures of parts and organs, to their actions and uses, or malfunctions in disease states, Galenic physicians linked the basic materiality of the parts with their healthy and morbid conditions. Anatomy provided them with this essential knowledge.

Academic physicians often described the four primary qualities as material properties (while Aristotelian philosophers would most often think of them as formal), and thought in terms of material mixtures. The best natural philosophy of the time, as Galenic physicians declared from Galen through the early seventeenth century, depended on the action of the primary qualities of hot, cold, wet, and dry in all material things. These mixtures or "temperaments" grounded the powers or "faculties" of body parts and drugs, in relation to different objects.

With this theory, they could connect the perceptible external signs, through inferences or conjectures, to the primary qualities of the interior organs and parts. Different organs and parts also had characteristic pains and diseases, based on their substance, the disease conditions or "affects," and the local distribution of nerves. As Otto Heurnius taught his students in a 1638 case and post-mortem dissection, it was of great importance in medical practice "to observe and distinguish the various kinds, size, and duration of pains, and from

---

49   For a clear introduction, see Distelzweig, "The Use of *Usus* and the Function of *Functio*." Also see Distelzweig, "Fabricius's Teleomechanics of Muscle." And Debru, "Physiology."

50   Cunningham, "Fabricius and the 'Aristotle Project.'" Siraisi, "Historia, actio, utilitas." Distelzweig, "Fabricius's Teleomechanics of Muscle," 71–72.

51   Galen, *On the Usefulness of the Parts* (*De usu partium*), trans. May, 17.1., 724.

52   Galen, *On the Usefulness of the Parts* (*De usu partium*), trans. May, 17.1., 724.

these we know the part affected, the cause of the affect, and the outcome."[53] A jabbing, point-like pain indicated a morbid membrane, a pulsating pain an affected part woven with arteries. In this, Otto Heurnius applied the teachings of Galen, and his father Johannes, who wrote "where there is *pain*, there most often the *disease* resides."[54] Anatomical and clinical expertise, structured by Galen's texts and method, joined with bedside experience to pinpoint diseased organs through their impairments and sensations.

2   **Disease Displayed in Private, Public, and Clinical Anatomies**

Anatomical dissections allowed professors and surgeons to display the hidden states of diseased parts they usually only inferred from signs and symptoms. This was not a marginal practice. Historians have marked the spread of making new pathological knowledge from the interrelation of clinical signs and post-mortem evidence across early modern Europe, from Italy to Spain, France, England, Germany, and the Low Countries.[55] By 1679, Theophile Bonet's *Graveyard* assembled thousands of post-mortem dissection reports from nearly *five hundred* different physicians and surgeons.[56]

Interpretation of surface signs, ejected matter, and excrements did not usually let the senses reach the hidden causes directly: post-mortem dissections did. Physicians could touch fevered or chilled patients while they lived and hear their reports of hot or cold sensations in different bodily locations, but they could not sense directly these qualitative variations of their patients' internal organs. Dissections allowed physicians and students to test and confirm their diagnoses via direct sensation, but not, of course, of the hot and cold primary qualities. They saw and touched the evidence of excess heat and cold in and around organs: cooked or congealed fluids, as well as blackened, shriveled, and palpably dry livers, kidneys, and other vital viscera. Of course, excessive dryness or wetness, as well as flabbiness or toughness, and other secondary qualities generated by the hot, cold, wet, and dry, remained open for direct sensation. They also saw, touched, and smelled the corrupt fluids,

---

53   Heurnius, *Historiae*, 16. Cf. Johannes Heurnius, *Nova ratio*, 468–9, 477–8. Galen, *De locis affectis*, bk. 2.

54   Johannes Heurnius, *Nova Ratio*, 468.

55   De Renzi et al, eds., *Pathology in Practice*. Skaarup, *Anatomy and Anatomists in Early Modern Spain*. Bylebyl, "Commentary." Bylebyl, "School of Padua." Ragland, "Experimental Clinical Medicine." Stolberg, "Bedside Teaching." Harley, "Political Post-Mortems."

56   Bonet, *Sepulchretum*. Irons, "Théophile Bonet." Rinaldi, "Organising Pathological Knowledge."

abscesses, pus, and ulcers in the lungs which caused pneumonia and phthisis. Although they did not use thermoscopes or thermometers to measure quantitatively these qualitative variations, they scrupulously measured the volume of morbid fluids found in cadavers.

At Leiden and for over a century, Professors Petrus Paaw, Otto Heurnius, Johannes Walaeus, Franciscus Dele Boë Sylvius, Johannes van Horne, and other anatomists emphasized the usefulness of anatomy for practicing physicians.[57] As the first longstanding anatomy professor, Paaw set up many institutions and practices of teaching. Tim Huisman has elegantly documented the institutional and moral or theological dimensions of Paaw's anatomy.[58] Here, we turn to the main purpose of his anatomy, medical training and practice. As Paaw put it in his major anatomical work, he reckoned that the profit of anatomical practice was the preparation of "practical physicians...who would thoroughly understand the affects and diseases of the individual parts of the whole body, and of those what is required for their curing."[59] Paaw's own autoptic practice, cultivated "diligently" (*diligenter*) in two to five human bodies a year, enabled him to critique his predecessors such as Vesalius and to make new observations about the number of bones in the inner ear.[60] Paaw performed about three documented post-mortem dissections per year and connected the study of pathological states from these cadavers with anatomical evidence from public anatomies and animal dissections.[61] In dissections from the anatomy theater to private rooms and the hospital dissecting room, Paaw demonstrated for students the causes of diseases in the lesions and morbid matter localized in various organs.

Paaw connected evidence from multiple post-mortems to argue for similar pathological states found in a range of cadavers displaying similar diseases. Some historians still assume that post-mortem dissection was necessarily a dishonorable fate for a dead body, shunned by the families of anyone not poor, marginal, or foreign to the local community.[62] Yet Paaw dissected a range of

---

57   For Walaeus, Sylvius, and Van Horne, see Schouten, *Johannes Walaeus*. Beukers, "Het Laboratorium." Beukers, "Mechanistische Principes." Beukers, "Acid Spirits and Alkaline Salts." Ragland, "Mechanism." Ragland, "Chymistry." Ragland, "Experimental Clinical Medicine."

58   Huisman, *Finger of God*, chs. 2 and 3.

59   Molhuysen, *Bronnen*, Vol. 1, 58. Paaw, *Primitiae Anatomicae*, unpag. preface.

60   Paaw, *Observationes*, 6.

61   The records we have give 33 dissections from 1591 to 1602, nearly 3 per year. Paaw, *Observationes*.

62   Huisman, *Finger of God*, 23, 28–29. But see Wear, *Knowledge & Practice*, 146–148, and De Renzi, et al., *Pathology in Practice*.

subjects, from the daughter of the local governor to the corpse of his colleague Johannes Heurnius.[63] In the bodies of phthisic or consumptive patients, Paaw found the lungs dotted with pus-producing abscesses and phlegm hardened into "stones."[64] He linked these morbid phenomena with the appearances from other patients' bodies, some with lungs full of abscesses. Later, as Harm Beukers and Tim Huisman have pointed out, Johannes's son Otto Heurnius extended the practice of post-mortem dissections, making it a regular feature of clinical teaching in the later 1630s.[65] In the following chapters, I excavate the writings of the professors, letters and notes from students, and the institutional records to detail this practice and put it in its place.

Even the public anatomies in the theater aimed at medical knowledge and practice, with moral or religious display a secondary purpose. Humanist erudition and theological or religious pieties certainly informed their work, as historians have emphasized. Paaw, in particular, often quoted Classical texts with humanist flair and occasionally mined the Bible as a source for anatomical knowledge. But in Paaw's publications on anatomy, he stressed the exemplars in anatomical practice from his own medical education, and especially the relevance of anatomical knowledge for the practices of physicians and surgeons.

To distinguish the professors' anatomical practices, I have chosen to categorize the dissections based on their locations and the sorts of people who could attend the procedure. I call dissections held in the anatomy theater, which were open to students, professors, and townspeople willing to pay a small fee, "public anatomies." Those in private homes or other private settings I mark out as "private anatomies," and those in the hospital "clinical anatomies" since they usually followed days or weeks of teaching, diagnosis, and treatment in the hospital. In distinguishing between public and private anatomies I am following in part the analysis of Katharine Park and Cynthia Klestinec.[66] But regular hospital teaching and post-mortem dissections allowed for professors and students to harvest more detailed and more frequent histories of symptoms and evidence from diseased cadavers, so I want to mark out the third category of "clinical anatomies." Like medical students at Padua, students and professors at Leiden expressed constant and eager interest in using all three sorts of anatomies for seeing the morbid states of bodies and so learning pathology from the

---

63   In 1566, professor Girolamo Cardano, who taught medical theory at Bologna, collaborated with his former student, the anatomist Volcher Coiter, to dissect the body of his colleague, Gianbattista Pellegrini. Siraisi, *The Clock and the Mirror*, 116–117.

64   Paaw, *Observationes*, 15.

65   Beukers, "Clinical Teaching," 142. Huisman, *Finger of God*, 141–143. Otto Heurnius, *Historiae*.

66   Park, *Secrets of Women* Klestinec, *Theaters of Anatomy*.

senses directly.[67] Of course, they could no longer sense directly the active qualities of hot and cold in the diseased organs of their dead, dissected patients' bodies. But they noted all of the preternatural appearances, or those "beyond nature" (*praeter naturam*), especially abscesses, ulcers, and corrupt fluids, as well as dry, blackened, and burnt organs apparently affected by excess heat, or parts congealed from cold. Recognizing these diseased appearances beyond nature depended in part on experience with healthy anatomical states.

Under Paaw and Heurnius' son, Otto, post-mortem dissections, or clinical anatomies, became institutionalized. They were a central part of what it meant to do medicine. Only through such dissections could professors and students locate every cause of the diseases, the internal lesions which injured the proper action of at least one organ or part. The celebrated 1636 establishment of regular clinical instruction in the hospital officially aimed at teaching students the nature of the diseases, the examination of their accidents, their treatment through surgery and medicines, and "the opening of all the dead bodies of the foreign or unbefriended persons, and showing the causes of death to the students."[68] Of course, as mentioned, surgeons and professors "opened" bodies from all sorts of social stations and locations.

Teaching practices followed the other parts of the official guidelines. Professors and surgeons carefully tracked down the perceptible causes of death and reconstructed the anatomical progress of diseases. As Otto Heurnius put it in his clinical diary in 1639, after the hospital dissection of the body of the young Sara Mente, killed by purulent wasting of the lungs, "With the Chest and Abdomen opened, we detected every cause of the malady."[69] Certainly, professors and students applied medical theory they took to be well-established by long experience—ancient Greek medicine from Hippocrates and Galen survived the centuries as the best general approach to understanding and curing diseases. But post-mortem dissections were no mere exercises in concocting likely stories. Sometimes they did not find local, preternatural lesions. In the body of Cathlyn Mathyloo, killed at only fifteen years of age by a wasting disease, they found no "exceptional cause of death of any visceral organ," but only a general drying and consumption of fat.[70] The limits and deliverances of their senses had greater epistemic weight than the pre-determined targets from medical theory.

---

67   Stolberg, "Post-mortems," 72–3, 79, *pace* Klestinec, *Theaters of Anatomy*, 169.
68   Molhuysen, *Bronnen*, II, 312*.
69   Otto Heurnius, *Historiae*, 19.
70   Otto Heurnius, *Historiae*, 18.

Professors and students frequently visited the poor, sick patients in the St. Caecilia Hospital and dissected those unfortunate enough to die. Throughout the post-mortems, anatomical dissection explicitly revealed to the senses the localized morbid matter or affected parts that caused or constituted patients' diseases. Through regular hospital teaching, they correlated this post-mortem evidence with days and weeks of observing patients' symptoms, signs, and treatment progressions. At times the Leiden professors and students made novel claims that persisted for centuries. For instance, Otto Heurnius discovered a range of morbid droplets, abscesses, and ulcers in the lungs of phthisis patients, from lungs "marbled with dark and pale droplets" to "many tiny tubercles [*tubercula*] from a crude, viscous matter."[71] Like his father Johannes, Otto Heurnius used newer chymical remedies such as sulphur compounds to treat his patients. He also tried remedies from global conquest and trade networks, notably when a soldier returned from the Dutch colonial headquarters in Brazil in 1637 with corrupted digits from the counter-invasion of tiny flea-like animals. Otto combined book learning and pharmacological skill to attempt a recreation of the indigenous "oil of Couroq" to treat the wounds.[72] By the 1660s, the Leiden pedagogical tradition of clinical anatomies flourished under the guidance of Franciscus Sylvius, who built his new theory of phthisis around the development of tubercles as revealed in dozens of dissections.

Thus from the early 1590s through the 1660s, at least, students at Leiden learned to seek the hidden, localized causes of diseases by correlating symptoms and local bodily changes revealed in post-mortem dissections. University statutes gave the professors the task of instructing the students at the public hospital and demonstrating "to ocular confidence the causes of death in dissected cadavers."[73] After the daily clinical teaching of diagnosis and treatment in the hospital and viewing the public post-mortems or experiments performed by their professors, students often could take up their own dissections on human and animal bodies. Only post-mortem dissections could reveal the sensory evidence, pinpointing the causes and progress of the disease, as professors in the 1650s and 1660s revived the pedagogical practice: "in the accurate opening and demonstration of their bodies it was revealed to all, whether they had judged rightly or wrongly about that Disease."[74] In this way, students could hone their skills and produce novel discoveries for credit, and put into practice the long Galenic-Hippocratic emphasis on *autopsia*—on seeing for oneself.

---

71   Otto Heurnius, *Historiae*, 10, 22
72   Otto Heurnius, *Historiae*, 8.
73   Molhuysen, *Bronnen*, Vol. 3, 150.
74   Sylvius, *Opera Medica* (1695), 907.

Post-mortem dissections appear as part of Leiden life from early on, embedded in legal systems and the education of physicians. Records of the dissections frequently name witnesses, especially the other professors or city officials present. No doubt, this buttressed the credibility of the findings for legal purposes. Many of the cases recorded involve suspected poisonings, infanticide, violence, and even suspected bewitchings. Public and private dissections could disenchant suspicions of witchcraft by finding material, localized disease instead. In each case, Paaw and Otto provided localized, material histories of the diseases over time, as revealed in the dissected bodies. These cases of suspected witchcraft appear side by side in the sources, arranged in a series by disease or suspected cause of death, as did others for patients who died of phthisis. This strongly suggests that, as in other practices in Italy and Spain, early modern physicians across Europe linked disease post-mortems in series to generate knowledge.[75] As mentioned, Bonet's 1679 *Graveyard* compiled nearly three thousand post-mortem reports from nearly five hundred physicians.[76] As I detailed below, other influential figures from William Harvey to Thomas Bartholin showed keen interest in pathological anatomy and post-mortem dissections. Early modern physicians, trained in pathological models stretching back to Galen, put into practice the search for the seats and causes of diseases.

With this new, revisionist, and comprehensive account of Galenic physicians' medicine in place, it is plain that the established view stressing the unimportance of anatomy for their practices of diagnosis and therapy is incorrect. Galenic physicians' humoral thinking did not conceal the organs and simple parts with vague talk of whole-body humoral imbalances, flows, and intractable individual idiosyncrasies. But the established view rightly points to the fact that the spread of anatomical dissection, the correction of Galen's anatomical errors (due to his dissection of animal rather than human bodies), and the accumulation of new discoveries in anatomy did not lead to equally widespread and *fundamental* changes in pathological theory or therapeutic practice. This may seem surprising to present-day presentist yearnings, but it makes good sense given the revised portrait of Galenic medicine presented here. In short, we should not expect major changes in early modern Galenic pathology and therapy since they were already anatomically oriented. Organ-based pathological theory and therapy in the 1500s and early 1600s built *from* Galenic and Hippocratic foundations, largely following Galen's methods and models.

---

75   Skaarup, *Anatomy and Anatomists in Early Modern Spain*. De Renzi, "Seats and Series."
76   Bonet, *Sepulchretum*. Irons, "Théophile Bonet." Rinaldi, "Organising Pathological Knowledge."

3   Reconstructing Intellectual Microcosms

To make the case for a revised and comprehensive account of early modern
Galenic medicine, I mine unstudied sources from professors and a few students
throughout the educational world of Leiden medicine in the first six decades,
from 1575 through the 1630s. In order to tell a story of change over time, the
breadth of medical culture demands attention, with a close focus on what was
worth knowing and the means for knowing it. Early modern physicians and
natural philosophers wrote books, letters, disputations, laudatory poems, lectures, and notes in such a deluge that it is difficult to keep your balance, let
alone recognize the patterns of the flow. The leading medical professor of the
early period at Leiden, Johannes Heurnius (or van Heurne, 1543–1601), wrote
at least eighteen works, treating chymistry, textbook medical theory and practice, and commentaries on the Hippocratic works, as well as separate works on
fevers, the diseases of women, and the diseases of the head, stomach, heart,
and chest. In order to understand this rich culture—its practices, ideas, modes
of communication, ideals, norms, and development over time—we must
immerse ourselves in its most extensive and complex products. As Anthony
Grafton insisted decades ago, to understand the history of education, or even
the history of science, we must take a perilous leap "and plunge into the vast
and terrifying Latin books that reveal these teachers' goals and methods in
detail."[77]

These texts demand close and even extended readings, rather than select
slices neatly ordered to the argument or plot of a thin history over time. A
central claim of this book is that we cannot understand the cultural practices
and intentional vision of students and professors building and living experimental lives by pulling out parts piecemeal, for instance separating faculty
theory or chymistry from pharmacology, pathology, or anatomical practices.
The weedy diversity of the texts, ideas, methods, apparatus, skills, and values
is visible only when viewed from a perspective that takes in the whole field.
Rather like a fractal pattern, or even the microcosm-macrocosm correspondence so prevalent in Renaissance academic thought, each text embeds and in
turn is embedded into the complex patterned life of the broader culture.

Books come first, but it would be rash to imagine that "bookish" learning
or humanist scholarship worked stolidly against experiential or even experimental practices. Books provided inspiring models of experiential inquiry
and targets for experience-based criticism. Questioning the claim of ancient

---

77   Anthony Grafton, "Civic Humanism," 74.

books often drove professors to use and celebrate personal, sense-based experience. Beginning at least in the 1490s, humanist physicians confronted apparent errors in ancient descriptions of medicinal plants with the reliability of their own experience.[78] At the same time, the recovery of ancient learning from authors such as Dioscorides, Galen, and Hippocratic writers inspired recreations of their activities, elaborations, and hands-on attempts to test or disconfirm their claims. Even the venerable commentary traditions in medicine showed increasing attention to critical evaluation of the claims about phenomena and causes in ancient texts.[79] Better methods, sharpened methodological discussions, and better *historiae* or descriptions of appearances spread across the 1500s, with learned medicine leading the way in many cases.[80] As Klaas van Berkel argues, this elevation of personal experience and first-hand descriptions developed in the Low Countries as well.[81] Here, we will explore these themes, and especially the growth of experience, in the broader context of early modern Dutch medicine, as seen through these sources from Leiden University.

Leiden medical culture in this period, roughly 1575–1639, also involved frequent tests and lines of investigation, especially in the three central areas of anatomy, clinical practice, and chymistry. Some of their practices, such as checking their diagnoses against the appearances in patients' bodies, trying different methods for growing plants, or their work making and testing remedies in practice, might well be called "experimental."[82] Yet professors and students in this period did *not* obviously embrace an *experimentalist* program either in rhetoric or sustained, coordinated practices. In other words, they did not set up intentional programs of using experiments to ground and test knowledge. These later programs and practices, though, developed *within* this medical culture and as elaborations or inflections of the existing practices of teaching, learning, knowing, and curing.[83]

---

78   Ogilvie, *Science of Describing*, 128–133. Nauert, "Humanists, Scientists, and Pliny." Palmer, "Medical Botany." Nutton, "The Rise of Medical Humanism."
79   Siraisi, *Avicenna in the Renaissance*, 201.
80   Pomata and Siraisi, eds., *Historia*. Ogilvie, *Science of Describing*. Pomata, "Observation Rising." Pomata, "A Word of the Empirics."
81   Van Berkel, *Citaten uit het boek der natuur*, ch. 2. Cf. Jorink, *Reading the Book of Nature*.
82   E.g., Egmond, "Experimenting with Living Nature."
83   I tell the more complete story of the emergence, development, and legacy of this experimentalist university medicine in a forthcoming book, which is complete, tentatively titled *Experimental Life*. For now, see Ragland, "Mechanism"; Ragland, "Chymistry"; and Ragland, "Experimental Clinical Medicine."

Humanist scholarly practices and pedagogical methods wove all of these threads together. They drove professors and students into constant contact with ancient sources, medieval and early modern commentaries and critiques, objects of knowledge, and the daily concern for their own research and scholarly reputations. In reconstructing this interplay of ancient texts, traditions and innovations, ideas and practices, and in a local setting over time, I take as exemplary the methods of scholars such as Domenico Bertoloni Meli, Robert Frank, Anita Guerrini, Dmitri Levitin, William Newman, Gianna Pomata, Rose-Mary Sargent, and especially Nancy Siraisi and Michael Stolberg.[84] My emphasis on pedagogical practices as sources for a conserved common culture and genuine innovations takes this humanistic intellectual historical approach on a different tack. This book also points to the vitality of its revisionist picture of early modern Galenism well beyond Leiden. My recovery of ancient models of anatomically-based pathology and therapy from texts widely used for teaching across Europe in the 1500s and 1600s and my reconstruction of the larger early modern context and pedagogical networks from Italy to the Low Countries strongly suggest that Leiden practices were a harvest and extension of widespread Renaissance pedagogical developments.

4   Pedagogy and Practices

Teaching, training, and learning link together the three themes of making physicians, making knowledge, and making trials. The development of experiments and experimentalism came about primarily through inflection points in pedagogy. Studies of pedagogy promise more robust, middle-level histories, between the idiosyncrasies of the very local and the broad strokes of big-picture generalizations. In large part, they do this by showing us how groups and generations of scientists are produced by pedagogical practices. As David Kaiser has emphasized for the modern period, "Scientists are not born, they are made."[85] Physicians and natural philosophers did not appear fully formed in early modern Europe, either. They were made most often in and around universities. The ideas, ideals, sources, practices,

---

84   Bertoloni Meli, *Mechanism, Experiment, Disease*. Frank, *William Harvey and the Oxford Physiologists*. Guerrini, *Courtier's Anatomists*. Levitin, *Ancient Wisdom*. Newman, *Atoms and Alchemy*. Pomata, "Observation Rising." Pomata, "A Word of the Empirics." Pomata, "*Praxis Historialis*." Sargent, *The Diffident Naturalist*. Siraisi, *Avicenna in the Renaissance*. Stolberg, *Experiencing Illness*. Stolberg, "Bedside Teaching." Stolberg, "Empiricism."

85   Kaiser, "Introduction," in *Pedagogy and the Practice of Science*. Warwick and Kaiser, "Kuhn, Foucault, and the Power of Pedagogy," in *Pedagogy and the Practice of Science*.

and human connections students cultivated and crafted in the process of becoming physicians at universities formed the cores of their ways of medical knowing and doing. After all, training students into professional practices through exercises, habit, and communal values was a major goal of education.

Historians of science have mined the riches of practice in the last few decades, but focused studies of early modern scientific training and pedagogy remain relatively rare prizes.[86] Even for medicine and the life sciences, scientific academies, courts, and museums still get a kingly share of scholarly investigations.[87] Clearly, historians of science now often self-consciously take practices, rather than ideas, as the privileged objects of study. But if we take practices in the rich sense, as complex, sustained, goal-oriented, and communally cultivated activities, rather than simply whatever people happened to do, then surely we must attend more carefully to the places and communities where people learned and developed such practices.[88] Universities as cultural institutions and communities cultivated robust practices and trained students and professors in them. Through repeated specialized activities and exercises, through acculturation in communities, and orientation toward the goals and norms of disciplines or traditions, education brings practices to be in the world.

Studies of pedagogy and practices in other disciplines and medicine have already borne important fruit. Mordechai Feingold and Peter Dear have elegantly argued for the importance of universities in their histories of mixed mathematics and philosophy.[89] Universities matter crucially for our histories of medicine and experimentation, too. The scope of university training naturally explains much of the shared intellectual culture of physicians, philosophers, humanist scholars, and other members of the emerging Republic of Letters.[90] If, then, we want to understand not only the work of the canonical

86 For a recent overview of "practice," see Hicks and Stapleford, "The Virtues of Scientific Practice." For pedagogy and early modern science and medicine, e.g,: Siraisi, *Avicenna in the Renaissance*. Stolberg, "Empiricism." Stolberg, "Bedside." Powers, *Inventing Chemistry*. Klestinec, *Theaters of Anatomy*.

87 E.g.: Findlen, *Possessing Nature*. Bertoloni Meli, *Mechanism, Experiment, Disease*. Rankin, *Panaceia's Daughters*. Guerrini, *Courtier's Anatomists*.

88 In my notion of practices in this richer sense, I am following and paraphrasing Hicks and Stapleford, "Virtues of Scientific Practice." Of course, historians have other definitions, but Hicks and Stapleford draw from an impressively ecumenical range of approaches and offer illumination for the way forward.

89 Feingold, *Mathematicians' Apprenticeship*. Dear, *Discipline and Experience*.

90 Levitin, *Ancient Wisdom*. Grafton, "A Sketch Map of a Lost Continent." Grafton, "The New Science and the Traditions of Humanism." Goldgar, *Impolite Learning*.

names in the history of science and medicine, but how broader intellectual, cultural, and practical shifts occurred, surely universities that trained thousands of students every year are a good place to look. From its founding in 1575 to 1650, Leiden University had over two thousand students matriculate in medicine.[91] Not all students, especially foreign students who studied with other medical faculties, stayed very long, but those who really studied for their degrees stayed for years.[92] In the middle of the 1500s—when Padua similarly embraced making trials of drugs and materials, innovative clinical teaching, anatomical research, systematic Galenic medicine, and some post-mortem dissections—three to five hundred students matriculated in medicine at Padua *each year*.[93] Physicians were not born, but made, and primarily in universities.

Luminaries such as Nancy Siraisi, Jerome Bylebyl, Charles Schmitt, and John Gascoigne have argued persuasively that the universities were the productive cultural sites for the great majority of the developments in the "life sciences" in the early modern period.[94] The case of anatomy is especially noteworthy. As Cynthia Klestinec argues powerfully, pedagogy shaped the teaching and learning of anatomy in Renaissance Italy.[95] Students pushed university administrators at Padua to encourage more practical anatomical demonstrations, and from the 1580s on eagerly sought out "private" anatomical demonstrations for developing their own practical skills and experience. Students spoke up and protested for better sight lines, closer engagement with bodies, useful anatomical knowledge, and kicking the gaping commoners out of the public anatomy theater.

Professors, too, developed influential innovations for pedagogical ends. As Allen Shotwell argues, Vesalius made sustained use of illustrations, skeletons, and animal bodies in order to remedy long-standing limitations in the public anatomy lessons.[96] And Vivian Nutton has revealed the importance of pedagogical practices and goals for stimulating critiques and revisions of Galenic anatomy in the work of Vesalius's teacher, Johann Guinter, and Vesalius's

91   Prögler, *English Students at Leiden University*, 293.
92   Prögler, *English Students at Leiden University*, 192–193, and 192 n. 355, reports that over half of English medical students at Leiden spent fewer than three months there, while those that stayed remained for over two years on average, though this is from a very small sample size based on incomplete records of student movements.
93   Ragland, "'Making Trials,'" 527.
94   Siraisi, "Medicine." "Bylebyl, "The School of Padua." Bylebyl, "Medicine, Philosophy, and Humanism." Schmitt, "Science in the Italian Universities." Gascoigne, "A Reappraisal of the Role of the Universities in the Scientific Revolution."
95   Klestinec, *Theaters of Anatomy*.
96   Shotwell, "Animals, Pictures, and Skeleton."

early work.[97] Leiden professors, as we will see, made gradual innovations in pathology and healthy anatomy through their use of anatomical and bedside teaching.

Looking to Leiden medicine from the later-sixteenth through the seventeenth century complements important studies of the early modern Low Countries. Historians of Dutch science have long emphasized the practical bent, democratic sentiments, and anti-speculative resistance of iconic investigators of nature, from Simon Stevin and Herman Boerhaave to Hendrik Lorentz.[98] Klaas van Berkel has argued that this should not be chalked up to a vague "national character," but the norms and values of institutions, especially universities.[99] Rienk Vermij's history of Copernicanism in the Low Countries recounts the importance of universities in the history of new astronomy and physics, as scholars gradually encountered then vigorously debated and taught Copernican, Cartesian, and Newtonian systems.[100] Eric Jorink has picked up on Van Berkel's call for a study of the idea of "the book of nature" in early modern Dutch thought and woven a reflective, magisterial survey: even the study of everyday *naturalia* such as silkworms—perhaps *especially* the littlest things—revealed the truths and splendors of Creation. Investigating, knowing, and representing nature merged what might appear to us as distinct scientific, moralizing, and religious pursuits.[101] In harmony with Van Berkel's suggestion, most of the wide cast of characters in Jorink's scintillating study came to know and create their shared culture through university training.[102]

Of course, the university thrived on student fees and some state support and developed as part of the wider world. Recent scholarly work on science and medicine in the Dutch Golden Age strongly suggests that Dutch global commerce shaped investigative practices and objects. Harold Cook's studies of incredible breadth and detail argue that we can find the cultural values and practices of modern investigative, communicative science in a global, commercial Dutch culture in which actors agreed to privilege things, facts, and useful information and to avoid theories.[103] Most recently, Dániel Margócsy shows that the competitive world of Dutch commerce, art, and science actually

---

97   Nutton, "Preface."
98   E.g., Dijksterhuis, *Simon Stevin*. Van Berkel, *Citaten uit het boek der natuur*, 11–23. Jorink, *Reading the Book of Nature*, 13.
99   Van Berkel, *Citaten uit het boek der natuur*, 21–23.
100   Vermij, *The Calvinist Copernicans*.
101   Jorink, *Reading the Book of Nature*.
102   Jorink, *Reading the Book of Nature*, esp. ch. 2, and *passim*.
103   Cook, *Matters of Exchange*. Cook, "The New Philosophy."

grew more from productive *disagreement* rather than normative consensus.[104] In my view, Margócsy is brilliantly persuasive that disagreement and competition drove the flourishing trade in anatomical representations and artifacts. Drives for reputation and novelty, as well as cultural contestations and patterns of critique, quickened the form of life in the university as well. Before the earthquake of William Harvey's experimental demonstration of the circulation of the blood in 1628, though, most of the innovation sprouted within well-tended, but increasingly eclectic, fields of Galenic-Hippocratic medicine.[105]

Humanist medicine, like more strictly literary forms of humanist scholarship, displayed a keen epistemological attention to particulars. The practices and patterns we have seen in Leiden academic medicine, 1575–1639, fit with larger trends across Europe. Humanist values and practices, especially among physicians, created Renaissance natural history. Richard Palmer, Charles Nauert, Nancy Siraisi, Vivian Nutton, Paula Findlen, Karen Reeds, and Brian Ogilvie, among others, have demonstrated in great detail how humanist scholarly culture motivated critiques of ancient authorities and cultivated the practices of sensory engagement, collection, description, communication, and testing that generated the new pedagogy of *materia medica* and the discipline of natural history.[106] Humanist culture continued to shape natural philosophy, anatomy, mechanics, and mixed mathematics in the seventeenth century.[107] The work of Gianna Pomata on academic medicine and the rise of *historia* and observation, of Dmitri Levitin on experimental natural philosophy and apothecaries, and of Peter Dear on mixed mathematics present a few noteworthy examples.[108]

In natural history, engagement with ancient texts and the emulation of ancient calls for personal experience of particulars motivated and structured the rise and spread of first-person, embodied encounters with things as the privileged means for knowing nature. Similarly, sixteenth-century anatomists' cultivation of epistemic reliance on their own sensory experiences of

104   Margócsy, *Commercial Visions.*
105   French, *William Harvey's Natural Philosophy.* Ragland, "Mechanism."
106   Palmer, "Medical Botany." Nauert, "Humanists, Scientists, and Pliny." Siraisi, *Avicenna in the Renaissance.* Siraisi, *The Clock and the Mirror.* Siraisi, "Medicine." Nutton, "Greek Science in the Sixteenth-Century Renaissance." Nutton, "The Rise of Medical Humanism." Findlen, *Possessing Nature.* Reeds, *Botany.* Ogilvie, *Science of Describing.*
107   For recent studies, see Levitin, *Ancient Wisdom*; Guerrini, *Courtiers' Anatomists*; Raphael, *Reading Galileo.*
108   Pomata, *"Praxis Historialis."* Pomata, "Observation Rising." Levitin, "Early Modern Experimental Philosophy." Levitin, *Ancient Wisdom.* Dear, *Discipline and Experience.* Levitin, "'Made Up from Many Experimentall Notions.'"

dissected bodies also echoed ancient models even as it gave anatomists, like the naturalists, the expertise to mount cutting criticisms of ancient errors.[109] Renaissance anatomy as a practice and as an important source of medical knowledge developed primarily within and around universities. University-based anatomists were not significantly playing catch-up to developments "moving rapidly ahead outside the schools."[110] Surgeons and apothecaries, too, embraced and interacted with humanist scholarly culture from Italy to England.[111] This shared humanist culture provided common ideas, language, and practices, including some toleration of religious differences, as at Leiden. But it also provided a common field for battles over facts and theories, and controversies and innovations based on practitioners' own experience did not end with their corrections of the ancients. Cycles of controversy appear throughout early modern natural history, anatomy, theory, and therapeutics. Increasingly, physicians, surgeons, apothecaries, and philosophers sought to ground their critical and novel claims in deliberate trials or experiments.[112]

Values of close description of materials, the investigation of useful effects, attempts at rational methods, and a reluctance to wrangle over theories were widely characteristic of Leiden academic teaching in this period. These themes call to mind Harold Cook's celebrated study of medicine, commerce, culture, and philosophy in the Dutch Golden Age. In this view, only with the European voyages of discovery and imperial expansion, the rise of global commerce, and the spread of the values of material description and material benefit could there have been a shift in values or practices away from philosophical contemplation and the pursuit of the Good toward modern materialist, empiricist, utilitarian science grounded on "materialism" and the pursuit of material goods.[113] In other words, the "intellectual activities we call science emerged from the ways of knowing valued most highly by the merchant-rulers of urban

---

109 Bylebyl, "School of Padua." Bylebyl, "Medicine, Philosophy, and Humanism." Klestinec, *Theaters.* French, "Berengario da Carpi." French, *Dissection and Vivisection.* Shotwell, "Animals, Pictures, and Skeletons." Shotwell, "Revival of Vivisection." Ragland, "'Making Trials.'"

110 *Pace* Cook, *Matters,* 36.

111 E.g., Savoia, "Skills, Knowledge, and Status." Levitin, "'Made Up from Many Experimentall Notions.'"

112 E.g., Dear, *Discipline and Experience.* Ragland, "'Making Trials.'" Levitin, "'Made Up from Many Experimentall Notions.'"

113 Cook, *Matters of Exchange,* 2, 39–41. Since very few of the figures Cook studies were avowed philosophical materialists, and pretty much all were pious Christians, it seems by the term "materialism" we should understand something like an emphasis on materials and material knowledge.

Europe."[114] Thus, the rise of global modern science and a global economy developed mutually, as co-productions.[115] Due to this shift in values from philosophical contemplation to detailed acquaintance with material particulars, "[e]ven the university professors had to start paying attention" to things like worldly objects, natural particulars, sensory details, careful description, and natural history.[116]

From our view in Leiden, though, it seems that Cook's impressive global survey has left out the sources and nature of many of the most important ideas and practices of academic medicine. So far as I can tell from the textbooks, lectures notes, letters, disputations, archival records, casebooks, and eyewitness reports from Leiden's medical school, there seems little need to invoke mercantile culture, or much evidence that the values and practices of such culture played a *significant* role in the explicit and implicit ways of knowing and cultivated practices of the professors and students. If we want to understand the origins of the values and ways of knowing of early modern physicians, why not look first to the pedagogical cultures that formed them?

Of course, the students and professors studied materials shipped along global trade networks, and fought imported and domestic diseases with new remedies from the New World and beyond. Professors such as Paaw also very occasionally used some mercantile language to express scholarly interests, as in his description of "the profit of this business" of anatomy, and his extended family amassed great commercial wealth and power.[117] But I can find no evidence to conclude that commercial culture had significant effects on his theory and practice, especially when compared to his years of study and daily teaching and research. Our evidence demonstrates that nearly every aspect of this medical culture—the activities, habits, virtues, practices, sources, ideas, goals, and language—was deeply and primarily scholarly. The fact that they mobilized their discursive scholarship in the service of administering and teaching a practical, supposedly results-oriented medicine shows them as practicing physicians and teachers of practitioners. Of course they lived connected to the wider world, especially through their natural historical work and search for God's remedies dispersed across the globe.

Dutch commerce exploded across the world mostly after the establishment of these academic medical practices and values. The core Leiden course on practice emphasizing the careful production of traditional and chymical

---

114   Cook, *Matters of Exchange*, 40.

115   Cook, *Matters of Exchange*, 416.

116   Cook, *Matters of Exchange*, 6, cf. 2.

117   Molhuysen, *Bronnen*, Vol. 1, 58. Paaw, *Primitiae Anatomicae*, unpag. preface.

remedies to treat anatomically-localized diseases began no later than 1587. (Similar courses in Italy, such as at Padua, date from the 1550s.) They founded the garden for sensory experience with plants and other medicinal ingredients in 1590, and developed it through 1594. The anatomy theater appeared in 1594, but professors held public anatomical demonstrations before then, likely as early as 1582. They also frequently performed post-mortem dissections, at least as early as 1591. Dutch trade began its rapid global expansion after the Spanish embargo on Dutch ships and goods in the Mediterranean in 1598. The first private expedition to the East Indies in 1595 brought little profit, and one or two years later returned with only a third of the crew and likewise generated little revenue. But the Second Maritime Expedition returned in 1599 laden with cloves, nutmeg, mace, and pepper, and Dutch ships began to outnumber Portuguese vessels on the trade route. A growing flood of Dutch private companies spread to Asia, Africa, and the Americas, and Dutch commerce openly took on imperial force with the United East India Company (VOC, chartered 1602, headquartered on Java in 1619) and the West India Company (WIC, chartered 1621, but headquartered in Recife, Brazil only by 1630).[118]

By the time the violent and profitable global trade and colonization programs began to succeed, Dutch academic medicine had institutionalized the pursuit of detailed, useful knowledge of material things for years. The European medical schools that shaped these Dutch professors had cultivated similar practices for decades, and ancient models and texts frequently supplied their exemplars. It is not at all clear that commercial values were the reason why "the material details of the world perceived by the senses became the foundation of a new approach to knowledge."[119] In academic medicine, in both theory and practice, educated sensation of the material details of the world already was the foundation of knowledge.

Beyond the universities, of course, early modern medicine embraced a dazzling range of practitioners, ideas, debates, genres, objects, and practices. Taking Groningen as representative of the common experience in the Low Countries in the sixteenth and seventeenth centuries, Frank Huisman shows how the handful of university-trained physicians gradually cultivated their civic and moral authority with the city magistrates, religious leaders, and townsfolk, gaining social status over the far more numerous itinerant healers and surgeons.[120] Before the second half of the 1600s, Groningen physicians did

---

118   Israel, *Dutch Republic*, 320–327.

119   Cook, *Matters of Exchange*, 41.

120   Huisman, *Stadsbelang en Standsbesef.* For a recent study of physicians negotiating their status and developing practices in sixteenth-century Nuremberg, see Murphy, *A New Order of Medicine.*

not establish their reputations through research, but rather in giving advice for public health measures and cultivating places in the religious-social networks.[121] Taking a bold wider view, as mentioned, Cook's capacious history puts Dutch medicine on the global stage and as the lead actor in the shift to the new science, linking colonial physicians and massacres with useful Chinese medical practices, tempered religious passions, and the flight from speculation to useful, factual knowledge.[122] Florike Egmond uses the natural historical correspondence of the Leiden professor Carolus Clusius to reconstruct his networks of experts and specimens, which spanned urban, regional, European, global, gendered, and class-based territories.[123] Alisha Rankin has beautifully demonstrated the important trial-making practices of German noblewomen in the 1500s, and the epistemic and cultural powers and dangers of trying poisons and antidotes on humans and animals.[124] Historians such as Elaine Leong, Sara Pennell, and Michelle DiMeo have revived the study of the most widespread medicinal practices, those of household medicine, especially as recorded and developed through recipe books.[125] The embodied, experiential practices of knowledge creation and healing among Caribbean healers takes welcome center stage in the recent work of Pablo Gomez.[126] The increasingly connected early modern world mixed local medical substances, ideas, and practices across scales and settings.

This larger world of medicine linked through Leiden, too. Professors traveled as medical students, often training in Italy and France, especially at the University of Padua. They participated in European or even global correspondence and specimen-sharing networks. Learned apothecaries such as Leiden's Dirck Cluyt helped to organize the first university garden and taught students medicinal botany. He also probably knew more about plants and their medicinal powers than many of the professors. His son Outgert Cluyt trained as a medical student at the university and traveled the Mediterranean, extending the established collection of specimens from across the globe. Similarly, professors relied on surgeons for their expertise in wound care and the removal of gangrenous digits and other dangerously morbid parts. By the later 1630s, Leiden students could see the effects of global diseases on the bodies of soldiers of the Dutch trading empire. Students, professors, and their surgeon

---

121   Huisman, *Stadsbelang en Standsbesef,* 210–217, 302, chs. 3 and 6.

122   Cook, *Matters of Exchange.*

123   Egmond, *The World of Carolus Clusius.*

124   Rankin, *Panacea's Daughters.* Rankin, *The Poison Trials.*

125   Leong, *Recipes and Everyday Knowledge.* DiMeo and Sara, eds. *Reading and Writing Recipe Books, 1550–1800.*

126   Gómez, *The Experiential Caribbean.*

colleagues inspected and investigated bodies of people from a wide range of social stations in their post-mortem dissections.

This book draws from these larger perspectives, and notes important connections between Leiden university medicine and the wider early modern world. But it aims to follow the methods of intellectual histories and histories of practices first of all, especially through close readings of the writings of professors and students. Reading closely across a range of pedagogical materials allows for a fine-grained and integrated portrait of medical thinking and acting. Of course, this is only possible by taking a single location as the site of integration and following professors and students through their massive textbooks (which served as lecture courses), disputations, study guides, garden notebooks, hospital teaching and anatomy observations, correspondence, and institutional records. Throughout, they blended new materials and concepts into ancient frameworks for knowing and treating bodies in disease and health. In the settings of university life—the lecture hall, library, garden, anatomy theater, clinical hospital teaching, and private rooms—ancient sources and new experiences together could even generate new knowledge and cures. Pedagogy made practitioners.

5   Making Medicines from Books, Gardens, and Chymistry

In the university garden and lecture halls, students learned to identify medicinal ingredients and their powers or "faculties," and how to make drugs for themselves and their future patients. In their lecture courses in the theory of practice, professors introduced students to the dizzying lists of medicinal simples or singular ingredients, their powers, means of preparation, uses, and therapeutic cautions. After 1590, students could see plants growing in the university garden and encounter natural-historical specimens in the Ambulacrum built in 1601. Once again, pedagogical practices and student interests brought embodied engagement with particulars together with sophisticated teaching schemes, book learning, and debate. Knowing medicines, too, began with experience and reason.

Recent scholarly interest in early modern medicines has built on earlier foundations and revealed the local communities and global networks involved in the search for useful medicines.[127] Historians are also giving more due

---

127   E.g., Cook, *Matters of Exchange*. Estes, "The European Reception of the First Drugs from the New World." Huguet-Termes, "New World Materia Medica." Barrera, "Local Herbs, Global Medicines." Wear, *Knowledge & Practice*, ch. 2.

attention to apothecaries and household medicine.[128] Current work on early modern practices of testing medicines and trying cures complements Paula Findlen's studies of sixteenth-century Italian testing and Andreas-Holger Maehle's pioneering focus on tests of drug substances in the long eighteenth century.[129] As Richard Palmer, Brian Ogilvie, and others have argued, learned physicians revived and emulated ancient models to lead a movement to improve pharmacy and medical botany.[130] These reforms combined humanist erudition and practical know-how.

Pharmacological teaching at Leiden enjoys brief mentions in older studies and some recent sustained treatment, especially in the largely yet-to-be published work of Saskia Klerk.[131] Klerk has already demonstrated some of the complexity and dynamism of pharmacological theory and teaching at Leiden, as part of a larger story of physicians' thinking about drugs in the early modern Low Countries. Here, I will add the hidden history of early chymical teaching, some student study practices in the garden, the model methods of knowing found in the ancient sources, especially Galen's works on drugs, and a sense of the earlier debate over knowing the faculties or powers of drugs and medicinal ingredients.

Galen's *On the Mixtures and Faculties of Simple Drugs* was a handy and much-cited source for knowing and using the powers of medicinal substances. Although it was not much used directly in the medieval period, adaptations and extracts by Arabic and Latin authors were standard teaching texts. Compared with these common extracts, Niccolò da Reggio's complete translation in the early 1300s did not reach a wide audience.[132] By the 1400s and 1500s, though, university professors increasingly relied on the text. *Simple Drugs* was mandated at Bologna in the early 1400s, and later translations helped to make it a favorite teaching text of the influential professors Luca Ghini and

---

128   For recent work, see, e.g.: Pugliano, "Pharmacy, Testing, and the Language of Truth in Renaissance Italy." Levitin, "'Made Up from Many Experimentall Notions.'" Newson, *Making Medicines in Early Colonial Lima.* Leong, *Recipes.* For earlier works, see Wall, *A History of of the Worshipful Society of Apothecaries of London.* Palmer, "Medical Botany." Palmer, "Pharmacy in the Republic of Venice."

129   Findlen, *Possessing Nature,* esp. chs. 5 and 6. Maehle, *Drugs on Trial.* Leong and Rankin, eds., "Testing Drugs and Trying Cures."

130   Palmer, "Pharmacy in the Republic of Venice," 100, argues that "the dynamic for change came largely from learned physicians." In corroboration, Pugliano, "Pharmacy, Testing, and the Language of Truth," argues that Italian apothecaries did not perform many tests, but rather lived out performances of sincerity and authenticity. Ogilvie, *Science of Describing,* 34–36, 128–133.

131   Klerk, "Galen Reconsidered." Klerk, "The Trouble with Opium."

132   Ventura, "Galenic Pharmacology in the Middle Ages."

Ulisse Aldrovandi at Bologna in the 1530s and 1550s, as well as professors at Montpellier and many other universities.[133]

To recover some of the riches and uses of this text, I provide a summary of major features of Galen's *Simple Drugs*, in part to remedy the lack of a translation. As always, humanist professors carefully mined these ancient veins of learning and studded their own lectures and textbooks with conceptual and practical gems. Dioscorides and Galen shone as models of the proper method of knowing medicines, through personal sensory experience. As in their theories and practices of bodies, professors taught that the hot, cold, wet, and dry mixtures or temperaments of substances generated their faculties, from the basic heating, cooling, etc. to the higher-order rarefying, thinning, attracting, or repelling effects.

Of course, professors also brought works by Galen and Dioscorides into conversation with new plants and other medicinal ingredients from across the globe, substances whose identities and powers necessarily far exceeded the ancient works of the Mediterranean region.[134] Under the apothecary Dirck Cluyt's guidance, the university set up a teaching garden in the early 1590s for growing and identifying medicinal ingredients. They soon added the preeminent naturalist Carolus Clusius's expertise, network, and specimens, while keeping Cluyt as a resource for physical simples, his set of illustrations of plants for teaching in the winter months, and his own learning and connections. His son Outgert Cluyt's university training informed his perilous travels in the Mediterranean and beyond, learning from Jewish and local healers and collecting and shipping specimens back to the university, while in Leiden professor Paaw took over the direction of the garden and field trips with students. Professors and students strove to gain first-hand knowledge of remedies from the ground up.

Surprisingly, this included chymistry. As I show, chymical teaching had deep pedagogical roots in Leiden University, with leading professors giving instruction in chymical operations, apparatus, materials, and some theory. By the later 1650s, chymistry formed the third major strand of experimental culture at Leiden, along with anatomy and clinical practice.[135] Yet classic and recent histories of chymistry at Leiden center on Hermann Boerhaave in the early eighteenth century. This is just as he wanted it. In fact, the standard histories

---

133   Grendler, *Universities*, 343, 346, 350. Findlen, *Possessing Nature*, 159, 250, 254.

134   Palmer, "Medical Botany." Estes, "European Reception." Ogilvie, *Science of Describing*. Cooper, *Inventing the Indigenous*.

135   Beukers, "Het Laboratorium." Beukers, "Mechanistische Principes." Ragland, "Chymistry." Ragland, "Experimental Clinical Medicine."

have missed the earliest chymical instruction and dedicated chymical courses entirely. Chymistry enjoyed a long and productive history at Leiden, despite the claims from Herman Boerhaave and his historians that it really begins with his program in the early eighteenth century.[136] In the most recent and force-ful statement, Boerhaave made a "discrete break" in the history of chemistry by transforming a "didactic" chymistry aimed at making things (especially medicines) into a philosophical, experimental discipline that equipped stu-dents for natural philosophical investigations.[137] In this view, even "didactic" chymical teaching began only in 1642, in a very marginal way, with the hiring of an apothecary to teach the production of chymical medicines.[138] *Making Physicians*, in contrast, recovers new histories of chymical teaching from new sources.

At least by October 1587, and almost certainly earlier, students in Johannes Heurnius' frequent course on the practice of medicine received instruction in chymistry. This course integrated making and knowing, practice and theory. Students learned the basic instruments and operations for making chymical distillations and remedies. They also heard Heurnius' praise of chymistry as a true part of the Galenic-Hippocratic tradition, an art Hippocrates suppos-edly learned from Democritus. These disciplinary histories staged depictions of the ideal physician for students. Rather than practice as mere Empirics who avoided reasoning to hidden causes, or Rationalists who privileged theory over shared and personal experience of curing, true physicians ought to combine experience and reason.

To do so, they ought to practice chymistry. For Heurnius, Paracelsus brought this art to even greater heights, so now chymistry was "not just *very useful*, but

---

136   Spronsen, "The Beginning of Chemistry." Knoeff, *Herman Boerhaave*, 116–117. Powers,
        Inventing Chemistry, esp. 6, 47–62, 197. Boerhaave, "Discourse on Chemistry Purging Itself
        of Its Own Errors."

137   Powers, *Inventing Chemistry*, 6–8, 62, 91, 169. Powers draws on Hannaway to characterize
        chymical pedagogy before Boerhaave as "didactic" or aimed at the production of medical
        remedies and not knowledge. Hannaway, *The Chemists and the Word*. For scholarship
        demonstrating the philosophical, experimental status of even academic chymistry
        beyond the "didactic" search for remedies, see the following. Clericuzio, "Teaching
        Chemistry and Chemical Textbooks in France." Newman, *Atoms and Alchemy*. Newman,
        "Elective Affinity before Geoffroy." For Sennert's debt to the medical humanists, see espe-
        cially Fortunio Liceti, see Hirai, *Medical Humanism and Natural Philosophy*. Klein, "Daniel
        Sennert." For experimental, philosophical chymistry at Leiden before Boerhaave, see
        Beukers, "Mechanistische Principes," Ragland, "Chymistry," and Ragland, "Experimental
        Clinical Medicine."

138   Powers, *Inventing Chemistry*, 47.

rather *necessary*" for life and medicine.[139] In his lectures on practical medicine, Heurnius continued his earlier enthusiasm for transmutational alchemy, expressed in a previously-unstudied Paracelsian preface to an edition of medieval alchemical texts. He freely referenced pseudo-Lull and other authors on chymical practice and the wonderful powers of *aqua vitae* to cure disease and prolong life. He made Hippocrates into an enthusiast for chymical operations and medicines. Yet he kept his basic medical theory largely within the prescribed confines of the official curriculum: instruction in the principles and method of Galenic-Hippocratic medicine, aimed at final exams focused on expounding Hippocratic aphorisms and applying Galenic teaching to a given disease. As at other universities, such as Marburg which set up more hands-on chymical *collegia* from 1608, at Leiden professors retroactively adopted chymical processes, medicines, and ideas into the Galenic-Hippocratic family tree.[140] This approach continued with other professors' lectures, such as those of Johannes Walaeus in the early 1630s, and reached a high point in the middle of 1600s with a confident program of experimental, philosophical chymical teaching.[141]

6   Experience, Empiricism, and Experiment

Medicine provided a fertile ground for the development of experimental practices. In the seventeenth century experimentalism took many forms, but investigators shared similar commitments to the programmatic use of experiments to ground and test knowledge claims.[142] This book aims to search out the ways of knowing that shaped physicians prior to experimentalism, cataloging both those that share a family resemblance with experimental practices and those that have more discursive features.[143] Scholarly physicians increasingly

---

139   Heurnius, *Nova Ratio*, 67.
140   Krafft, "The Magic Word Chymiatria." Moran, *Chemical Pharmacy Enters the University.* Moran, *Andreas Libavius and the Transformation of Alchemy.*
141   Beukers, "Mechanistische Principes." Beukers, "Het Laboratorium." Ragland, "Chymistry." Ragland, "Mechanism." Ragland, "Experimental Clinical Medicine." I mention Walaeus' teaching briefly in chapter seven below.
142   For differences in experimentalisms, see Schickore, *About Method.* For a comparative analysis of experimental philosophies, see Sargent, *The Diffident Naturalist* and Levitin, "Early Modern Experimental Philosophy."
143   Without, of course, neatly separating the two, since humanist methods of reading, thinking, collecting, and writing informed experimental science, and vice versa. Grafton, "The New Science." Levitin, "The Experimentalist as Humanist." Levitin, *Ancient Wisdom.* Raphael, *Reading Galileo.*

cultivated experiential and even experimental practices across the sixteenth century. By the end of the sixteenth century and the beginning of the seventeenth, Leiden University medical education drew on rich pedagogical traditions and models to train thousands of students in such practices.

Historians have crafted many excellent histories that trace the rise or origins of early modern experimentation across a huge range of traditions or communities.[144] It seems that wherever historians have looked, they have found the origins of early modern experimental methods or practices. Together, they make a fascinating tapestry of early modern historical complexity. Not all of these histories are compatible, though. Four decades ago, scholars placed influential emphasis on gentlemanly culture, politics, and courtly sociability as the grounds for "the" experimental philosophy.[145] This approach has met with both pointed critiques and expeditions in new directions.[146] Similarly, Kuhn's postulation of two contrasting "traditions" of experimental practice,

---

144   For example, some historians have found the origins in medieval discussions of method, per Crombie, *Robert Grosseteste and the Origins of Experimental Science*; in mixed mathematics, especially as reconstituted and taught by Jesuits, per Dear, *Discipline and Experience*; in the work of the "superior craftsmen" of the craft or artisanal traditions, per Zilsel, "The Sociological Roots of Science"; in an embodied "artisanal epistemology" which is appropriated by elite gentlemen, per Smith, *The Body of the Artisan*; in the creation of "trading zones" and hybrid cultures by artisans, scholars, and patrons, per Long, *Artisan/Practitioners and the Rise of the New Science*; in the reaction to William Harvey's work, per French, *William Harvey's Natural Philosophy*; in alchemy, per Newman, *Atoms and Alchemy*; and Newman, "The Place of Alchemy in the Current Literature on Experiment"; in the optical traditions from at least Ibn al-Haytham through Kepler, per Sabra, *The Optics of Ibn Al-Haytham*, pp. 3–19; and Hackett, "Roger Bacon on Scientia Experimentalis"; and Dupré, "Inside the 'Camera Obscura'"; in the work of mechanics, per Bennett, "The Mechanics' Philosophy and the Mechanical Philosophy"; across a range of disciplines (but omitting the life sciences), but in two different forms, per Kuhn, "Mathematical vs. Experimental Traditions in the Development of Physical Science"; in reformed religion, per Harrison, *The Fall of Man and the Foundations of Modern Science*; and in the natural magic tradition, per Thorndike, *A History of Magic and Experimental Science*; and Rossi, *Francis Bacon*; and Henry, *The Scientific Revolution and the Origins of Modern Science*, Ch. 4. For a summary of the increasing pace of investigators setting up sustained experimentation around 1600, see Cohen, *How Modern Science Came into the World*, p. 245. For a recent overview, see Steinle, Pastorino, and Ragland, "Experiment in Renaissance Science."

145   Shapin and Schaffer, *Leviathan and the Air-Pump*. Shapin, *A Social History of Truth*. Findlen, "Controlling the Experiment." Beretta, Feingold, Findlen and Boschiero, "Regress and Rhetoric at the Tuscan court." Daston, "Baconian Facts, Academic Civility, and the Prehistory of Objectivity," on 348–349.

146   Sargent, *The Diffident Naturalist*. Hunter, ed., *Robert Boyle Reconsidered*. Schuster and Taylor, "Blind Trust." Guerrini, "The Truth about Truth." Lux and Cook, "Closed Circles or Open Networks?"

with open-ended experimentation in "Baconian" sciences of electricity, magnetism, etc. and confirmation experiments in mathematical sciences, is explicitly contradicted by historians such as J. A. Bennett and Domenico Bertoloni Meli (and, as Kuhn himself noted, his story left out the life sciences entirely).[147]

Other exemplary recent histories of artisanal cultures cover similar figures but present contrasting theses. Pamela Smith's far richer history largely agrees with Edgar Zilsel's thesis that gentlemanly elites "appropriated" the "empirical experiential knowledge" and expertise of the artisans and elevated it to generate the new philosophy.[148] In contrast, Pamela Long discusses many similar figures and sources to describe the new literate, artisanal, experiential, utilitarian philosophy as the product of the *shared* trading zones in which scholars and artisans shared goals and developed new outlooks, methods, and artifacts. In detailing the blending of scholarly and artisanal cultures and communities with shared goals, interests, and methods, Long explicitly rejects the idea that "superior artisans" alone or primarily influenced the new sciences in these ways, "as Zilsel and the other Marxists would have it."[149] Long's history again demonstrates the complexity of historical interactions, as well as the importance of scholars, even in the history of artisanal ways of knowing.[150]

Like most historians, I am happy to embrace explanatory pluralism for the complex rise and development of experimental practices across the early modern world. Given the fruitfulness of so many different approaches and the complexity of the increasingly interconnected globe in this period, it would be absurd to claim that any one history could capture the singular or privileged story of how we got early modern experimental science. Still, how people came to be trained to experiment seems a promising direction for understanding the rise and especially the *spread* of making trials and experiments.

In this book and its forthcoming companion, I would like to emphasize the university training of thousands of physicians in the grand weave of many threads and themes. This should come as no surprise, whether we look backwards or forwards. Looking ahead to the experimentalist societies of the later

---

147   Bennett, "Mechanics' Philosophy," is the most direct: "Whatever its heuristic value, there are no historical grounds for the distinction drawn by Kuhn" (6). Bertoloni Meli, *Thinking with Objects*, 12.

148   Smith, *The Body of the Artisan*, 238–239. Zilsel, "The Origins of Gilbert's Scientific Method," argues that William Gilbert's "spirit of observing and experimenting was taken over not from scholars but from manual workers" (15). Zilsel, "Sociological Roots," 558, argues that manual workers alone developed and added "experimentation" to "the genesis of science."

149   Long, *Artisan/Practitioners*, 129. Cf. Long, *Openness, Secrecy, Authorship*, esp. 244–250.

150   For the humanism of apothecaries, see Levitin, "'Made Up of Many Experimentall Notions.'"

seventeenth century, we can see physicians forming large or even predominant cohorts in the English Royal Society, the French Académie des Sciences, and especially the German Academia Naturae Curiosorum.[151] In his magisterial study, Robert Frank demonstrated over four decades ago that university professors and students in Oxford, through their institutional and extracurricular associations, developed a vibrant experimental research program to tackle the pressing questions left by Harvey's circulation of the blood doctrine. In so doing, they gradually formed the core of the Royal Society experimentalists.[152]

Turning to past exemplars, Galen and his works were often the leading exemplars of knowing by personal experience, testing claims by sense perceptions, limiting explanations to what one can sense, and confirming and refuting theories by making deliberate, sophisticated experiments or trials.[153] Galen explicitly founded his medicine on experience and reason (*peira kai logos*) and argued that all things had to be submitted to the test of experience.[154]

It is impossible to discuss learning from experience without introducing the term "empiricism," though the ambiguities and many meanings of the term pose perils to understanding. We may as well begin with the thought of the ancient Empirics, which demands a strict reliance on phenomena without recourse to causal explanations. In this skeptical rejection of knowledge about hidden causes, the Empirics (*empeirikoi*) denied the claims of the Rationalists (*logikoi*) and Dogmatists (*dogmatikoi*) to knowledge of qualities, humors, body parts, corruption, and other hypothesized causes of diseases. The Empirics relied on three sources as guides to effect cures: experience, history, and imitation. History consisted in reports that described phenomena. Imitation, in the use of similar cures on similar diseases in similar patients. Empirics divided experience (*empeiria*) into three sorts of trial (*peira*): involuntary, voluntary, and imitative. In no case, as Heinrich von Staden argues, do we find any sense of deliberately making a test, let alone setting up complex artificial conditions.[155]

In the early modern period, as Gianna Pomata has shown, physicians and philosophers drew on Galen's works and those of other ancient writers to

---

151   Cook, "New Philosophy and Medicine in Seventeenth-Century England," 403–404; Stroup, *A Company of Scientists*, 172; and Barnett, "Medical Authority and Princely Patronage."

152   Frank, *Harvey and the Oxford Physiologists*.

153   Hankinson, "Epistemology." Tieleman, "Galen on the Seat of the Intellect." Lloyd, "Experiment in Early Greek Philosophy and Medicine." Von Staden, "Experiment and Experience in Hellenistic Medicine." Stolberg, "Empiricism," 588, 493–495.

154   Hankinson, "Epistemology," 169–177. Wear, *Knowledge & Practice*, 130–133 and Maclean, *Logic, Signs, and Nature*, 191–203.

155   Von Staden, "Experiment and Experience in Hellenistic Medicine," 188–192.

recover the ideals and methods of the ancient Empiric medical sect.[156] From the Empirics' models, physicians drew out a notion of "observation" (*observatio*) with a "clear-cut distinction between direct and indirect experience, and the separation of observation from theory."[157] This Empiric-inspired empiricism mutually strengthened physicians' elevation of *historia* from simple knowledge without causes to "knowledge as preparatory to the investigation of causes" and the "cognitive value and dignity of experience."[158]

In comparison, Galen advocated a rational empiricism, in which the phenomena perceived by the senses ground and test knowledge claims, and experience or tests make discoveries, but reason must condition experience and develop knowledge with rigor and consistency. The best philosophers and physicians, after all, admired the certainty of geometric demonstrations and endorsed the hot, cold, wet, and dry qualities as the fundamental stuff of the mixtures of things.

Quite different again is the empiricism of chymist and medical reformer Paracelsus (1493–1541), who relied on his senses for knowledge of things, at times in the direct manner of artisans, but also elevated a form of "experience" (*Erfahrung*) as contemplative, divinely guided intuition of essences and the union of the knower and the known.[159] In further contrast, as Ann Blair has shown, the "bookish" empiricism of the natural philosopher, historian, and lawyer Jean Bodin freely mixed "facts" drawn from a vast treasury of books, nuggets of erudition sifted out through his commonplacing method of notetaking, alongside some of his own first-hand observations and sense experiences.[160] Bodin's program of measuring specific gravities for a range of substances brings us to yet another "empiricism" notable in the early modern period from canonical figures such as Galileo, Kepler, and Newton: the use of instrument-mediated measurement and experiments to construct mathematical theories. This empiricism, far removed from those of Paracelsus and the Empirics, had only limited appearances in medicine in this period, notably in Santorio Santorio's attempt to attack the errors in medicine with rigorous quantification of Galenic qualities and weights.

In all of these empiricisms, knowers make significant use of sensory phenomena—supposedly or actually perceived by themselves or others—to

---

156 Pomata, "A Word of the Empirics." Pomata, "Observation Rising."
157 Pomata, "Observation Rising," 69.
158 Pomata, "*Praxis Historialis*," 111, 137.
159 Smith, *The Body of the Artisan*, 82–89. Weeks, *Paracelsus*, 182–183, argues that Paracelsus's "'experience' suggests something altogether different from and very nearly opposite of the quantifying empirical analysis and experiment of the scientist."
160 Blair, *Theater*, 96–99, 228.

generate, support, or test knowledge claims. Yet the Empirics themselves would reject every one that rises from the phenomena toward theories or causes. In contrast, early modern physicians often followed Galen's slogan and method of joining together a reasoned understanding of causes with long personal experience in anatomy, pharmacology, diagnosis, pathology, and therapy.

By the middle of the 1500s, medical professors and students deemed Galen "the major authority" for a new, "positive attitude toward empirical approaches," as Michael Stolberg concludes from his review of student notes.[161] Riding the wave of Greek texts and translations that revealed a more direct, complete "new Galen" of the 1520s and 1530s, physicians began explicitly following Galen's example in making trials.[162] In anatomy, Vesalius replicated Galen's experiments on the pulse, including replacing part of an artery in a living animal with a tube, as well as Galen's sections of the recurrent nerves, and performed his own experiments on the male organs of generation.[163] Later anatomists such as Realdo Colombo and William Harvey also followed Galen's methods and replicated his experiments, even as they advanced anatomical discoveries against Galen's anatomical system.[164]

Physicians put even greater reliance on experience and tests in making and knowing medicines. As Philip van der Eijk demonstrates, Galen relied on systematic and reflective methodology for testing medicinal substances. His notion of "qualified experience" articulated conditions for the careful assessment of possible causal connections between the powers of drugs and foods and changes in human bodies. Galen used this experimental methodology for testing extant claims about the powers of substances and making new discoveries, and stressed replicability as a requirement for trials, as well as what look like parallel trials.[165] Dioscorides, the other major ancient authority on medicinal substances, also emphasized the importance of personal experience for knowing the identities and powers of ingredients. As we will see, in the 1500s Galen's works on drugs, especially *On the Mixtures and Faculties of Simple Drugs*, were widely popular teaching texts and provided models for experience-based testing.

Discursive pedagogical activities and ideals still structured much of university life. Core practices of reading ancient texts, taking notes in lectures,

---

161   Stolberg, "Empiricism," 495.
162   Nutton, "Greek Science in the Sixteenth-Century Renaissance."
163   Ragland, "'Making Trials,'" 521.
164   Shotwell, "The Revival of Vivisection." Galen's trials on the urinary system probably
        provided models for Harvey. See Shank, "From Galen's Ureters to Harvey's Veins."
165   Van der Eijk, *Medicine and Philosophy*, ch. 10.

developing skills of argument, passing the examinations, and defending a public disputation flourished throughout the period of this study. In the first half of the century, professors Johannes Heurnius and Albert Kyper wrote guides for students that spent page after page recommending the best books to read on various subjects, and methods for reading them. Heurnius also noted the necessity of anatomical and botanical study. Hippocratic texts, and especially the version of Hippocratic medicine codified by Galen, occupied the high seat. Kyper, writing decades later, added more recent authors to the list such as William Harvey and even René Descartes, and praised the recent revival of clinical instruction by his colleague Otto Heurnius.

Reason and experience remained the twin pillars of true medicine, from the Galenic physician Johannes Heurnius to the later chymical physician and Leiden professor Franciscus Sylvius and beyond.[166] The meaning of academic practices of "reason" remained relatively stable, rooted in Aristotelian logic and ongoing practices of argument and disputation. Logical fallacies of contradiction and begging the question remained the same. Working out consequences or effects from principles, and from effects back to principles or fundamental qualities, or inferring hidden causes from clusters of signs persisted as iconic activities of reason.

"Experience" shifted to include more and more local or individual forms, and especially the making of deliberate trials to test claims and discover new knowledge. Through the sixteenth century, Italian universities, especially Padua, had already developed frequent practices of testing claims and making new knowledge by "making trials."[167] Professors, students, apothecaries, and museum naturalists learned that arguments based on authority were weak and that personal experience in clinical practice, testing drugs, anatomy, uroscopy, and more active practices was essential for real knowledge and a successful medical practice.[168]

In making medicines, physicians increasingly had to rely on their own experience and the communicated reports of other experts. The teeming numbers of local and northern European plants and other medicinal ingredients had already far exceeded the hundreds of ingredients listed in the pharmacopoias of ancient authorities such as Dioscorides and Galen.[169] As European global empires uprooted more and more plants and peoples from their native lands and brought specimens and knowledge back to commercial and imperial

---

166 Ragland, "Experimental Clinical Medicine," Ragland, "Chymistry," and Ragland, "Mechanism."
167 Ragland, "'Making Trials.'"
168 Stolberg, "Empiricism." Findlen, *Possessing Nature*. Ragland, "'Making Trials.'"
169 Ogilvie, *Science of Describing*. Cooper, *Inventing the Indigenous*.

centers, physicians and naturalists had to contend with thousands of new samples and simples, as well as new diseases.[170]

In the early texts from Leiden, such as those of Johannes Heurnius and Paaw, "experience" most often stood for the general "long experience" of physicians in their construction of the Galenic-Hippocratic tradition. At times, it included individual "experience." Johannes Heurnius included reports from his own clinical experience and occasionally referenced anatomical post-mortems, and even some animal vivisections. He also referenced experience with chy-mistry in his lectures on chymical procedures and medicines. But he built his system of localized Galenic medicine almost entirely from the materials available in ancient and early modern *texts*. The "experience" that warranted the use of his recommended medicines "proven by use" was his own anecdotal experience and the "long experience" of physicians in his own envisioned, textual tradition. Paaw, in some contrast, followed the model of late-Renaissance anatomists and emphasized more his own experience—*autopsia*—and even contributed here and there to new discoveries and critiques of anatomical authorities.

An individual's sense-based experience, directed but not determined by discursive learning, stood as the foundation of knowledge in both epistemological theory and, increasingly, in pedagogical practice. Scholars and physicians drew on Galen's constant emphasis on the primacy of the senses for grounding and testing claims, as well as the common Aristotelian philosophy in which knowledge formation began with the senses, then memories, experience, and finally universals. Properly trained, the senses really revealed the fundamental principles of the natural world, especially the qualities hot, cold, wet, and dry, as well as the regular actions of faculties of different substances.

These values and practices of personal observation and sense-based investigation, coupled with deep humanist book-learning in recovering the true Galenic and Hippocratic medicine, drew on sixteenth-century academic pedagogy. Like the Leiden professors, other medical students at Padua learned to meet arguments from authority with suspicion, that personal sensation of bodies and medicinal substances was the proper foundation for knowledge, and that the good physician tested remedies and anatomical claims.[171] Contrary to assumptions about the straitjacket rigors of stale or bookish Galenism, early modern academic medicine taught thousands of students to learn from and question ancient authorities—even Galen—and make knowledge from

---

170   Estes, "The European Reception." Huguet-Termes, "New World Materia Medica." Barrera, "Local Herbs." Arrizabalaga, Henderson, and French, *The Great Pox.*

171   Stolberg, "Empiricism," 493–504, 512.

their own experience and trials. Galen became an icon of experience-based knowledge and his writings inspired experimental trials and innovations in anatomy and pharmacology.[172] Even for innovators such as Santorio Santorio (1561–1636), who pioneered instruments and methods for quantifying bodily states, and William Harvey, whose experimental investigations struck at the core of Galenic physiology, Galen was the leading exemplar of experimentation in medicine.[173]

Taking the case of mixed mathematics, Peter Dear has argued brilliantly that the widespread pedagogical institutions of the Jesuits reconstituted general experience toward the particular experiments of modern science, with mathematics supplying epistemic universality.[174] Similarly, looking to the period after the focus of this present study, Gerhard Wiesenfeldt has shown how demonstration experiments in physics and chymistry gained a home at Leiden University.[175] Like mixed mathematics, medicine and natural philosophy increasingly embraced exemplary cases of trials or experiments, stretching from at least the time of Galen and Ptolemy to the proliferation of making trials in the sixteenth century.[176] By the 1570s, committed Aristotelian philosophers such as Girolamo Borro at Pisa, where Galileo studied, made deliberate trials of theories of weight and the elements by dropping lead and wood balls from high windows, following "experience, the teacher of all things."[177] In the seventeenth century, explicitly experimentalist rhetoric and programs appear in the Aristotelian natural philosophy of universities at least by the 1640s.[178] Strikingly, this is true in university medical cultures as well, and well before the founding of experimentalist societies such as the Royal Society.

At the same time, academic medicine increasingly elevated accounts of particulars and facts.[179] Well before Boyle's supposed invention of the "literary technology" of detailed experimental narratives and communal witnessing to establish facts, physicians and students credited novel phenomena with witnessed reports.[180] Anatomical practices, taught and learned in communities,

---

172   Ragland, "'Making Trials.'" Stolberg, "Empiricism." Pomata, "*Praxis Historialis.*" Siraisi, *Avicenna in the Renaissance,* esp. 299, 323.

173   Siraisi, *Avicenna in the Renaissance,* 323. Ragland, "'Making Trials,'" 524–525.

174   Dear, *Discipline and Experience.* See also Raphael, *Reading Galileo.* Ragland, "Reading Galileo in Conversation with Other Scholars."

175   Wiesenfeldt, *Leerer Raum.*

176   Ragland, "'Making Trials.'"

177   Borro, quoted in Ragland, "'Making Trials,'" 506, n. 15.

178   Martin, "With Aristotelians Like These, Who Needs Anti-Aristotelians?"

179   Pomata, "*Praxis Historialis.*"

180   Shapin and Schaffer, *Leviathan and the Air-Pump.*

remained necessarily social activities. This is clear not only in the pedagogical routines of anatomical demonstration, post-mortem autopsies, experimentation, and student anatomical explorations, but also in the "literary technologies" developed to establish credit for novel experiments and phenomena. Just as sixteenth-century alchemists established detailed, historical, witnessed narratives of alchemical transmutations, anatomists too shared forms of historical narratives of experiments and novel observations, witnessed by anatomical experts.[181] Realdo Colombo's 1559 *De re anatomica*, for example, included witnesses for many of the "things rarely found in anatomy" (except for the rarest, hermaphrodites).[182] Leiden students and professors of medicine established norms of witnessing and historical descriptions for experiments around 1640. In these demonstrations to professors and students, which drew on earlier forms of post-mortem witnessing practiced by Paaw and Heurnius, witnesses viewed and "were befouled" by the bloody anatomical experiments.[183]

Setting the stage for the medical culture and practices of pedagogy before experimentalism is essential. Only in this way can we have any good sense of what changed and what stayed the same over time, as well as the resources with which students and professors worked and the ideals motivating and guiding them in their practices. Only in its connections with the theoretical-practical *Institutes* courses, and the rational *practica* courses, does the frequent practice of clinical anatomy or post-mortem dissection make full sense. The professors' and students' own histories of medicine wove these strands together into ideal images of the best sort of medicine and the good physician. All of these major threads of practice—even chymistry—formed a seemingly coherent whole in the narratives that presented Galenic-Hippocratic medicine as the true, effective art of healing.

Although this book is the first volume of a broader study of the emergence of experimentalism in university medicine, it stands on its own as a reasonably complete, integrated history of later Renaissance, university-based medical education. This sort of history necessarily attends to the core teachings and practices, as well as to a sense of what it was like to teach and learn. It is also a story of what happened before systematic experimentation and experimentalism, which emerged when professors and students in the late 1630s, 1640s, and especially the 1660s elaborated and re-arranged older ideals, methods, and practices, and added a few new ones, to create an experimentalist medicine.

---

181   Principe, *Aspiring Adept*, 106–110.

182   Ragland, "Making Trials," 522.

183   Ragland, "Mechanism," 183.

7   Plan of Chapters

Although the parts are all interconnected, I have organized the chapters by their practices and their sites of learning: first, the context and founding of medical learning at the university in chapter one. Then, we look to the ideals, curricula, practices of disputation, bookish study guides, and embodied student life in chapter two. Next, we visit the lecture hall as the site for learning philosophical medical theory in chapter three. In chapter four, we will stay for a while in the lecture hall to learn about chymistry in the course on medical practice, then head out the back of the lecture hall to visit the university garden where students learned to identify plants, and learned of ancient and early modern methods for tasting or testing them to know their qualities and medicinal faculties or powers. Chapter five looks to books, lectures, and patients' bedsides to recover the central place of organs and simple body parts in Galenic disease theory, diagnosis, and treatment. Chapter six attends to different sites for anatomy: dissections in private homes to find the causes of disease and death, as well as public dissections in the anatomy theater. Finally, chapter seven draws the various practices together to reconstruct the clinical teaching and clinical anatomies performed as a regular part of instruction in the city hospital after 1636. There is also some chronological progression, as we move from the founding of the university and the education of the professors in chapter one to the core theory and practice courses in the middle chapters, and then to the development of anatomical and clinical practices over time in chapters six and seven. As I show, the combination of ancient knowledge and new pedagogical practices, driven by the desire for new knowledge and scholarly glory won through research, produced gradual innovations in pathology and therapy.

This integrated portrait of ideas and practices goes well beyond existing treatments, such as J. E. Kroon's excellent institutional and prosopographical survey from a century ago, in its new evidence and close readings of texts from a range of sites and topics: the garden, drug theory, chymistry, medical philosophy, and the extensive practices of anatomy.[184] Attention to the shared sources and texts from other medical schools and professors has allowed me to suggest that Leiden should be representative of medical culture at other universities, too. The integrated approach here offers the first relatively comprehensive

---

184   Kroon, *Bijgraden*. Kroon's concise, learned book gives short but effective institutional histories of clinical teaching, anatomy, and botany, as well as very useful short biographies and extensive bibliographies of the professors.

history of academic medicine for this period, fitting into a clear gap among canonical secondary works.[185]

Chapter one situates academic medical culture in Leiden, and in relation to the ideals of the university and practices of making trials or experiments in other medical schools and among Leiden mathematical practitioners. Here, I give a short summary of the founding of the university and the republican and classical ideals that shaped it. Maps of the city, reports of its climate, and a series of four engravings of important spaces of the university introduce academic life in the city. Drawing on my previous work, I sketch the history of making trials in sixteenth-century academic medicine, especially at Italian universities. Responding to historians' long emphasis on Dutch mixed mathematics, I also note evidence for some experimentation among the mathematical practitioners in Leiden, especially Simon Stevin and Willebrord Snel (or Snell or Snellius). Unlike the practices in medicine, though, it does not appear that Leiden University mathematicians developed pedagogical programs that depended on making trials or experiments. The chapter closes with a summary of early plans for medical teaching and official lecture series, showing how professors built on ancient foundations with new teaching and practice, including their own methods and texts.

Chapter two moves to the lecture hall, and shows how students and professors disciplined their brains and bodies in learning to be physicians. It draws primarily on unstudied published works by the leading teaching physician Johannes Heurnius, as well as the anatomists Petrus Paaw and Otto Heurnius, university records, and several students' disputations. Reason and experience were the watchwords of Leiden medicine, as they were for the prince of medicine, Galen, over a thousand years earlier. Students studied Hippocratic and Galenic sources, often through their professors' textbooks and lectures, and practiced disputing with an eye toward their exams and public doctoral disputation. They trained to be alert, quick, and well-spoken, and to make arguments free of logical fallacies. All this study with the right authors sharpened the "wit" or *ingenium*, making students' brains quicker and finer in their

---

185   Siraisi, *Medieval and Early Renaissance Medicine* stops short of this period. Similarly, Maclean, *Logic, Signs, and Nature* concentrates brilliantly on logical categories, operations, and semiotics, but does not address pedagogical practices, chymistry, natural history, or anatomy in much detail. For philosophy and physiology, Siraisi, *Avicenna in the Renaissance* is excellent and indispensable, but limited to a rich set of commentaries on the first fen of Avicenna's *Canon*. Other works tend to address one subdiscipline or tradition, for instance these studies of anatomy and chymistry: Klestinec, *Theaters of Anatomy*. Moran, *Andreas Libavius*. Moran, *Chemical Pharmacy*. Krafft, "The Magic Word." Powers, *Inventing Chemistry*.

substance. Yet drunkenness and "manly" violence slowed students' wits, and corrupted their morals. Unruly students needed discipline, but their social status in the minor nobility and the upper bourgeoisie allowed for resistance and even occasional riots against the rule of the university and city administrators.

Books and lectures on the *Institutes of Medicine* and its ancient sources formed the foundation of medical theory and fill our chapter three. As Galen emphasized throughout his works, the best natural philosophy taught that the four qualities of heat, cold, wetness, and dryness tempered into the elemental and qualitative mixture of each thing. I show that faculties—the capacities for drugs, lodestones, organs, organ systems, or whole bodies to perform actions on objects—were not understood as mysterious or metaphysical inhabitants of material bodies, but as the dispositional, relative, and emergent properties of the temperament or basic qualitative mixture and material structure of a given thing. Increasingly, early modern physicians followed Galen to describe faculties working through the local anatomical structures of organs, especially their different contractile fibers. The regular activities of organs and parts, revealed through repeated close inspections, indicated their faculties. To identify the faculties of drugs, in particular, physicians had to try them out, on their own bodies or those of patients, and note their effects. Seventeenth-century philosophers with rival ontologies, such as John Locke, passed on to historians the errors of thinking about faculties as mysterious entities added to the material composition of things.

In chapter four, I turn to explore how students learned about plants and other medicinal ingredients in and around the garden. This included practical experimentation for growing the splendid varieties of plants available from local and global networks. New substances seized during imperial expeditions and commerce, newly popular natural historical practices, and the rise of chymistry drove this pedagogy of personal trying, but ancient models may well have played an even greater role. By giving a novel history of Galenic drug theory and testing, based on widely-used textbooks, I show that Galen's works provided models of sophisticated experiments for drug-testing, as well as an explicitly experimentalist methodology. Only by first-person sensory experience of ingredients and making trials of drugs in themselves and their patients could physicians build knowledge of the complex actions of the drugs' faculties in living bodies. Yet this very sophistication, combined with widespread confidence in traditional drugs supposedly "proven by long use," often dissuaded practitioners from making their own exhausting, systematic trials of simple ingredients and all the myriad compound drugs.

Increasingly, those drugs included chymical productions. Professors such as Johannes Heurnius eagerly adopted new ideas and practices from the burgeoning traditions of chymistry. In his youth, Johannes publicly called for a Paracelsian investigation of the chymical *semina* of things, and celebrated medieval treatises on the transmutation of base metals into gold. As a professor, he brought chymical apparatus, operations, medicines, and some theory into his lectures and textbooks, describing how students could use distillation apparatus to extract small, pure, pleasing, and effective samples from medicinal ingredients.

Chapter five goes back to Galen and his early modern followers to reconstruct their systems of diagnosis, pathology, and therapy that put impaired organs and the causes of impairment at the center of medicine. I give close readings of the main texts and lectures used for decades in the courses on practical medicine in order to show that Leiden professors and students, like those at Padua earlier, focused their attention on local diseases, seated in individual parts of the patients' bodies. They frequently wrote about the "sick part" students had to identify as the "seat" of the disease. Johannes Heurnius combined the longstanding quest for a rational, qualitative medicine with the head-to-toe organization of practical medicine by mapping healthy and diseased organs and parts. For him, each organ had a proper temperament and structure, and departures from this healthy material temperament or structure interfered with a part's action. Like Galen and other physicians, Leiden professors and students defined diseases in terms of these impairments to the actions and functions of body parts. General humors or total body balance mattered little, and Johannes developed a method for dosing the sick parts of patients' bodies with precisely-formulated remedies. This rational theory of practice mapped well onto actual bedside care and practices of frequent post-mortem dissections embraced by these Galenic-Hippocratic teaching physicians.

Dissections displayed the causes of diseases and death in patients' bodies, as I show first in chapter six. Professor Petrus Paaw pursued his own anatomical and pathological research through his performance of frequent public anatomies in the anatomy theater and private anatomies in patients' homes. Just as he displayed diseased organs and morbid matter preserved in the anatomy theater—from his colleague Johannes Heurnius' kidney stones to the bladder of humanist scholar Isaac Casaubon—Paaw displayed the causes and seats of diseases to his students in his public and private anatomies. I also show that Paaw performed original anatomical research, and critiqued previous anatomists' claims. His medical diary records dozens of post-mortem dissections of the bodies of patients from a wide range of social standings, not just the poor or foreign bodies commonly allowed in secondary scholarship. In each case, he precisely located the material cause of the disease in an organ or part.

Paaw taught students to note morbid changes in color, size, texture, swollenness or flaccidity, and other characteristics of organs. Morbid concretions and local fluid buildup often attracted his attention, and he examined the color, consistency, smell, and even quantitative volume of these fluids. These qualitative and quantitative changes revealed the hidden states students learned to infer from external signs, as the temperament and structures of organs and parts became changed and impaired.

Professors collected, collated, reported, and attested to their public and private anatomies in increasingly standardized and productive ways. Paaw also put some cases in series, and connected his observations to understand types of diseases as generalizations from an expanding set of observed cases. Paaw and his colleagues took great care to identify the causes of disease that had arrested the mysterious processes of human generation. They also frequently determined the legal cause of death by distinguishing between organs corroded by caustic poison and those corrupted by morbid matter. Even eminent physicians such as Johannes Heurnius received accusations of murder-by-poisoning, charges Paaw could refute with the mute witness of the cadaver's interior states made visible and the expert credibility of himself and his collaborators. Frequent collaboration with the learned surgeons and physicians of the city and the legal demands for establishing official causes of death generated standard reporting practices. As experimentalist anatomists and philosophers did throughout the later seventeenth century, the Leiden professors gave detailed historical narratives of the common or even marvelous sights revealed in dissected bodies, described carefully their interventions, and attested to the truth of their accounts by naming expert witnesses.

Chapter seven details how students and professors engaged with innovations in healthy anatomy and pathology. It shows how professors cautiously approached radical innovations such as Aselli's experimental discovery of the lacteals and Harvey's demonstration of the circulation of the blood. Students often took a more enthusiastic stance toward even revolutionary changes. In pathology, Otto Heurnius extended the Leiden pedagogical tradition of pathological anatomy with regular hospital teaching. He dissected patients' bodies after he had displayed proper practices of diagnosis and treatment for students as part of the official program of clinical teaching. This allowed students and professors to correlate different patients' symptoms and treatments with the evidence of the seats and causes of diseases revealed in clinical anatomies.

Otto Heurnius' decades-long sensory experience with a range of morbid and healthy bodies allowed him to describe the common and rare perceptible states discovered in the anatomical seats of diseases. Following Galenic and Hippocratic diagnostic methods, he taught students to detect the variations of patients' pulse, excreta, faces, feet, hands, and at times the more private areas covered by clothing. These external signs directed students' inferences to the hidden causes of diseases, and guided their treatment regimens, according to the schemes for purging morbid matter and restoring impaired organ temperaments taught by Johannes Heurnius and other professors. They tried out drugs from the New World and Asia, or at least attempted to replicate indigenous peoples' remedies, embraced chymical remedies, experienced the actions of medicines on their own bodies, and changed treatment plans as patients recovered or declined.

Studying the extensive records on the treatment and clinical anatomies of patients who suffered from phthisis (or consumption) shows how these institutionalized pedagogical practices fostered the gradual development of innovations in pathology. Otto Heurnius and other early modern physicians drew from Hippocratic and Galenic ancient sources to focus on ulcers or the ulceration of the lungs as the primary cause of phthisis. They applied ancient methods of diagnosis, but added new forms of treatment such as the chymical remedy flowers of Sulphur. Locations of pain indicated by patients, as well as coughing up pus, fever, and whole-body wasting, pointed to the anatomical sites of the accumulation and corruption of phlegm. This process produced "tubercles" or swellings like tiny drops throughout patients' lungs. Over time, ulcers formed which grew into purulent sores. Two decades later, a Leiden student and professor, Franciscus Sylvius, would take up these new threads of pathology, make the development of tubercles central to phthisis, and weave them into his experimentalist chymical-anatomical medicine. Striking new innovations built on old traditions, as pedagogy shaped practitioners.

The history of early modern Galenic medicine and the roots of seventeenth-century medical experimentalism are right in front of us, although buried by the centuries and the layers of complex scholarship long past. These roots are ready to be unearthed in the texts and practices of professors, students, surgeons, and apothecaries in and around early modern universities. We just have to take a break from the scientific societies, courts, and other fashionable settings, and go back to school.

Contexts for the Medical Curriculum

Leiden University appeared rather suddenly in 1575. Its fresh founding amid war and political crisis drew on a humanist scholarly culture of discursive erudition and practical training. Founded by the leader of the Dutch rebellion against Spain as a "strong blockhouse" or bulwark for the "maintenance of freedom," the university sought first of all to train officers for battles and governing, and preachers and theologians for the preservation of orthodoxy.[1] In these pursuits and in medicine, as well as mathematics, philosophy, and other fields of study, professors' humanist linguistic and bookish skills guided and inspired their practical interests and exercises. Revived, rigorous learning in ancient texts and practical pedagogy blended together in the training of officers with the military methods of the ancient Romans, the extension of ancient surveying practices to local geographies, and the recovery and expansion of anatomy, medical botany, and clinical teaching. Surrounded by razed buildings and flooded fields, and faced with further Spanish violence, the initial scholarly culture at the new university still tolerated Christian confessional differences among faculty and students, and embraced the best scholarship and teaching from across Europe.

This chapter briefly situates the professors and pedagogical practices of the medical faculty of the new university in several contexts. First, the founding and the surrounding city, then the longer rise of making trials or experiments in academic medicine, the humanist experimental projects of Leiden mathematicians and engineers, and the education of the first generations of medical professors. It concludes with an overview of the medical curricula over the first several decades, as preserved in official series-of-lectures lists. These contexts and maps of places and teaching should provide a short orientation for new students, especially present-day readers, in the teaching and learning of medicine at Leiden.

The city and university grew quickly, but the medical faculty started slowly, with only one professor for the first six years. The other two higher faculties, theology and law, started with many more professors and students, as well as higher pay and status. But by the mid-1590s, the medical faculty flourished in discursive scholarship *and* in the direct sensory experience of particulars, with

---

1   Molhuysen, *Bronnen*, I, 1*–2*.

© EVAN R. RAGLAND, 2022 | DOI:10.1163/9789004515727_003

a burgeoning garden for teaching medicinal ingredients or *materia medica* and a permanent anatomy theater. Professors modeled these pedagogical institutions and their practices on Italian, notably Paduan, exemplars.

Throughout the sixteenth century, medical faculties across Europe felt the spurs of ancient achievements and ancient errors. With the ancient authorities as models to match and then correct and surpass, humanist scholars sought to refine their own discursive learning and engagement with the particular objects of medicine: plants, bodies living and dead, animal subjects, and chymical ingredients and processes. They made a range of trials or tests of ancient and contemporary claims about medicinal ingredients and bodies. Leiden professors trained in Italian and other European medical faculties, notably the University of Padua, and then cultivated similar traditions of wide and precise textual expertise combined with sensory engagement with the objects of discursive claims. In mathematics and engineering, too, Leiden scholars celebrated and surpassed the techniques and programs of the ancients in the study of falling objects, surveying, and optics.

The early curricula of the medical faculty display a similar critical enthusiasm for the ancients, as well as new developments in rational diagnosis and therapy, medical botany, and anatomy. By the late 1580s, professors increasingly taught their own syntheses and systems of the medical theory and practice courses, as well as new approaches to anatomy and pharmacology gathered from other professors or their own practices. The books of Johannes Heurnius, especially, formed the foundation of lectures and teaching on the philosophical and rational theory and practice of medicine. Over the following chapters, we will unpack these books and those of other professors, in conversation with their ancient, medieval, and early modern sources, and reassemble their practices of making students into learned, practical physicians.

1 Medicine for a Young Republic in the 1575 Founding

In early 1575, the gutted ruins of homes and barns loomed here and there among the fields still dotted with debris from the floods. Breaking the dykes had loosed the waters, but only a providential torrent of heavy rain finally helped to wash away the Spanish army besieging the city of Leiden from 1573 to October 1574. Reminders of the revolt persisted for Leideners and other locals who had survived starvation and disease during the siege, and also avoided the fate of hundreds massacred at Mechelen, Zutphen, and Naarden in the fall and winter of 1572. Spanish destruction only incensed and consolidated support for the revolt in the north and west, Holland and Zeeland, where institutional

Protestantism and refugees from the southern territories stiffened the rebels' resolve. When relief came to the city in early October 1574, the Leiden people, already thinned by months of siege, had been starving for weeks.[2]

Nearly three months later, William of Orange, the leader of the opposition against the Spanish, wrote a letter calling for the formation of a new, pious, free university in the northern Low Countries. William rushed the official founding to precede peace talks with Spanish representatives, intent on sending a message to the Spanish King Philip II about Dutch resistance and renewal. The January 6, 1575 founding patent forged Philip's seal and approval, not in a laughable attempt at fraud, but as a signal communicating the rebels' continued reverence for a king's sovereignty.[3]

William intended the university as a stronghold for his people: an institution training God's soldiers, either as orthodox Protestant theologians and pastors or as military officers. At that time, the Low Countries counted only the famed Leuven as a university of their own, and for Protestant rebels the deeply Catholic Leuven (founded in 1425), which remained in Spanish hands, offered no warm welcome. William proclaimed that the prospective university would support the "maintenance of freedom" against tyranny, standing as a "strong blockhouse" and an unbreakable tie of unity for the people of the provinces. In this vision, a fighting and uniting spirit inspired the pedagogical practices of the university, an academic fortress and training ground for the "true knowledge of God" as well as the arts and sciences (*wetenschappen*).[4]

The university realized much of William's vision, and reached well beyond it. Until 1581, the entire university operated within two former Catholic convents seized by the Protestant rebels. Theology initially excelled in the size of its matriculating classes, the number of its faculty, the larger holdings in the library, the two colleges for students, and the scholarships for students to live on. Even Leiden's European fame for philology and language training in Hebrew, Arabic, Greek, and more came in the service of building confessional strength and theological truth.

Still, as Willem Otterspeer argues persuasively, it is difficult to style Leiden as a strongly Calvinist university in its first several decades.[5] The city itself and its council did not express strong Calvinist piety in its early years, with comparatively few on the council regularly attending the congregational communions. Across several early conflicts, the university let go or passed over more

---

2 Israel, *The Dutch Republic*, 178–182.
3 Otterspeer, *Groepsportret*, 1, 63.
4 Molhuysen, *Bronnen*, 1*–2*.
5 Otterspeer, *Groepsportret*, 1, 137–158.

stridently Calvinist faculty and retained more conciliatory or even Catholic faculty. In the early 1580s, the eminent Calvinist theologian Lambert Daneau objected to the activities of the more high-church Caspar Coolhaes among the students. The magistrates responded that they had not escaped a Spanish inquisition only to suffer under a new one from Geneva. Danaeu resigned, and moved on to more rigorous settings. In the end, three aggressively Calvinist faculty moved on, at least two Catholic professors remained (Dodonaeus or Dodoens and Sosius), and Catholic students could be taught the Catholic catechism.[6]

After the Arminian controversy in 1618–1619, and again in the 1650s, though, the university administrators and some professors tightened the rigors of orthodoxy. In the wake of the conflict, two of three Curators were dismissed.[7] In the 1650s, opponents of less-rigorous religiosity among the faculty also attacked Cartesian philosophy as a threat to orthodoxy. The specter of Catholicism loomed behind Descartes's philosophy as well. In 1672, the Curators apparently found the Catholic Reinier de Graaf unfit to succeed his teacher Sylvius as a professor at the university, although he was recognized as an outstanding anatomist and chymical physician in Sylvius' mold.

Of course, theological motivations also generated new knowledge. This was obviously the case in the ongoing humanist attempts to recover the original text and meanings of the books of the Bible by Leiden scholars such as Louis de Dieu, Daniel Heinsius, and Joseph Scaliger.[8] The defensive efforts of scholars to use new learning in the service of orthodoxy and Biblical authority also generated material for a wealth of theological and social debates, from the controversy over Arminius's teachings to public disputes over the proper length of men's hair in the 1640s.[9] Theological visions also generated a striking novel philosophy. The brilliant Leiden student David Gorlaeus (1591–1612) articulated a speculative atomist metaphysics—including God and the angels—which he hoped would resolve the ongoing theological disputes and provide a philosophy favorable to Arminianism.[10]

The embrace of old texts and new research marked the symbolism of the founding. To celebrate the founding, officials of the city and university declared a holiday for rich and poor alike, and slapped together an inaugural procession.

---

6   Otterspeer, *Groepsportet*, 1, 147–148.
7   Otterspeer, *Groepsportet*, 1: 159–162, 281.
8   Otterspeer, *Groepsportet*, 1, 361–370. De Jonge, "The Study of the New Testament, 65–109. Grafton, *Joseph Scaliger*, vol. 2.
9   Otterspeer, *Groepsportet*, 1, 320–321.
10   Lüthy, *David Gorlaeus*.

Proper theology and military display led the founding procession. First came the clergy and theologians, escorted by officers and soldiers. The personification of medicine, *Medicina*, made her appearance with the other faculties, significantly attended by the icons of the best, true medicine: Hippocrates and Galen. The best of the old buttressed the ambitions of the new.

2   University, City, State

Leiden University and the city of Leiden grew rapidly together, feeding and fighting each other through the first four decades after the defeat of the Spanish siege in 1574. Ensconced in the medieval walls, threaded with canals, and open to the flow of immigrants, especially Protestants from the southern Low Countries, Leiden still embraced many Catholics and the majority of the city officials were from the seated bourgeoisie rather than the patrician class. With the steady flow of immigrants and the growing eminence of the Leiden wool textiles industry, the population of the city doubled from 1580 to 1600, then nearly doubled again over roughly the next two decades, going from around 12,000 inhabitants in 1581 to almost 45,000 in 1622.[11] Taking into account sharp decreases in student residence during epidemics, such as when thousands of local citizens died in the fever epidemic of 1669, students most often made up about two to three percent of the city's growing population.[12]

Climate and bodily constitutions mattered, and in early modern Europe everyone knew the former shaped the latter. The Anglo-Welsh traveler, historian, and writer James Howell complained of his 1619 visit, "The Heaven here has always some Cloud in his Countenance, and from this grossness and spissitude of Air proceeds the slow nature of the Inhabitants."[13] Yet he conceded the intellectual keenness of the scholars, noting that "Apollo hath a strong influence here." He even echoed Cicero's praise of Athens, that the place had a dense air, but the Leideners displayed "thin subtle wits (some of them)." Howell's snobbery was not obviously widespread. Many others from abroad praised the erudition, research vigor, and humanist toleration of the faculty.

Four famous prints will help to situate us among the students of Leiden University. Engraved by Willem Swanenbrugh based on drawings by Jan

11   Otterspeer, *Groepsportret*, 1, 56, 259.
12   The Leiden doctor Franciscus Sylvius identified the disease as epidemic fever, not plague. Otterspeer, *Groepsportret*, 1, 431.
13   Quoted in Grafton, "Civic Humanism," 59.

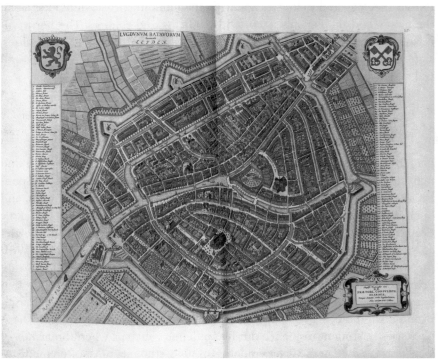

FIGURE 1   1652 Map of Leiden by Joan Blaeu (1596–1673). The small academic building with
            small garden behind is toward the bottom, just left of the middle, on the opposite
            side of the large Rapenburg canal from the large Pieterskerk in the lower middle,
            and just below the Pieterskerk and the smaller Faliedebegijnkerk, which housed
            the library, anatomy theater, and fencing school after 1590. Joan Blaeu, *Toonneel der*
            steden van de Vereenighde Nederlanden, met hare beschrivingen (Amsterdam, 1652).
            COURTESY, LIBRARY OF CONGRESS, WASHINGTON, D.C., CONTROL NUMBER
            76516940.

Cornelisz. van 't Woud, Leiden publisher Andreas Cloucq issued them in 1610.
They have enjoyed a long and ongoing life in reproductions.[14]

First, the 1594 medical and botanical gardens where medical students
viewed medicinal and collectors' plants first-hand for a few hours a week.
Below, the print shows close-ups of notable rarities, and in the back there is
the Ambulacrum, or gallery, where anatomical experiments occurred at least
around 1640. Later on our historical tour, we will take a more leisurely stroll
through the plants there.

---

14   Otterspeer, *Groepsportret*, 1, 180.

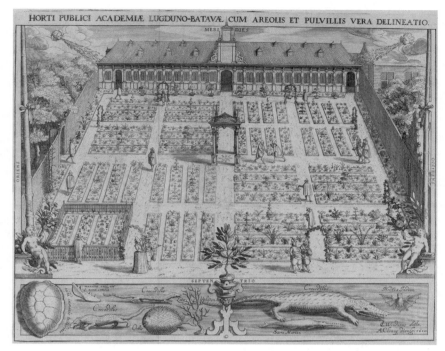

FIGURE 2   Engraving of the Leiden botanical garden (est. 1591), by Willem Swanenburg based
on drawings by Jan Cornelisz. van 't Woud (Johannes Woudanus) (1610).
COURTESY, THE BRITISH MUSEUM.

Across the Rapenburg canal in the old Catholic church and religious sisters'
compound, we come to the 1593 anatomy theater. It boasted comparative animal and human skeletons, anatomical instruments in the back, messages of
human mortality, and, in this illustration, a curiously sparse and nonchalant
audience. We will spend much more time here in later chapters, situating the
theater not in the moralizing messages of the banners and art, but in its explicit
pedagogical context of cultivating learned and effective medical practice.

Third, the fencing school for training officers of the Republic, following the
vision of Prince William of Orange. The geometric forms traced on the floor
and enacted by the students point to the rising importance of mixed mathematics in shaping soldiers and citizens. The combatants are also plainly not
low-class young men, as they skillfully use rapiers rather than knives along
well-reasoned geometric lines and in good dress. These well-trained, decorous
soldiers represent the new image of disciplined, masculine military might
advertised by Maurits of Nassau (1567–1625), stadtholder of the Republic and
leader of the rebel armies, as well as the success of the Dutch armies in holding

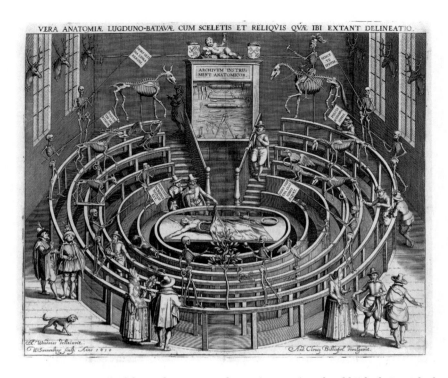

VERA ANATOMIÆ LUGDUNO-BATAVÆ, CUM SCELETIS ET RELIQVIS QVÆ IBI EXTANT DELINEATIO.

FIGURE 3   Engraving of the Leiden anatomy theater (est. 1593), in the old Faliede Begijnkerk,
            by Willem Swanenburg based on drawings by Jan Cornelisz. van 't Woud
            (Johannes Woudanus) (1610).
            PUBLIC DOMAIN. CC BY.

off the massive Spanish empire.[15] Maurits studied with the humanist Stoic philosopher Justus Lipsius at Leiden and persisted in reforming the Dutch soldiers
to fit the model of the ancient Roman military. Lipsius had reconstructed the
Romans' organizations, discipline, uniforms, diet, chains of command, and
quick-deploying, adaptive units by mining Greek sources, especially Polybius's
history. As Anthony Grafton shows, Maurits embraced Lipsius's recommendation to follow the Roman model, applying harsh discipline and steady training.
But Maurits continued forcing his soldiers into the ancient Roman mold, even
testing their weapons by arming one troop with ancient-style weapons versus
another troop armed as Spaniards.[16] As Lipsius pointed out in reply, sometimes
useful bookish ideals went too far in practice.

15   Roberts, *Sex and Drugs*, 221–222.
16   Grafton, "Civic Humanism," 68–9.

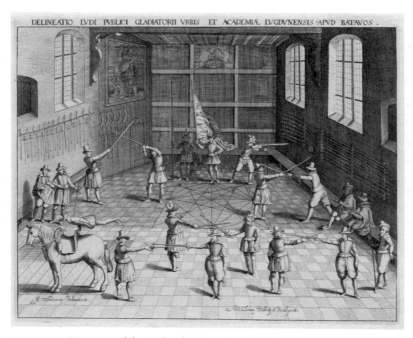

FIGURE 4   Engraving of the Leiden fencing school, in the old Faliede Begijnkerk, by
Willem Swanenburg based on drawings by Jan Cornelisz. van 't Woud
(Johannes Woudanus) (1610).

Fourth, and last, the library. They moved the growing, and moldering, collection from the Academic Building across the Rapenburg canal to the old
convent, the Faliedebegijnkerk, in 1591.[17] The collections assembled slowly,
with repeated difficulties over professors lending out keys, and students and
others using copies of keys and books too freely. After 1597, the library finally
had regular, and meager, hours: Wednesdays and Saturdays, four to six in the
afternoon. Then, in 1605, the university administrators announced that, "due
to the misuse of the books by some," the library was now closed to students.
It would remain closed to the possibilities of student misuse for twenty-five
years, until 1630.[18] Even before this closure, it is more likely that students relied
on their private collections of books and university lectures, copied by themselves or by paid transcribers.[19] By 1618, the library stocked important and quite

17   Hulshoff Pol, "The Library," 404.
18   Hulshoff Pol, "The Library," 410–411.
19   Otterspeer, *Groepsportet*, I, 264–5.

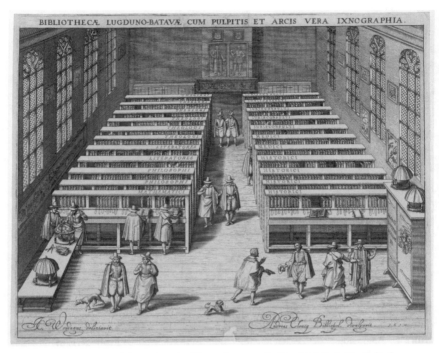

FIGURE 5   Engraving of the university library (est. 1591 in the old Faliede Begijnkerk
            chapel), by Willem Swanenburg based on drawings by Jan Cornelisz. van 't Woud
            (Johannes Woudanus) (1610).
            PUBLIC DOMAIN. CC BY.

recent books on anatomy, such as Jean Riolan's eminent *Osteologia* (1614), the
Opera omnia (1606) of Gabriele Falloppia, and Caspar Bauhin's *Anatomes*
(1591–1597).[20] But the anatomists and students likely relied more on the books
housed in the anatomy theater itself, the lecture room of the academic building, or the covered gallery of the garden. In 1618, the anatomy theater supplied works by Hippocrates, Falloppio, Cardano, Platter, Fabricius Hildanus,
Colombo, Riolan, Bauhin, Van Foreest, and Johannes Heurnius, as well as eight
different surgery books by authors such as Tagliacozzi, Van Foreest, and Hieronymus Fabricius (Girolamo Fabrizi or Fabrici).[21] This friendly association of
anatomical and surgical books points to the close ties and practical collabora-
tions of the anatomists and surgeons in public, private, and clinical anatomies,
as we will see in later chapters.

---

20   Barge, *De Oudste Inventaris*, 28–29.
21   Barge, *De Oudste Inventaris*, 58–61.

Leiden University combined long tradition with new ventures, in its spaces and in its prospects. This was no less true in its medical culture, as suggested by the first two prints. It also appears strongly in the humanist mixed mathematics practiced by professors there, some of whom combined their revival of ancient methods with experimental techniques. To get a sense of the broader interplay of the old and new in making medical and mathematical knowledge and trials, through some diachronic and synchronic context, we will look over snapshots of the heritage of academic medical trials and Leiden mathematics in the next two sections.

3   The Harvest of Trials from Earlier Sixteenth-Century Academic Medicine

Early modern medicine became an extremely fruitful set of traditions for the development of new categories and practices of observation and experimentation. The productive interrelation of these threads was not neat, however, but complex and contested. Academic medicine also involved sophisticated developments in a range of areas: anatomy, chymistry, drug testing, clinical experience, semiotics, humanism, philosophy, and theology. Here, we will concentrate on the first three. More broadly, early modern academic physicians shaped and popularized the two epistemic categories of *historia* and *observatio*.[22] Galenic texts supplied a notion of *historia* as *autopsia*, or the narration of what one has seen, while Aristotelian tradition set out a distinction between *to hoti* ("the that"), description without causes, and *to dioti* ("the reason why"), knowledge of causes. By the second half of the sixteenth century, humanist physicians crafted a category of *historia* as autoptic descriptive knowledge preparatory to causal explanation. Seventeenth-century philosophers and physicians broadened the notion of *historia* to "a descriptive account of observational knowledge in any field."[23]

Sixteenth-century physicians increasingly made hands-on tests or trials of phenomena and claims.[24] Drug testing, natural history, and anatomy were the central fields for this development. From Galen through the seventeenth century, most physicians and philosophers agreed that one had to make trials of drugs in order to know their properties. Even though the primary, secondary,

---

22   Pomata and Siraisi, eds. *Historia*. Pomata, "*Praxis Historialis*"; Pomata, "A Word of the Empirics"; Pomata, "Observation Rising."

23   Pomata, "Observation Rising" 67.

24   Findlen, *Possessing Nature*; Stolberg, "Empiricism"; Ragland, "'Making Trials.'"

tertiary, and quaternary levels of a drug's faculties or capacities in the body ought to work according to the elemental qualities (e.g., predominantly hot drugs should dry), this did not always work out in practice. Making careful trials remained the only way reliably to know a drug's faculties. For Galen, all use of reason to infer the faculties of drugs from the qualities of their ingredients had to be confirmed by trial (*peira*) carried out by "qualified" experience. Only by this sort of experience could one control for interfering factors and isolate causes, and so really test whether foods or drugs had certain faculties, and make new discoveries. Influential texts ascribed to Galen also describe setting up parallel trials with roosters to test the efficacy of theriac, a purported antidote for poisons.[25] Developing Galen's rules, the Persian physician and philosopher Avicenna (ca. 970–1037) articulated seven conditions for generating knowledge of a drug's medical properties from the "footpath" of experience.[26] These rules aimed for the isolation of cause-effect relations based on the testing of drugs under various conditions, and carried on into the early modern period, where they increasingly faced the challenge of the hidden or "occult" powers of drugs. The nature of these powers, such as the virulence of even a small amount of poison, seemed to elude the senses in much the same way the magnetic power of a lodestone seemed perceptible only from its effects on iron and other magnets.

Engagement with texts and controversies over facts and explanations repeatedly drove physicians and philosophers to make trials.[27] In the 1490s, controversies over the accuracy of Pliny's natural history, contradicted by other texts and physicians' own experience, led to increasing emphasis on personal sensation and experience of things, in conjunction with humanist textual scholarship.[28] In this reaction, humanist physicians also followed the ancient herbalist Dioscorides' exhortation to personal experience of plants, as they would Galen's constant call for autoptic engagement with bodies to learn anatomy. From the 1520s and 1530s, the wave of newly-available texts by Galen allowed anatomists to adopt and critique Galen's anatomical procedures and claims. In many cases, Galen's texts provided detailed models for making anatomical trials, especially his *On Anatomical Procedures*, first translated into Latin in 1529, but published in a much better translation by Johann Guinter von Andernach in 1531. Anatomists such as Guinter and his student Vesalius,

---

25   Rankin, "Of Antidote and Anecdote," 284–285, citing Pseudo-Galen, *On Theriac to Piso*. Rankin, *The Poison Trials*.

26   Avicenna, *Liber canonis Avicenne revisus*, fol. 82r.

27   Ragland, "Making Trials."

28   Ogilvie, *Science of Describing*, 122–133.

like earlier investigators such as Berengario da Carpi, emulated and critiqued ancient and medieval authors, increasingly building criticism and innovation from their own, personal experience.[29]

In the 1550s and 1560s, the next generation of anatomists and physician-naturalists performed trials to test ancient or "modern" claims, or to make new discoveries. Paracelsian texts became more widely published in the 1570s, provoking further controversies and recourse to hands-on trials. Ample evidence for this increasingly widespread trial-making in medicine comes from universities, especially the University of Padua. Three to five hundred students matriculated in medicine each year at Padua, throughout the mid-1500s. Students learned that arguments based on authority were weak, and that personal experience of medicinals, clinical practice, the efficacy of drugs, anatomy, and uroscopy could be essential for a successful and thriving medical practice.[30]

The sixteenth-century practice of making trials had even clearer philosophical significance in anatomy. Across the century, leading anatomists increasingly made trials to establish structures, actions, and uses of the parts. Early in the sixteenth century the humanist surgeon Berengario da Carpi made careful trials of the action of the kidneys—did they filter passively?—and fetal urine flow. Similarly, Vesalius followed Galen in critiquing Aristotle's claim that the testes served only as counterweights for the seminal vessels, and produced no semen. In the two editions, Vesalius noted that he had "experienced/tried" and "made a trial" through a careful castration specifically to test Aristotle's claim.[31] In this case, making a trial or experience allowed Vesalius to gain knowledge of the philosophical "use" (*usus*) of the testes. Importantly, Vesalius defined anatomy as a "branch of natural philosophy" offering contemplative knowledge, even *scientia*. Similarly, his successor Realdo Colombo dissected a wide range of bodies, deliberately noting and seeking out the boundaries of human anatomical variation. In this way, he could move toward a more universal anatomy based on accumulated particular dissections, rather than Vesalius's idealized constructions with occasional variations.[32] He also made trials of Galen's claim that finger bones had internal cavities, and trials to discover that the pulmonary vein remained full of blood carried from the lungs to the heart. Colombo's student Hieronymus Fabricius (or Girolamo Fabrizi or Fabrici) made trials to test the action of a new structure, the "little doors" or valves in the veins, and other trials to determine the transparency of the vitreous humor of the eye.

29   Shotwell, "The Revival of Vivisection." Ragland, "'Making Trials.'"
30   Stolberg, "Empiricism." Ragland, "'Making Trials'."
31   Ragland, "'Making Trials,'" 521.
32   Moes and O'Malley, "Realdo Colombo." Siraisi, "Vesalius and Human Diversity."

Finally, Fabricius's student William Harvey discussed Galen's trials (*experimenta*) in detail, and performed sophisticated experiments to establish a revolutionary finding: the circulation of the blood. After Harvey's 1628 book on the circulation, physicians and philosophers increasingly made experimental tests on a wide range of animals, living and dead, while noting the challenges of correlating anatomical observations from dead or living bodies, individual variations, ephemeral activity, and the sensitivity and complexity of living things.

In their own ways and context, Leiden professors and students continued this productive, humanist blend of erudition and practical experience. A very similar confluence of humanism and hands-on trials also drove innovation in Leiden in mixed mathematics and engineering. We will tour these practices in mathematics and engineering first, since they represent the more canonical focus of stories of the development of experimentation, and then we will return to the teaching of medicine.

4   Experience and Experiment in Early Leiden Mixed Mathematics and Engineering

There were other disciplines and traditions surrounding and interweaving with medicine in this time and place. Historians of Dutch science have long emphasized the practical bent, republican sentiments, and anti-speculative resistance of early modern investigators of nature and mathematics in the Low Countries.[33] This is not the whole story, of course, since natural historians, philosophers, philologists, physicians, and astronomers at times blended what we often distinguish as moral, religious, and "scientific" motivations for knowing nature. As Eric Jorink and others have argued, there is certainly ample evidence of religiously-infused practices of collecting and investigating nature at Leiden, especially in its first six decades.[34] For many physicians, astronomers, collectors, poets, and other scholars, the cosmos offered the open "Book of Nature" for reading evidence of God's glory and goodness, alongside Scripture. The city also hosted important examples of practical, mathematical work, and two celebrated figures who employed experiments to good effect: Simon Stevin (1548–1620) and Willebrord Snel (1580–1626). It is worth spending some

---

33   Van Berkel, *Cit Citaten uit het boek der natuur aten*, 11–23. Van Bunge, *From Stevin to Spinoza*, 1–9.

34   Jorink, *Reading the Book of Nature*, 278–288. Lunsingh Scheurleer, "Un Amphithéâtre." Vermij, *The Calvinist Copernicans*.

time in the Leiden engineering school and mathematical faculty to get a sense of the experimental practices used there

The history of Dutch early modern science usually begins with the hero of engineering, mathematics, and vernacular practicality, Simon Stevin. He settled in Leiden in 1581 and matriculated at the university in 1583, later traveling to Delft in 1590 and to Den Haag before 1600. Stevin taught mathematics useful for a ruler and military leader to Prince Maurits of Nassau, then the stadtholder and commander of the States Army, and in 1600 helped to establish a school for engineers in Leiden (though he did not teach there). His major works intervened in and argued over an impressive range of topics, from offering tables of interest rates for merchants, advocating for decimal notation, celebrating arithmetic and algebra, and mathematically treating artists' perspective, to reviving and expanding Archimedean statics, developing methods of navigation, planning efficient mills, proposing musical tuning, and defending the "burgerly" or bourgeois life of order and deference to political authority. In his 1608 *De Hemelloop* (*The Heavenly Course*), he also defended Copernican theory. Publishing in Dutch allowed Stevin to spread his new knowledge to every Dutch reader with enough wit to understand it. He hoped to recover and celebrate the Dutch language he claimed the "sages" spoke in the most ancient period. Stevin also reached back to antiquity in his revival of Archimedean methods in mechanics and hydraulics. Properly understood through mathematics and mechanics, Stevin's motto insisted, "a wonder is really no wonder (*wonder en is gheen wonder*)."[35]

In his work on the science of weights and mechanics, *De Beghinselen der Weeghconst* (*The Elements of the Art of Weighing*, 1586) Stevin described a manual test of a theoretical claim in mechanics as an "experience" (*ervaring*).[36] He adduced a historical experiment against Aristotle's venerable, and long-controversial, explanation of falling objects. Arguing against the possibility of a vacuum, Aristotle had claimed that objects of different weights fell in times inversely proportional to their weights, and proportional to their impediments or the resistance of the medium.[37] Stevin joined the current debate over Archimedean and Aristotelian theories of fall, and attacked both the recent book of Jean Taisnier, who had plagiarized the Venetian mathematician Giovanni Battista Benedetti, and Aristotle himself.[38] Against Aristotle, Stevin declared,

---

35   Stevin, *De Beghinselen der Weeghconst*, title page.
36   Stevin, *Anhang, De Beghinselen der Weeghconst*, trans. Dijksterhuis, 511 [66]. Dijksterhuis, *Simon Stevin*, 59–60.
37   Aristotle, *Physics*, IV 215a–216a in *The Complete Works of Aristotle*, vol. 1, 365–367.
38   Bertoloni Meli, *Thinking with Objects*, 48, 62–63.

"The experience [*ervaring*] against Aristotle is the following: Let us take (as the very learned Mr. Jan Cornets de Groot, most industrious investigator of the secrets of Nature, and myself have done) two spheres of lead, the one ten times larger and heavier than the other, and drop them from a height of 30 feet on to a board...."[39] So arranged, the sounds of the spheres hitting the board will be simultaneous. This "experience" is clearly a historical, singular event, which Stevin described in the traditional subjunctive or imperative mood of mathematical proofs, but anchored to historical reality by the report of his own actual performance. Importantly, he also added the witness of his collaborator, Jan Cornets de Groot, who held both social authority as the burgomaster of Delft, and skilled authority or expertise as an "industrious investigator of the secrets of Nature."

Stevin's experimental practices and reports provide us with an important exemplar for local experiments in mixed mathematics. Though he did not teach officially in the university, Stevin's use of experiment to refute a long-debated Aristotelian claim and establish his own counter-claim no doubt circulated among local practitioners of mixed mathematics. He clearly made the trial in order to test Aristotle's claim. His reporting format is worth noting, too. Stevin gave his own witness, and pointed readers to the testimony of his skilled and upstanding colleague, De Groot, if they wanted further corroboration of his iconoclastic claim. Strikingly, these same reporting characteristics of making an intentional test, reporting some details of the historical event, and adding the names of expert witnesses also featured prominently in earlier tests, especially those performed by Vesalius and Colombo in anatomy, mentioned in the previous section.[40]

Stevin intervened in philosophical debates with set-piece experiences or trials from the position of a practitioner of mixed mathematics and engineering. Aristotelian philosophers, even those deeply opposed to the use of mathematics in philosophy, could make conclusive experiments, too. Galileo's trials of weights dropped from a tower are more famous, but already in 1575, one of Galileo's Aristotelian philosophy professors at Pisa, Girolamo Borro, had published an account of a historical trial of lead and wood balls dropped from a high window.[41] Borro and his colleagues resorted to "experience, the teacher of all things" and "made a trial" of lead and wood balls of apparently equal weight. They sought to resolve the ancient controversy over whether the air or other elements had weight in their own natural places. After noting that

---

39   Stevin, *Anhang, De Beghinselen der Weeghconst*, trans. Dikshoorn, 511 [66].
40   Ragland, "'Making Trials.'"
41   Ragland, "'Making Trials,'" 506.

the wood balls, with more elemental air, hit the ground before the lead, they affirmed that elements had weight in their own place, a general philosophical truth taught by their novel, historical "experience."[42] In his text, Borro made a deliberate linguistic distinction between "making a trial" (*periculum facere*) and "experience" (*experientia*) constituted by repeated trials. Galileo's later use of just this distinction in his own discussion of falling objects almost certainly carries on Borro's Aristotelian practice and language.[43]

Practical interests heightened by the rapid rise of Dutch sea trade in the late 1590s, as well as the ongoing rebellion and frequent wars, heightened local interest in mathematics, from Prince Maurits to local merchants. At the Leiden engineering school Maurits established with Stevin's curricular advice in 1600, teachers received the title "professor" and participated in the university's academic senate. The university Curators ran the school and in 1600 appointed the German mathematician Ludolph van Ceulen (1540–1610) as a professor of arithmetic, surveying, and fortification. Mathematical instruction appealed to some practical artisans; in 1611, the school included some local carpenters and masons, as well as surveyors, engineers, and navigators.[44]

But Van Ceulen was also a dedicated calculator and like his fellow mathematicians sought to revive and extend the best mathematics of the ancients. He elaborated on Archimedes's method of calculating the circumference of a circle by inscribing and circumscribing polygons, allowing him to calculate the value of pi to twenty and then thirty-five decimal places. He applied new algebraic methods, assigning numbers, even symbols for unknowns, to the lengths of geometric line segments and manipulating numbers and symbols.[45]

Scintillating pieces of mathematical experimentation at Leiden University proper come from the work of Willebrord Snel (or Snell or Snellius) (1580–1626). Willebrord wrote about contrived, manual "experience" with mirrors teaching new findings in optics, notably something like the sine law of refraction. (Willebrord is often credited with formulating the sine law of refraction, though Thomas Harriot articulated it first in his own manuscripts and Descartes published a formulation in 1637.[46]) With support from Stevin, Willebrord followed his father Rudolph Snel as a mathematics professor at the university in 1613, though he had been teaching as early as 1600. Both Rudolph and Willebrord

42   Borro, quoted in Ragland, "'Making Trials,'" 506–507, n. 15.
43   Ragland, "'Making Trials,'" 506–507. Schmitt, "Experience and Experiment." Camerota and Helbing, "Galileo and Pisan Aristotelianism."
44   Struik, "Ceulen, Ludolph van," 181. Van Berkel, *Citaten uit het boek der natuur*, 47–48.
45   De Wreede, "Willebrord Snellius (1580–1626)," 1, 12, 20, 28–29.
46   Goulding, "Thomas Harriot's Optics, Between Experiment and Imagination."

emphasized clarity of instruction and the practicality of mathematics, interests shaped by the pedagogical program of Petrus Ramus and a lively subculture of Ramist enthusiasts at Leiden.[47] All told, Willebrord published twenty-one works, fulfilling the aspirations of like-minded mathematicians to elevate the pedagogical status of mathematics into a fully humanist, learned endeavor.

On the recommendation of Stevin and others, and before he received a doctoral arts degree, Willebrord taught mathematics briefly at the university in Leiden. Later in 1600, he traveled and studied, staying in Denmark with Tycho Brahe, a friend of his father Rudolph, and performing astronomical observations.[48] He also met Kepler and Kepler's teacher Mästlin, as well as Prince Maurice of Hesse, alongside his father Rudolph. Back in Leiden in 1604, Willebrord began an energetic program of publication, including some translations from Dutch into Latin, such as his edition of Stevin's lengthy record of his mathematical instruction of the Prince.[49]

Even the titles of Willebrord's works express his humanist project, especially his 1608 *Apollonius Batavus* and his 1617 *Eratosthenes Batavus* which revived and extended the programs of the ancient Greek mathematicians Apollonius and Eratosthenes into the Low Countries. The famed Leiden University humanist J. J. Scaliger wrote a laudatory poem for his student Willebrord's 1608 work, speaking as the voice of Apollonius, thanking Willebrord for giving him eternal life.[50] Like other mathematicians, Willebrord used the evidence from Pappus to reconstruct mathematically the lost work of Apollonius. He became the "Batavian Eratosthenes" when he published his account of using a two-meter iron quadrant to measure the angles among some thirteen different towns, relating those to the lengths of surveyor's chains, then calculating the distance between two towns on a meridian, and so the finding circumference of the earth—within 4% of the present-day value.[51]

Mathematical experiments appear in Willebrord's work on weights and optics. Like Stevin and Borro, Snel wrote of "making experience." In his discussion of the proper length of the Rhenish foot in *Eratosthenes Batavus*, Willebrord recorded an experimental determination of the weight of water filling the volume of a cubic Rhenish foot. Willebrord designed a special container of two connected bronze cylinders which he could fill completely. He compared the weights of various waters filling this container: rainwater, well water, and

47   Van Berkel, *Isaac Beeckman*, 153–156.
48   De Wreede, *Willebrord Snellius*, 47.
49   De Wreede, *Willebrord Snellius*, 54.
50   De Wreede, *Willebrord Snellius*, 56.
51   De Wreede, *Willebrord Snellius*, 101, 118–130.

distilled rainwater. This allowed him to calculate the weight of "pure" water filling the container as completely as possible. As Liesbeth de Wreede suggests, Willebrord distilled rainwater in a chymical apparatus with gentle heat, a *balneum Mariae*, to purify it, which may indicate some familiarity with chymistry.[52]

In optics, Willebrord famously articulated the sine law for refraction at least by the end of 1621. Willebrord's manuscript treatise on refraction remains lost to the hazards of history, but a few notes remain which attest to his experimental approach. In December of 1621 he rejected his earlier purely geometrical speculations about how radiant points meet the eye by "solid experience/experiment [*experimentiam (sic)*] which I have explored with the highest diligence in mirrors, both concave and convex."[53] A solid experience or experiment refuted his earlier geometric constructions. The slip of "*experimentiam*" for "*experientiam*" or "*experimentum*," might reveal the continuing interchangeability of these terms.[54]

Like others working in optics, Willebrord drew on a long tradition of experimentation, as preserved in texts from Ibn al-Haytham (c. 965-c.1040) through Kepler.[55] He also tested the transmission of candlelight through a semicylinder of ice. Other experiments with a convex mirror and glass allowed him to establish the geometry of refraction that today often bears his name. Reports of optical experiments around the same time could even take on the form of historical narratives, "event-experiments" which could establish or disconfirm general theoretical claims. Sven Dupré has shown that Kepler's 1604 *Parilipomena* narrated in detail a historical experiment in a Dresden Kunstkammer, which he used to criticize Della Porta's general claims about the formation of images, as well as to distinguish perspectivist, geometrical images and experimentally-produced projected images.[56]

Back in Leiden, Snel may well have discussed some of his experimental methods in his classes, as he taught optics from at least 1605. He demonstrated a telescope to students in 1609, just a year after its invention. One student, David Fabritius, used the new instrument to look at the sky, mirroring Galileo himself.[57] When the university built what may have been the first academic astronomical observatory in 1633, it continued an early tradition of practical

52   De Wreede, *Willebrord Snellius*, 121–122.
53   Vollgraff, "Snellius' Notes on the Reflection and Refraction of Rays," 722.
54   Schmitt, "Experience and Experiment."
55   E.g, Sabra, *The Optics of Ibn Al-Haytham*, vol. 1, pp. 3–19; Hackett, "Roger Bacon on *Scientia Experimentalis*." Dupré, "Inside the 'Camera Obscura.'" Against Sabra's interpretation, see Dear, *Discipline and Experience*, 52–53.
56   Dupré, "Inside the 'Camera Obscura.'"
57   Van Berkel, "The Dutch Republic," 97.

experience in mixed mathematics.[58] Given the rich and widespread practices of making trials and experiments in both medicine and mixed mathematics around 1600, there may well have been cross-fertilization of investigative programs. Unlike the established medical instruction at the university, though, it seems Leiden professors of mathematics did not set up curricula that depended on students learning to experience, try, and even experiment with different objects of knowledge. As we will see, medical students gained first-hand experience with plants, other drug ingredients, dissected healthy and diseased cadavers, and the bodies of living patients.

5   The Humanist, Practical Education of Medical Professors

Like other academic medical institutions, Leiden University trained students through acculturation in communal practices, disciplinary histories, practitioner networks, and objects of study. Of course, the professors had to go through similar pedagogical formation first. Most of the first generation of professors experienced important formation at the University of Padua, then probably the leading physician-training school in Europe, and they set out to emulate and extend the sites and practices of Paduan medical education at Leiden. As many historians have noted, the Leiden anatomy theater, garden, and clinical teaching programs followed practices and spaces established at Padua and other Italian universities.[59] In their student years, Leiden professors had followed the common academic practice of traveling to many universities. Most began at Leuven, the leading university in the southern Low Countries, and then made their academic pilgrimages to Italian institutions such as Ferrara, Bologna, and Pavia. Some learned surgery and anatomy at the universities of Paris and Rostock.

Across European medical faculties in the 1500s, humanist pedagogy transformed medical education, elevating personal experience with the particulars of botany and anatomy, and this came about primarily through scholars' bookish goals and practices. First, professors sought to use book learning to establish and restore the proper ancient texts. Next, when persistent errors clashed with the physician-scholars' own experience with plants and dissected bodies,

---

58   Van Bunge, *From Stevin to Spinoza*, 6.

59   See especially Luyendijk-Elshout, "Der Einfluss der italienischen Universitäten auf die medizinische Facultät Leiden." Lunsingh Scheurleer, "Un Amphithéâtre," 218. Beukers, "Clinical Teaching," 139–140. For an overview of Italian university medical teaching, see Grendler, *Universities*, ch. 9.

their desire for true, accurate knowledge and scholarly renown pushed them beyond the ancient authorities.

As many historians have shown, the productive and lively interaction of scholarly, philological expertise in reading and restoring ancient texts drove physicians working on medical botany and anatomy to rely on their own experience.[60] The humanist reform of medical botany appeared vibrantly in the 1490s among the medical faculty at the University of Ferrara, a movement spearheaded by Niccolò Leoniceno. The "single largest collection of Greek scientific, philosophical, and medical writings in Western Europe" allowed Leoniceno to hone his philological and textual excisions of supposed Arabic accretions and corruptions.[61] The attacks of Leoniceno and like-minded scholars on Avicenna's *Canon* took aim at perceived problems for medical practice introduced by Arabic terminology and translations.[62] If students became confused about how body parts worked, they could not preserve or restore their health. And Leoniceno coupled more than twenty chapters criticizing Avicenna's *Canon* to a much more extended catalogue of Pliny's personal errors of identifying and describing plants.[63] Strikingly, the humanist, bookish work of restoring the original, accurate words of Pliny's *Natural History* sparked Leoniceno's call for scholars to live out the epistemology of Aristotle and Galen and "investigate the truth" with their own eyes, noses, ears, and minds rather than rely on the judgment of others.[64] Leoniceno experienced and knew the plants from nearby swamps, riverbanks, hillsides, and forests.

Even as Avicenna's *Canon* and other sources of Arabic medicine, such as Rhazes' works, continued to be used in Italian universites, especially Padua, the humanist return to Galen as the basis for medicine spread throughout Europe.[65] Leoniceno committed himself to teaching, and inspired and shaped a generation of disciples. One student, Antonio Musa Brasavola (1500–1555) wrote vast humanist treatises on Hippocratic works and a still-useful index for Galen's sprawling corpus. Brasavola taught from the herbal (or compendium of medicinal ingredients) of Dioscorides, which he thought the more accurate ancient source for medical botany, but also traveled about, applying his own senses and experience to over 2,000 plants, versus some 1,000 in

---

60   Nutton, "The Rise of Medical Humanism." Nauert, "Humanists, Scientists, and Pliny." Bylebyl, "The School of Padua," 345–346 Findlen, *Possessing Nature*. Ogilvie, *Science of Describing*, esp. 122–133, and ch. 3.

61   Nutton, "The Rise of Medical Humanism," 7

62   Siraisi, *Avicenna in the Renaissance*, 74–75.

63   Siraisi, *Avicenna in the Renaissance*, 68–69.

64   Leoniceno, trans. in Ogilvie, *Science of Describing*, 129.

65   Siraisi, *Avicenna in the Renaissance*.

Pliny and about 850 in Dioscorides' text.[66] Brasavola extended the marriage of philology and practicality to post-mortem dissections. Just as in the case of botany, Brasavola used dissections of diseased cadavers to resolve philological disputes about the meanings of words in ancient texts and to extend medical knowledge based on his own sensory experiences of disease states in bodies.[67]

At Padua, administrators recognized the formal teaching of medical botany or *materia medica* more broadly in 1533 with the appointment of a professor of medicine to a lectureship in simples. They also opened a large, ornate teaching garden in 1546 to display and grow the burgeoning stores of medicinals.[68] Other universities, such as Bologna, Pisa, and Montpellier, instituted similar courses combining humanist learning of ancient texts and the direct sensation of particular samples of medicinal ingredients, especially plants.

Humanist motives and practices also inspired the restoration of the original Galenic corpus as the foundation and arbiter of Galenic medicine among other students of Leoniceno. Giambattista da Monte (1498–1551) continued the project of textual reform and practical instruction.[69] Although he was the most eminent physician in Europe, Da Monte spurned the wealth of a court appointment and dedicated his life to teaching future physicians. He sought a return to the original, rational method of Galen, in which the physician learned to reason from all the signs and evidence available, including the individual temperament of the patient and all the complex causes of the patient's life, to identify the nature and cause of the disease and the precise remedies for proper treatment. As Jerome Bylebyl and Michael Stolberg have shown in detail, Da Monte combined this sophisticated method of diagnosis and treatment, which he recovered from his humanist reading of Galen's texts, with the actual practice of Galenic medicine, especially through vigorous bedside teaching.[70]

At least by 1542, when the arts school moved next door to the Hospital of San Francesco, Da Monte regularly brought students to see patients in the hospital, discuss their diagnoses and treatments, and observe the outcomes. This practice continued into the 1550s, when students visited hospital patients with Antonio Fracanzani, probably persisted in the 1560s since many of the

---

66   Nutton, "The Rise of Medical Humanism," 15.

67   Liboni, "Humanist Post-mortems," 29–35.

68   Ogilvie, *Science of Describing*, 33. Bylebyl, "The School of Padua," 352.

69   Bylebyl, "The School of Padua," 346. Nutton, "The Rise of Medical Humanism," 8–9, also describes the Galenism of Leoniceno's pupil Giovanni Manardi (1462–1536).

70   Bylebyl, "The School of Padua," 348–349. Bylebyl, "Teaching *Methodus Medendi* in the Renaissance." Bylebyl, "The Manifest and the Hidden." Stolberg, "Bedside Teaching."

hospital physicians were also university faculty, and gained official status in 1578, with professors Albertino Bottoni and Marco Oddi.[71] Students learned a vital array of practices: uroscopy, stool analysis, the inspection of sputum and blood, feeling for the pulse, assessing the qualities of patients' skin, techniques of abdominal palpation, some surgical procedures, and the administration of drugs.[72] In this hospital teaching, professors continued and refined practices of bedside instruction in private homes that were embraced widely in Italy. Students came for this practical instruction most of all. In their own words, foreign students traveled across "so many mountains" not for books, which they had at home, but for "the study of practice," especially "the constant inspection of the sick, and careful observation of the daily changes of diseases and their symptoms."[73] At times, under Falloppio in the 1550s and other professors later in the 1570s and early 1600s, the hospital teaching ended in post-mortem dissections to view the internal states of diseases.[74] Similar training in techniques of palpation and examination occurred in anatomy classes, too, such as Vesalius's 1540 lectures in Bologna.[75]

Students also demanded practical skills and knowledge from anatomical instruction. As Cynthia Klestinec details, students throughout the second half of the sixteenth century praised accurate, diligent anatomists who could use their technical skill and expertise to show clearly body parts and even disease states.[76] In the early 1550s, students demanded that Falloppio be allowed to continue acting as both the demonstrator and the dissector, combining in one person his careful search for distinct anatomical structures.[77] They eagerly attended public and especially private anatomies by physicians and surgeons who could show them structures and techniques up close. The more philosophical, Aristotelian lectures of Hieronymous Fabricius, who held the primary anatomy teaching duties at Padua from 1565 to 1612, seem to have annoyed students for their comparative lack of a practical focus.[78] Yet Fabricius also established the first permanent anatomy theater in 1584 as a tranquil,

---

71   Stolberg, "Bedside Teaching," 642, 645, 657. Klestinec, *Theaters of Anatomy*, 84. Bylebyl, "School of Padua," 349.

72   Stolberg, "Bedside Teaching," 642–647, 652–659. Bylebyl, "The Manifest and the Hidden."

73   Student from the German nation at Padua, in 1597, quoted and translated in Bylebyl, "School of Padua," 351.

74   Stolberg, "Post-mortems," 72–73. Bylebyl, "School of Padua," 363.

75   Heseler, *Andreas Vesalius' First Public Anatomy at Bologna*, 224–225. I thank R. Allen Shotwell for this reference.

76   Klestinec, *Theaters of Anatomy, passim*. Cf. Stolberg, "Post-mortems"; Stolberg, "Bedside."

77   Bylebyl, "School of Padua," 362. Klestinec, *Theaters of Anatomy*, 42–53.

78   Klestinec, *Theaters of Anatomy*, chs. 2 and 5.

scholarly space for seeing and especially hearing, and he served as the ordinary professor of anatomy and surgery, amassing wealth and success as a surgeon.[79] Fabricius applied his dissecting skill and expertise to Aristotelian-Galenic philosophical projects, moving from detailed descriptions or *historiae* to the philosophical understanding of the uses of various parts and anatomical systems.[80] After Fabricius, though, Santorio Santorio, teaching at Padua from 1611 to 1624, joined the wider campaign of physicians to make a reformed Galenism triumphant over speculative Aristotelian philosophy. Joining a chorus of other professors and students, he followed Galen to insist that the physician, "who is a sensate philosopher, deals only with those things that are submitted to the senses: truly, the physician always despises insensible dogma."[81]

Students and professors followed Galen and Italian tradition in finding a close connection between anatomy and surgery, and the numerous (three to seven) lecturers in surgery at Bologna also had medical degrees. The reform of anatomy began at least by the 1490s, when anatomists and physicians, especially at Bologna, began to use their humanist erudition and experience to correct texts and claims. From the origins of Bologna anatomy teaching around 1316, professors revived the practice of dissection as an explicit return to the methods and texts of Galen, especially *On the Usefulness of the Parts*.[82] By the first two decades of the 1500s, the surgeon and physician Berengario da Carpi (c. 1460-c. 1530) lectured on surgery at Bologna, using his own experiences with hundreds of dissected bodies to ground and generate anatomical knowledge.[83] His massive 1521 *Commentary* used anatomical demonstration (*demonstratio*) according to the senses (*ad sensum*) to make new claims about the muscles, bones, and vessels, as well as to reject Galen's claims about the existence of the *rete mirabile*, a network of blood vessels found in the brains of ungulates but not in the brains of humans. As we have seen, Berengario explicitly set out to make tests of authorities' claims.

At Padua, professors of surgery often had medical degrees as well, at least after the rushed appointment of Vesalius as the sole holder of the two lectureships in surgery at the end of 1537.[84] Vesalius, of course, first achieved fame

---

79   Klestinec, *Theaters of Anatomy*, 73, *passim*. Bylebyl, "School of Padua," 367.
80   Klestinec, *Theaters of Anatomy*, ch. 2. Cunningham, "Fabricius and the 'Aristotle Project.'" Distelzweig, "Fabricius's Galeno-Aristotelian Teleomechanics of Muscle." Siraisi, "Historia, actio, utilitas."
81   Santorio, *Commentaria in primam fen primi libri canonis Avicennae*, col. 62. Latin quotation in Bylebyl, "Medicine, Philosophy, and Humanism," 49 n. 123. Cf. Stolberg, "Empiricism," 493, 495.
82   Park, *Secrets of Women*, 106. Robison, *Healers in the Making*, ch. 4.
83   French, "Berengario da Carpi," 42–74.
84   Bylebyl, "School of Padua," 355, 359–360.

for his combination of humanist linguistic skill and his manual ability in dissection. Humanist anatomists like Vesalius and his professor Johann Guinter
moved toward hands-on anatomical practice and critique in response to the
publication in the 1520s and 1530s of major anatomical manuals and treatises
by Galen which had been previously unknown, such as *On Anatomical Procedures* and *On the Doctrines of Hippocrates and Plato*. These works offered first
models and then targets, as they stimulated Vesalius to establish Galen's texts
and then gradually critique them based on his own experience.[85] Even in his
polemical preface, Vesalius styled Galen "easily the chief of all the professors
of dissection," while in the same breath criticizing his "false doctrines" and
over two hundred errors generated by his dissection of animals alone, and not
human bodies.[86] Although he had little surgical skill initially, Vesalius taught
anatomy and surgery at Padua until 1544, when the surgeon and anatomist
Realdo Colombo succeeded him.

The institutionalized and celebrated combination of surgical expertise and
academic medical training extended to other institutional traditions as well,
for example in the fact that the ordinary physicians of the Paduan hospital
were often physician-surgeons. As Paolo Savoia shows, "graduate surgeons,"
with degrees in surgery, may have had less official status but they often enjoyed
fluid careers of rapid ascent, and combined academic book learning, surgical
apprenticeships and skill, and recognition as published authorities.[87]

In brief, the Italian schools and especially Padua constituted the most
influential pedagogical culture that shaped Leiden's own medical professors.
So who were the first professors? Here it will be helpful to introduce some of
those professors with snapshot resumes.[88] After the first, solitary professor, we
will concentrate our attention on those professors whose practices and writings we will examine in greater detail throughout the chapters.

At first, there was only Bontius. Gerardus Bontius (or Geraert de Bondt, 1536–
1599) began teaching medicine at Leiden University as a professor of medicine
from the beginning, with an appointment in July 1575. His arts and medical education drove his initial selection for teaching mathematics and astronomy, but
he likely did not teach those subjects.[89] After all, he would have been busy with

---

85   Nutton, ed., *Principles of Anatomy*. Bylebyl, "The School of Padua," 358–359.
86   Vesalius, *De Humani Corporis Fabrica Libri Septem* (1543), *3v, correcting "principijs" as
      "principii" as in the 1555 edition: Andreas Vesalius, *De Humani Corporis Fabrica Libri Sep-
      tem* (1555), a4r.
87   Savoia, "Skills, Knowledge, and Status." 27–54.
88   Throughout, I am drawing from Kroon, *Bijdragen*; Lindeboom, *Dutch Medical Biography*;
      and Adamus, *Vitae Germanorum Medicorum*, as well as other works as noted.
89   Kroon, *Bijdragen*, 91. Lindeboom, *Dutch Medical Biography*, col. 208.

his duties as the lone professor in the art and science of medicine. Although his father had left the military life for the honest pleasures of farming, "in the manner of the ancients," Bontius traveled to Italy, to the universities of Ferrara and especially Padua for a cutting-edge medical education.[90] He brought his keen knowledge of Greek and the practice of medicine to Leiden. There, he read Galen and Hippocrates in the Greek originals for his lectures, enjoyed a successful medical practice, and taught anatomy. In 1582, his student Petrus Paaw later reported, he "presented an anatomy" to students, well before his formal appointment as a professor of anatomy and medical botany in 1587.[91] Despite his recognized erudition and practical success, Bontius embraced modesty and published nothing.

Another early professor shaped Leiden medical pedagogy deeply. Johannes Heurnius (Jan van Heurne, 1543–1601) crafted the main teaching texts and lectures of Leiden's instruction in theoretical and practical medicine, and so established the core of instruction for six decades. Although he came from noble stock, his relatives had eaten up much of his patrimony while his father traveled, and at first he was a slow learner in school. But he later excelled in mathematics, philosophy, and medicine at the University of Leuven, living and studying with the famed mathematician Cornelius Gemma. After two years at Leuven, at the age of twenty-one, he traveled to the University of Paris. There Heurnius impressed the eminent humanist physician Louis Duret so much that Duret urged him to teach medicine.[92] Of course, Heurnius also gained practical knowledge, training in the ability to cut for bladder stones safely and skillfully. He also excelled in philosophy at Paris, and grew close to the philospher, mathematician, and pedagogical reformer Petrus Ramus.

Naturally, Heurnius headed to Italy around 1567, and learned from the University of Padua's eminent medical faculty. There, he joined a circle of dedicated students with Pieter van Foreest, later one of the most famous Dutch physicians and surgeons. Heurnius embraced the lecture-hall and book learning as well as the bedside practical instruction of physicians such as Girolamo Capivacca, Girolamo Mercuriale, and Bernardino Paterno.[93] He learned anatomy under Hieronymous Fabricius, then arguably the most eminent anatomist in Europe, who elevated anatomy toward Aristotelian philosophical contemplation of the uses of the parts.[94] Further cultivating his practical education,

---

90   Adamus, *Vitae Germanorum Medicorum*, 366.

91   Paaw, *Primitiae Anatomicae*, 130. Huisman, *Finger of God*, 19, dates the beginning of Bontius' anatomical teaching to 1584 and Kroon, *Bijdragen*, 92, dates it to 1587.

92   [Otto Heurnius], "Vita Auctoris."

93   [Otto Heurnius], "Vita Auctoris."

94   Cunningham, "Fabricius and the 'Aristotle Project.'" Klestinec, *Theaters of Anatomy*. Distelzweig, "Fabricius's Galeno-Aristotelian Teleomechanics of Muscle." Siraisi, "Historia, actio, utilitas."

Heurnius studied botany in the university garden, first opened in 1546. After four years at Padua, Heurnius traveled to Pavia, where he finally received his doctorate in medicine after only a short time there, a common practice for medical students on their academic travels.[95]

Back in the Low Countries in 1573, Johannes Heurnius gained practical experience as a physician to aristocrats, including Prince William and Prince Maurits, as well as other patients from France, Utrecht, and Leiden. Heurnius gained renown for his Galen-like diagnosis of the fatal poisoning of a local lord, then married and served in the Utrecht senate. When Heurnius was thirty-eight, in September 1581, the Curators of the young Leiden University called him to a professorship in medicine, and he began his lectures on the theory of medicine, or the *Institutes of Medicine*, soon after.

Another professor, the venerable Rembertus Dodonaeus (Rembert Dodoens, 1517–1585) joined the Leiden faculty just over a year after Heurnius but did not stay long. He grew up in a merchant family in Mechelen (Mechlin) and like many other scholars in the Low Countries he started his studies at the University of Leuven, obtaining a licentiate to practice medicine in 1535, at the age of only seventeen. Dodonaeus then studied in France, Italy, and German lands. He displayed his humanist linguistic skills in his first publication, a revision and correction of Johann Guinter's Latin translation of Paul of Aegina's seventh-century medical encyclopedia. Back in Mechelen as a city physician, he oversaw the town apothecaries, and expressed a humanist physician's skepticism about their knowledge and honesty.[96] From his book learning and wide experience, he published a vernacular herbal, the *Cruydeboek*, first in 1554 and then in many subsequent editions, and his massive *Six Quintuplets of the History of Plants (Stirpium Historiae Pemptades Sex)*, with over 1300 figures. From 1574, he served as physician and counselor to the Emperor Maximilian II, and then to his successor Rudolph II until 1580. Dodonaeus described cases and remedies from his long practice in his published *observationes*, including some post-mortem pathological dissections.[97] Although he turned down an offer to teach at Leuven, he taught medicine and natural philosophy at Leiden from late 1582 to early 1585.

Once Leiden's medical faculty had gained their discursive and practical expertise in established faculties elsewhere, they could train future professors. Petrus Paaw (or Pieter Pauw or Paeuw or Pavius, 1564–1617) came from a wealthy and powerful Amsterdam family of merchants and government officials. He matriculated to study medicine at Leiden in 1581, just about the time Johannes

95   E.g., Cunningham, "The Bartholins, the Platters and Laurentius Gryllus."
96   Klerk, "Galen Reconsidered," 65.
97   Stolberg, "Post-mortems," 76–77.

Heurnius arrived to teach.[98] After three years learning from Heurnius, Bontius, and Dodonaeus, he traveled to Paris and studied and practiced anatomy. Then he moved on to the University of Rostock, where he continued his anatomical education with Henricus Brucaeus, an anatomist as well as a prolific mathematician and successful court physician, and took his medical degree in 1587. He began to teach anatomy publicly at Rostock and published two short works, including notes on Galen on dietetics. From there he traveled to Italy and saw Fabricius dissect cadavers in Padua. By the time he returned to Leiden to practice medicine, in 1589, he readily took on an appointment as extraordinary professor at the university.

Our last major character from among the Leiden professors is the eldest son of Johannes Heurnius, Otto Heurnius (or van Heurne, 1577–1652). Like Paaw, he matriculated at Leiden University to begin his studies, and he remained there, working through degrees in law and philosophy by 1599, and then medicine in 1601. Otto Heurnius, too, embraced the pedagogical traditions passed on through Leiden professors, notably helping to establish regular clinical teaching and post-mortem dissections in the hospital.

Other professors from the earlier generations, such as Aelius Everhardus Vorstius (1565–1624) could study at Leiden as well as other universities, with Vorstius traveling to Padua, Bologna, Ferrara, and even more universities in the 1580s and 1590s before returning to Leiden.[99] Once established, Leiden professors also followed common European practice and kept many teaching positions in the family. Otto Heurnius became an extraordinary professor after his father's death, Reinier Bontius followed his father Rembert, and Adolph Vorstius his father Aelius. Pedagogical lines of formation and acculturation linked universities and generations.

6 Early Medical Curricula

A few months after the founding of the university in February 1575, the highest-paid new professor, theologian Guilielmus Feugueraeus, submitted a hypothetical curriculum to the university Curators.[100] For the forming of the physician, "that most faithful helper of nature," he recommended allotting just

---

98   *Album Studiosorum*, col. 11 shows Paaw matriculating on 2 November and Heurnius also registering on 7 November.

99   Luyendijk-Elshout, "Der Einfluss der italienischen Universitäten auf die medizinische Facultät Leiden," 341, 347–348.

100   In Molhuysen, *Bronnen*, 1, 39*–43*.

a little time to oration and disputation in the early years. In the later years, these practitioners-in-training should study "the inspection, dissection, dissolution, and transmutation of living bodies, plants, and metals; to the three former labors, he joins the fourth, by far of richer fruit." This bold call for the "richer fruit" of alchemical transmutations found an echo in the earliest publication of the Leiden professor of medicine, Johannes Heurnius, as we will see. But even from the founding, hands-on learning, practical goals, and bodily engagement with materials and objects appeared as primary goals for medical students. It seems that Leiden professors and students did not follow the specifics of this plan, though as we will see there was far more teaching of chymistry than has been noticed.[101] A strong interest in practical learning, allied with humanist erudition and ancient knowledge, remained a characteristic feature of Leiden medical training from the beginning.

Medical students getting their bearings around the university academic building in 1587 depended on posted sheets displaying the series of lectures. Wednesdays and Saturdays generally remained free for disputations, processions, promotions, inaugural lectures, and, for two hours at a time, perhaps even use of the library.[102] Lectures began early and continued through the afternoon. At the eighth hour of the morning, Johannes Heurnius began the day's lectures on medicine, "the practice of the art composed by himself."[103] In the second hour after noon, the other medical professor, Gerardus Bontius (1536–1599), lectured alternately on the Hippocratic *Prognostics* and Jean Fernel's *Physiologia*, or philosophical medical theory of bodily causes and actions, with some anatomy.

This instruction came interspersed with teaching by the law faculty, theology professors, and the arts instructors. Throughout the day, thirteen other professors gave four different lectures on law, with three on ancient Roman law, the minor Hebrew prophets, the "Epistle of Paul to the Hebrews," the *Logic* and *Physics* of Aristotle, the Gospel of Matthew, the prophet Isaiah, the letters of Cicero, the Greek of Homer and the Aristotelian *De mundo*, the *Politics* of Aristotle, and cosmography and astronomy (by the mathematician Rudolph Snel).

Around five years later in 1592, sixteen professors lectured on a wider range of topics. The new professor of medicine Petrus Paaw, hired to teach medical botany first in 1589 but appointed as a more-secure ordinary professor in 1592, added instruction on plants and other *materia medica*. Paaw likely taught using Pietro Andrea Mattioli's more recent correction, expansion, and commentary

---

101 Kroon, *Bijdragen*, 13
102 Hulshoff Pol, "The Library," 425.
103 Molhuysen, *Bronnen*, 1, 157*.

on Dioscorides' ancient Greek herbal. At the same time, Heurnius interpreted the Hippocratic texts on the rule of sustenance in acute diseases, and Bontius used the encyclopedic work on diseases of the seventh-century Byzantine physician Paul of Aegina to teach the method of recognizing and curing diseases of the individual parts.[104]

In 1599, Paaw taught from more recent anatomical texts, such as Realdo Colombo's *De re anatomica* of 1559, beginning with Colombo's important innovations on the liver, veins, and blood.[105] After lecturing on recent anatomy in the ninth hour of the morning, Paaw taught first-hand knowledge about medicinal ingredients through the plants in the university's public garden. Bontius, in turn, lectured on the Hippocratic works on the diseases of women, and on Galen's *Simple Drugs*. Just two years later, we find Paaw set to teach his *own* botanical method on Mondays and Tuesdays, and from the first book of Dioscorides on Thursdays and Fridays. By then, Heurnius taught from the books of Galen on the differentia, causes, and symptoms of diseases. Everardus Vorstius, hired as an ordinary professor of medicine in 1601, taught the course on medical theory, the "Institutes of Medicine," likely using Heurnius' new textbook, *Institutes of Medicine*, in the corrected editions from 1592 or 1593.[106] According to his son's biographical account, Heurnius had started teaching from his own *Institutes of Medicine* in 1581, when he began his first lecture at Leiden on November 7th, at eight in the morning.[107] Heurnius' book and lectures formed the continuous core of medical theory at Leiden for over half a century; professors used his textbook at least through the 1640s.[108] From around 1600 on, then, Leiden medical professors formally taught their own methods and textbooks, incorporating the best of ancient and modern learning and relying on their own expertise in ancient languages and texts, as well as their own experiences with human bodies and medicines.

Courses over the decades showed their dedication to the best of the ancient experts, from Galen's *Simple Drugs* to Paul of Aegina's compendium of medicine. But they also drew readily from choice recent authors such as Jean Fernel, especially his textbook on human bodies, *Physiologia*, which covered basic anatomy and then moved on to philosophical discussions of the elements and humors, and then to bodily faculties, spirits, and generation. They used

---

104   Molhuysen, *Bronnen* 1, 191*.

105   Molhuysen, *Bronnen*, 1, 384*.

106   Molhuysen, *Bronnen*, 400–401*.

107   [Otto Heurnius], "Vita Auctoris," in Johannes Heurnius, *Opera Omnia*.

108   Molhuysen, *Bronnen*, 3, 14.

Mattioli's greatly expanded commentary on Dioscorides' ancient herbal, as well as Realdo Colombo's new anatomy book, which updated both Galen and his modern rival, Vesalius. Increasingly, Leiden professors taught from their own textbooks and methods, especially Johannes Heurnius' comprehensive texts and courses on medical theory and practice, the *Institutes of Medicine* and *New Method of the Practice of Medicine*. Over the next several chapters, we will mine these books and many others to get a sense of what professors taught and students learned in order to make students into new physicians.

7   Conclusions

The quick founding of the university in the setting of war puts the humanist openness to religious difference (at least until the theological-political battles of the Remonstrants and Counter-Remonstrants, roughly 1610–1619) and scholarly innovation in sharper relief. At first, a shared humanist scholarly culture tempered any demands for confessional conformity and Protestant uniformity, and rewarded research into ancient texts *and* the making of new devices, trials or experiments, and mathematical tools. Clearly, this drive for research and innovation did not spark a rejection of ancient knowledge, but in many cases, from Stevin and Snel to the medical professors Johannes Heurnius and Pieter Paaw, motivated professors to recover, appropriate, and build upon the works of the ancients. After all, the ancients excelled in innovation for their own time and left tantalizing riches of learning and utility for scholars with the right mining tools. Increasingly, scholars at Leiden and elsewhere sought to surpass the ancients' achievements.

In mathematics, Willebrord Snel's humanist erudition fueled his practical trials. Reviving the projects of ancient mathematicians, he added practical tests: he measured the weight and density of water with special containers, "made experience" with mirrors and lenses, and measured the circumference of the earth through surveying the local geography. Though innovative and important for the history of optics and geodesy, Willebrord's teaching and work do not seem to have advertised or cultivated practices of experimentation among the students.

In contrast, the increasingly widespread practice of making trials or experiments in sixteenth-century academic medicine carried directly into Leiden medical education by the traditional routes of pedagogical transmission. As students, Leiden professors studied in hotspots for the humanist recovery and intellectual and manual test of ancient claims. As the premier university for academic medicine, Padua attracted many of the early cohort of Leiden medical professors. The Leiden garden and anatomy theater clearly imitated those similar sites of medical learning established at Padua. There, as well as at patients' bedsides, students continued the revived tradition of learning medicine through a close marriage of reason and experience.

CHAPTER 2

Ideals of Learning and Reading

Reason and experience were the watchwords of the Leiden professors and other academic practitioners of Galenic medicine.[1] In this chapter, we are concerned mainly with the ideals and practices of reason. Over the next two chapters, we are moving to the lectures and books of the university's main academic structure, the Academy Building (*Academiegebouw*). Like the lectures themselves, our tour travels through a range of courses, texts, subjects, and ideas. But there is no other way to recover the richness and patterns of early modern medical education.

In the Academy Building, Johannes Heurnius and other professors told mythic histories of the founding of the true medicine, the "Asclepian" tradition, which ran from Asclepius, through Hippocrates, and especially through Galen's revival and synthesis. Though they sharpened their philological and philosophical tools to mine the insights of Hippocratics texts such as the *Aphorisms*, they did so largely through the filters of Galen.[2] Like his followers, Galen often stressed the predominance of experience over reason. In early modern Galenic medicine, the wise, effective physician always organized and refined experience with reason, and grounded and tested reason with experience.

Students and professors prized hands-on and practical exercises, but much of the book-learning aimed at passing the private exams and public disputations required for a medical degree. Concentrating on the Hippocratic *Aphorisms* and practicing the writing and oral defense of mock theses, students developed the virtues of performing and writing formal disputations. They trained to be systematic readers, laying out etymologies, definitions, diagnoses, indications, and recipes, and replying with sharp, alert, ready responses to objections.

Bookish study guides from leading professors give us a vision of exemplary ideals, texts, and methods of study. But it is important to emphasize that these scholars were self-consciously *embodied* teachers and learners. Bodily death and impairment crowded their daily lives. Even the Stoic philosopher Lipsius sat rapt in study too long, and thought he had passed near to death. After Johannes Heurnius' death, biographical anecdotes framed him as a new, Dutch

---

1 For references beyond Leiden, see, e.g., Wear, *Knowledge & Practice*, 130–133 and Maclean, *Logic, Signs, and Nature*, 191–203.
2 *Pace* Cook, *Matters of Exchange*, 111.

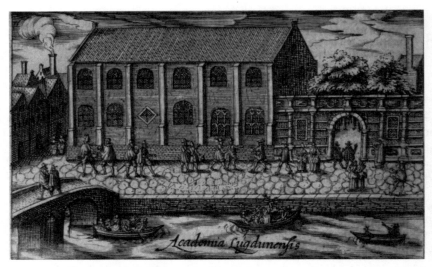

FIGURE 6   The Academic Building on the Rapenburg canal was the main lecture space of
the university. J. J. Orlers, *Beschrijvinge der Stadt Leyden* (Leiden, 1614), 128.
COURTESY, BAYERISCHE STAATSBIBLIOTHEK MÜNCHEN, 4 BELG. 137 M,
P. 128, URN:NBN:DE:BVB:12-BSB10224648-3.

Galen diagnosing a ruler's fatal symptoms. His own family, like so many others,
suffered heavy losses of life from epidemics.

Through the best books and classes, and especially through philosophical
reading and discussion, professors taught that students ought to literally shape
their brains and bodies for sharp thinking. They again followed Galen in thinking that the *ingenium*, the faculty of the brain responsible for distinguishing
differences among things and connecting true similarities, depended on a fine
substance of the brain. The faculty of memory depended on a stable and firm
substance. These sons of bourgeois merchants, and some aristocratic families,
enhanced their *ingenia* (wits) through their bookish studies. Alas, professors
and students alike often succumbed to the lures of drink and violence, which
dulled the wit. Perils to bodies were perils to learning.

1   Ideals of Curing Bodies by Reason and Experience

Reason and experience, knowing and doing, formed the two chief rhetorical
and practical supports of medicine at late-Renaissance Leiden. The institution
flourished in the seventeenth century, growing into a popular medical school,
and thus can be taken as representative of the trained knowing and doing

of many hundreds of physicians. The integrations of knowing and doing (or making) attempted and practiced there are also significant for our historiography, since historians of medicine and science have cast doubt on the reality of "reason and experience" slogans, at times splitting the century's innovative theorizing from any substantial practical effects.[3] As we will see here and in the following chapters, the message of the medical school's 1670 seal, "*experientia et ratione*" (by experience and by reason) was not so much a Baconian break with the bookish past as the continuation of a long tradition in Galenic medicine.[4]

Across the sixteenth and seventeenth centuries, physicians performed anatomical dissections and made anatomical discoveries, systematized schemes for diagnosis and drugs, and incorporated chymical procedures and theories into their work.[5] By the early seventeenth century, anatomy and chymistry, in particular, emphasized the necessity of long experience and careful attention.[6] But the novelties of the seventeenth century should not distract us from important continuities perpetuated by pedagogical institutions and shared textual resources, especially those found in universities. In ancient, medieval, and early modern sources, the integration of *ratio et experientia*, *logos kai peira*, remained especially prominent and essential in the making and testing of drugs.[7] The ancient "prince" of the Roman physicians, Galen, and his medieval Arabic heir and commentator, Avicenna, agreed: only trial-making or experimentation (*peira*) could teach the more complex properties and faculties of materials, especially drugs.[8] As Galen argued, physicians and philosophers needed both reason and experience working together to produce and support theory.[9] In his view, reason supplies explanations, usually in terms of philosophical causes such as the primary qualities. It allows the physician to understand the natures of patients—constituted as this or that temperament of their bodies and organs, constituted by the proportions in their mixtures of the elementary

---

3 Even Frank's *Harvey and the Oxford Physiologists*, though still an excellent and exemplary work in the history of science and medicine, pays scant attention to the interests of the physicians in medical practice. For a recent argument for Marcello Malpighi's integration of new mechanical philosophizing and medical practice, see Bertoloni Meli, *Mechanism, Experiment, Disease*.

4 Beukers, "Acid Spirits and Alkaline Salts," 40–41.

5 Ragland, "'Making Trials.'" Andrew Wear, *Knowledge & Practice*. Bertoloni Meli, *Mechanism, Experiment, Disease*.

6 Goldberg, "William Harvey." Klein, "Daniel Sennert."

7 Ragland, "'Making Trials,'" 509–510. Ragland, "Mechanism."

8 Van der Eijk, *Medicine and Philosophy*, 298, 282, 287.

9 Hankinson, "Epistemology," 169–177.

qualities hot, cold, wet, and dry—and to make inferences about a patient's natural temperament, the causes of a disease, its course, and the proper cure.

For Galen, experience confirms or disconfirms the inferences of reason, judges the phenomena, and tests the explanations of reason about the hidden states in the body. Specifically, experience is the "teacher" of the faculties or powers of foods and drugs, and the ultimate judge of the claims of reason.[10] In well-known works such as *On the Natural Faculties*, and *Simple Drugs*, Galen repeatedly evaluated philosophical conclusions of reason by reference to experience, trials, or the obvious phenomena (*phainomena*), practices he asserted were necessary to confirm or deny the conclusions of reason.[11] These works enjoyed widespread publication and reading in the sixteenth and seventeenth centuries, with *On the Natural Faculties* appearing in ten editions from 1537 to 1596, and *Simple Drugs* (*De simplicium medicamentorum facultatibus ac temperamentis*) reaching 16 editions from 1530 to 1592.[12]

Physicians carried this program into the sixteenth and seventeenth centuries, and across the sixteenth century increasingly made tests to adjudicate various rational claims and discover new phenomena.[13] The integration of experience and reason framed the core courses in medical theory and the most influential medical textbooks, such as Johannes Heurnius' textbook *Institutes of Medicine* (*Institutiones Medicinae*), published from 1592 to 1658.[14] As the title page of the first edition declared, the book presented his lectures, "taken from his mouth while teaching."[15] Heurnius' innovative and influential book combined the best of medical theory and rational practice in one volume or one course of lectures.

As Heurnius put it, all good "rationalists" ought to integrate deeply the two sources of medical knowledge and practice. The rationalists "embrace experience, and join reason to it. Beyond this, they hunted knowledge of the human body, and they dissected it, judging necessary the investigation of the elements

---

10   Van der Eijk, *Medicine and Philosophy*, 280.

11   E.g., Galen, *On the Natural Faculties*, trans. A. J. Brock, vol. 1, 48–49, 68–69, 80–81, 226–227. Frede, "On Galen's Epistemology," 82. Hankinson, "Epistemology," 176–180.

12   Durling, "Chronological Census."

13   Ragland, "'Making Trials.'"

14   Johannes Heurnius, *Institutiones Medicinae* (1592). Lindeboom, *Dutch Medical Biography*, col. 858.

15   Petrus Paaw insisted they are his own notes from Heurnius' lectures, lightly edited, and checked versus the memories of other students. See Paaw's unpag. preface in Johannes Heurnius, *Institutiones Medicinae* (1638). Unless otherwise noted, references to Heurnius' *Institutiones* are to the 1638 edition. The editions after Otto Heurnius' corrected version of 1609 appear nearly identical, with some typos fixed and new ones introduced.

and causes by which the body could be changed. We ourselves embrace this, brought together from reason and experience."[16] Starting from philosophical first principles, such as the nature of the elements and qualities, then the temperaments and humors, a physician could establish important truths. But these derived from experience, and experience remained necessary: "Many individual things persuade by reason, which finally convinces by use. For which reason Sallust says rightly, *Each by itself lacking, the one needs the help of the other.*"[17] The endeavor of academic physicians to integrate experience and reason stood out in the early modern period, such that even in 1553 Richard Eden, an alchemist and translator, invoked their example in his vernacular presentation of the novelties of the New World: "that experience to be most certayn which is ioyned with reason or speculacion, and that reason to be most sure which is confirmed with experience, accordinge as the Phisicians determen theyr science."[18]

Histories of medicine taught at Leiden and elsewhere emphasized the necessity of combining reason and experience, and helped to articulate what should be included in those two categories. In this marriage of reason and experience, reason illuminated the hidden causes of health and disease in bodies, while experience provided the phenomena and regular correlations of clusters of signs and symptoms (which marked out most diseases) and cures. Johannes Heurnius presented an oration of such a history in 1589, which appeared in print later.[19] His narrative stuck with some of his students, too, indicated by the thin but similar history in Johan van Beverwijck's 1644 *Treasury of Unhealthiness (Schat der Ongesontheyt).*[20]

In Heurnius' history, medicine's earliest shoots appeared in the mists of myth. Chiron the centaur invented the art of medicine and then taught Asclepius, the true father of the best, legitimate medicine.[21] At least, such was the story by the Greek poet Pindar, reiterated by Pliny. Hippocrates "the Great" descended on his father's side from Asclepius (the seventeenth generation), and on his mother's side from Hercules (the twentieth generation). During the great plague of Athens during the wars with Sparta, "Hippocrates, skilled to know the hidden causes of things, destroyed the sacred plague by fire."[22] Here,

---

16   Johannes Heurnius, *Institutiones Medicinae*, 7.
17   *Ibid.*, italics in original. Sallust, *The War with Catiline*, 20. Sallust insists the necessity of the strength of the body and the excellence of the mind together, for waging war.
18   Eden, "Richard Eden to the Reader," in *A treatyse of the newe India*, Aiii.
19   Johannes Heurnius, *De morbis ventriculi liber.*
20   Van Beverwijck, *Schat der Ongesontheyt*, *5r–*6r, 7–9.
21   Johannes Heurnius, *Institutiones*, *2–*3. Pliny, *Historia mundi naturalis*, 105, 368, 427.
22   Johannes Heurnius, *Institutiones*, *4r. Pinault, "How Hippocrates Cured the Plague."

Heurnius drew on a venerable tradition from Pliny, Galen, and other ancient authors crediting Hippocrates with the cure of an epidemic through purifying and fumigating fires.

Hippocrates, foremost of the later Asclepians, went well beyond the Empiric sect, which sought only to treat similar diseases with similar remedies, without speculating about hidden causes. Even before Hippocrates, "since men wanted to confirm the experiences [*experientias*] with causes, and since they could see that the observation of effects from unknown causes was not confirmed, they began to turn toward their contemplation."[23] Interestingly, Heurnius positioned the philosopher Democritus as the teacher of Hippocrates himself. As Christoph Lüthy demonstrates so well, in the late Renaissance Democritus appeared in four guises, as an atomist, an anatomist, a laughing philosopher, and an alchemist—as the philosophical teacher of Hippocrates.[24] As we will see in chapter four, putting Democritus as the teacher of even the great Hippocrates fit well with Heurnius' elevation of chymistry into an essential part of medical history and practice. In his oration on the origin of medicine, Heurnius idealized Democritus as one given over "wholly to the contemplation of nature," as well as someone skilled in the use of the violent purgative, hellebore. Democritus's student, Hippocrates, had the ancestry, education, experience, and emphasis on action—"he speaks for the sake of doing things" in laconic aphorisms—to practice the best medicine and merit more honors than any living mortal. Even after his death, Heurnius wrote, bees made honey in his tomb, and nurses used the honey to cure the ulcers of their infants, "as if Nature is shouting, 'this man showed the true medicine of the Gods to men.'"[25]

Then the sectarian schismatics ruined things. Herophilus, the ancient Alexandrian anatomist, turned aside from true Hippocratic medicine, and so did his heir Erasistratus. The harmony of Hippocratic reason and experience fractured into camps of Rationalists, Methodists, and new Empirics. These Empirics rejected the investigation of causes and natures. Instead, they only observed the concourses of signs in diagnosing diseases, and observed the effects of medicines, trusting in the medicinal trials (*experimenta*) of others.[26] Happily, Galen later restored the Hippocratic light in the darkness, shining the brilliant light of truth, and threw out the unhealthy rubbish of the Empirics and Methodists.

---

23   Johannes Heurnius, *Institutiones*, *3r.

24   Lüthy, "The Fourfold Democritus," 473.

25   Johannes Heurnius, *Institutiones*, *4r.

26   Johannes Heurnius, *Institutiones*, 6. For these sects and their methods, see Von Staden, "Experiment and Experience in Hellenistic Medicine."

As with all of his published works, Heurnius ended with a hymn to God's handiwork: "Indeed this study of nature, in this hard nature, softens the mind toward piety, and by the contemplation of things calls forth veneration toward Holy God. Certainly, in so great a fabric and economy of the human body, which perpetually runs with the wisdom of the architect, it is not possible for it to happen that religious fear does not occupy minds."[27] This short history, then, given in public orations and multiple printed editions, presented students with ideals and a stirring history of the "true" and even "divine" medicine, one which always integrated reason and experience.

Medicine for Heurnius, as for many other early modern physicians, remained a factive art, aimed at *making* healthy patients. Yet it also involved knowing, even systematic theoretical knowledge, or *scientia*. At the time Heurnius wrote his major works, around 1600, influential physicians such as Daniel Sennert, drawing on earlier precedent, emphasized the factive status of the art of medicine, while others, such as the philosopher Jacopo Zabarella, sought to claim all of the theoretical parts of medicine for natural philosophy.[28] Across this period, physicians and philosophers vigorously debated the status of medicine as an art (*ars*), a science (*scientia*), or both.[29] Galen could claim medicine as a science, at least in the broad sense of the term, but treat it most often as an art. Vesalius claimed for anatomy the status of contemplative *scientia*, while Giovanni Argenterio denied the status of demonstrative science to both medicine and natural philosophy, arguing that "lazy philosophers" should not hold the honest hands-on activity of healing as inferior to philosophizing.[30] The range and vehemence of this debate suggests two things: that a single, controlling definition did not exert hegemonic force, and yet early modern physicians and philosophers persistently placed medicine in relation to the categories of *ars* and *scientia*.

Among arts and sciences, medicine promised its own perils. Physicians took the human body, its health and disease, as the subject of their study. Early modern physicians returned again and again to the aphorisms of the legendary founder or fountainhead of the true medicine, the Greek healer Hippocrates. These brief, pithy guides to diagnosis, prognosis, and therapy offered a distillation of the art of medicine, the knowledge of which exceeded any one lifetime. They began with a famous summary of the physician's experience: "Life is short, the Art is long, opportunity fleeting, trial [*peira*] dangerous, judgment

---

27   Johannes Heurnius, *Institutiones*, *5v.
28   Maclean, *Logic, Signs, and Nature*, 74. Mikkeli, "The Status of the Mechanical Arts," 118.
29   Maclean, *Logic, Signs, and Nature*, 68–84.
30   Siraisi, "Vesalius and Human Diversity." Siraisi, "Giovanni Argenterio," 174–175.

difficult."[31] Heurnius turned his humanist training in Greek to a detailed commentary on the aphorisms, producing a popular translation and commentary appearing in fourteen editions across the seventeenth century.[32] Here, he drew on his strong appreciation for Hippocratic texts and the lexical skill he had learned in Paris, especially from Louis Duret (1527–1586), who produced the first edition of the *Coan Prognoses* and whom Heurnius reportedly reverenced as "first among physicians after Galen."[33] Galen, of course, came first.

Hippocratic aphorisms also formed a strong pillar in the core of Leiden pedagogy, since student exams and lecture courses aimed at their explanation and application to practical cases. For the first aphorism, Heurnius emphasized the labor and dangers of medicine: "Arduous is the contemplation of our nature: and the economy of the body is known laboriously."[34] Given the dangers of distinguishing the causes of diseases, and the complexity of bodies, the demands of the art vastly exceeded the length of a human life. Physicians had to rely on the long experience of past healers, often as preserved in choice books, as well as the cultivation of their own long experience.[35]

Epistemic and vital dangers resisted even long experience. Identifying diseases and reasoning to their causes embraced not only vexing variability, but hidden variables. Experience or trial-making aimed to overcome these limitations, but always imperfectly. Heurnius, for example, used his humanist language training to unpack the Greek term *peira* in three directions. First, it represented Aristotelian experience, in which many repeated sense perceptions give rise to memory, and memory to experience.[36] Second, it is experience which imitates nature. Third, and most perilously, *peira* "signifies trial-making." Sometimes making trials rendered reliable practice fairly directly, such as the observation that mead given to a series of patients with pleurisy helped them, and so should be given to patients with pleurisy in general.

But a strict Empiric approach offered no easy solution. Empirics attended only to outward appearances, or the phenomena. As he explained elsewhere, Empirics sought "the art from use alone" and not from understanding causes, especially hidden ones.[37] Yet similar diseases could have opposite causes, such as in colic caused by cold or hot juices. The remedies for each would be their

31   Hippocrates, *Aphorisms*, 1, trans. W. H. S. Jones, 99. I have rendered *peira* as "trial" rather than "experiment."

32   Johannes Heurnius, *Hippocratis Coi Aphorismi Graecè, & Latinè*. Kroon, *Bijdragen*, 94.

33   [Otto Heurnius], "Vita Auctoris." For Duret, see Lonie, "'Paris Hippocrates.'"

34   Johannes Heurnius, *Aphorismi*, 6: "*corporis oeconomia*."

35   Cf. Maclean, *Logic, Signs, and Nature*, 79.

36   Ragland, "Making Trials," 504. Heurnius, *Aphorismi*, 6.

37   Johannes Heurnius, *Institutiones*, 2.

qualitative opposites: hot or cold medicines. How could an Empiric judge the proper cure from only the outward appearances? "Certainly, I know that I myself would not want to give a cure from these, I who, as often as I eat a [cold] radish or a [hot] pepper, on that very spot am dragged into a very severe colic pain....Clearly experience is dangerously fallacious, and fallaciously dangerous, as long as it tries these things in human fabric, which for a long time are not proved."[38]

Inexperienced drug trials in human patients merited only condemnation, since rash experience or trials meant certain death. "Plainly, it is the most atrocious crime to rashly try the human body, the domicile of the eternal soul, and dwelling place of the holy spirit." These were no mere academic worries. As Alisha Rankin has recently described, from the 1520s on, rulers across Europe tested poisons and antidotes on condemned criminals, with physicians assisting, directing, and, by the 1560s, narrating the progress of the poison and the effects of the supposed antidotes in close historical detail.[39] Whether Heurnius counted those trials as "rash" is not clear, but he repeatedly insisted on the importance of the use of reason, well-trained in philosophy, along with experience. Without such reason, the resulting experience could only be rash and hence "the teacher of the stupid."[40]

2   The Virtues of Disputation for Learning and Exams

As ever, students studied to pass their exams. Formal and informal practices, from hearing and noting down lectures, to highly regimented extracurricular "colleges" for practicing oral disputations, all shaped the students into candidates who could pass these examinations. The requirements of these exams kept Leiden students and faculty oriented toward a core of more traditional Hippocratic and Galenic medicine, even as they innovated in the details and forms of instruction. A 1576 proposal, likely also by the theologian Feugueraeus, who had drafted the first ideal curriculum statement, detailed examination requirements for the higher degrees.[41] The examinations and disputations emphasized understanding of ancient Hippocratic and Galenic texts. Candidates for a doctor of medicine title had to provide evidence of their erudition in two public disputations prior to promotion. After interpreting

---

38   Johannes Heurnius, *Aphorismi*, 8.
39   Rankin, *The Poison Trials*. Cf. Palmer, "Medical Botany."
40   Johannes Heurnius, *Nova Ratio*, 463.
41   Molhuysen, *Bronnen*, 1, 48*. Otterspeer, *Groepsportret*, 1, 239.

how an aphorism of Hippocrates related to the method of curing generally, the student had to explain the cure of a given disease from either Hippocrates or Galen, in order to see how well he understood the proper use of therapeutic theory on individuals. After this interpretation, the examiners would give some objections, and the candidate would respond. If satisfied, the examiners would choose a thesis for a later public defense.

A less-rigorous examination procedure allowed students to leave with a license or licentiate to practice medicine. After a private examination involving set theses, the student could leave, avoid paying the heavier fee for the doctoral promotion, and still practice medicine.[42] In contrast to these seemingly bookish examinations, earlier surgeons' exams held by the guilds required clear hands-on knowledge of how to sharpen scalpels, and where to cut for bloodletting.[43]

Professors took these university exams seriously, and expected students to practice and prepare. So did the university Curators, who recorded absentee teachers and their excuses, and fined professors for unduly neglecting the required lectures.[44] In 1592, the anatomy professor and physician Petrus Paaw objected to the promotion of the student Laurentius Brant, claiming he was ignorant and nearly infamous.[45] The university senate set up an inquiry into his character, and found nothing incriminating. Eventually, professors Paaw and Bontius agreed to let Brant proceed with the disputation, on the condition that Johannes Heurnius declared him suitable, which he did. In response, the senate decreed that each candidate had to be examined privately by the respective faculty before the public disputation, according to their own formula which they also shared with the Curators.

Learning, logic, and quickness marked out a good disputant. In the diary of Everardus Bronckhorst (or Bronchorst), a professor of law from 1587 to 1627, evaluations of student performances in disputations turned on their ability to display their learning: "smart and eager," "accurate and prompt," "learned and subtle" praises contrast with criticisms such as "almost cold," and "shy and insufficiently prepared."[46] These disputation performances rewarded book learning, attention to professors' and students' predilections and objections, and skills of logic and debate.

---

42   Kroon, *Bijdragen*, 14–15, 12.

43   Kroon, *Bijdragen*, 4–5, citing exams from Amsterdam in the 1550s.

44   Kroon, *Bijdragen*, 25–7.

45   Molhuysen, *Bronnen*, 1, 68.

46   Bronckhorst (Bronchorst) quoted in Otterspeer, *Groepsportet*, 237.

Student authorship of the theses for disputation varied by discipline and over time, but until the 1630s and 1640s, students usually relied on textbooks and professors, or professors wrote the theses.[47] Medical students developed theses under the direction of a professor, and practiced disputing in extracurricular groups in the early 1600s.[48] In the printed disputations, students self-identified as "Author" and not merely "Respondent" as early as 1634.[49] By the 1660s, students in medicine wrote most of the disputations, and each student wrote at least one of his own, even if he defended another authored by a professor.[50]

In other disciplines, student authorship varied. Law students were expected to formulate their own theses earlier, perhaps around 1600, though assigning authorship is often difficult.[51] Generally, theology and philosophy students had fewer chances to author their own theses, especially if their writing touched near any perilous points of confessional divisions. Theology students occasionally generated their own theses to defend, but this appears to have been an unusual, and likely risky, venture given the confessional divisions and strife in and around the Low Countries.[52] Despite some real humanist, scholarly latitude defended by professors and students, some topics were too divisive to allow regular disputation by unruly or inventive students.

Professors' works of natural philosophy often appeared in the form of a series of student-defended theses or disputations. Leiden philosophy professor Franco Burgersdijk's influential textbooks of philosophy from the 1620s and 1630s exemplify this pattern.[53] Even Johannes de Raey's innovative attempt to give a Cartesian re-interpretation of the official Aristotelian natural philosophy in the 1650s began with a series of disputations. Given the bans on mentioning Descartes's name, instituted a few years earlier by the university Curators in an attempt to ward off theological and personal fighting, it is no surprise that De Raey's deeply Cartesian public disputations avoid mentioning "Descartes." Yet even these are clearly the work of the presiding professor, De Raey, and not

---

47   Schlegelmilch, "Andreas Hiltebrands Protokoll."

48   Schlegelmilch, "Andreas Hiltebrands Protokoll," 58, 69.

49   Sylvius, *Positiones Variae Medicae*. This is the first explictly student-authored medical disputation I have found.

50   Ragland, "Experimental Clinical."

51   Ahsmann, *Collegia en Colleges*, 274–323. Otterspeer extends Ahsmann's conclusions to the entire university: Otterspeer, *Groepsportret met Dame*, 1, 236–238.

52   Stanglin, *Arminius on the Assurance of Salvation*, 44–58.

53   Ruestow, *Physics*, 16–17.

the students publicly defending them, each identified only as "Respondent."[54] With some exceptions, the strong trend of professors writing the theology and philosophy disputation theses continued into the 1660s.[55]

Even for famously direct Dutch students, these formal, scholarly disputations required practice. Petrus Paaw, the professor of medicine, anatomy, and medical botany, held an informal college for practicing disputations among the students, at least around 1603–4.[56] Taking on different roles and pitting textual sources against each other, students learned to identify contradictions and question textual authorities. In student notes, use of two columns allowed them to place theses from other students or even the presiding professor in one column, and then oppose them with objections and additions in the other. Most of these objections came on logical grounds, such as when one student, Hendrik, begged the question by assuming tempering in his definition of temperament.[57] As elsewhere in the medical curriculum, students in the disputation group used Heurnius' *Institutes of Medicine* as a textbook.

Of course, students could settle for less than a doctorate, finish coursework elsewhere, or take courses at Leiden and then move on for a final degree at another university. Given the formal practice and learning required for the public performance of a doctoral disputation in medicine, it is no accident that in the first few decades, more students matriculating in medicine took the licentiate degree. With that, one could still practice medicine and earn a living, though without some of the honors and status of a doctoral degree. Foreign students, particularly the two dozen English medical students studied in detail by Daniela Prögler, often came to Leiden as "degree collectors," with over half staying less than three months before taking their degree.[58] Most of the students studying medicine at Leiden were Dutch young men, making up over half the student population, while students from German lands were the next largest group at about one fifth of the medical matriculations.[59] Dutch

---

54   Verbeek, *Descartes and the Dutch*, 72. [Johannes De Raey], *Disputationum physicarum ad Problemata Aristotelis*. The main text is the same as the main sections of De Raey's major work, *Clavis philosophiae naturalis*.

55   E.g., see the contrasting disputations—all authored by the professors—of the Cartesian De Raey, the self-consciously eclectic Heerboord, and the likely anti-Cartesian Stuart (he opposed Henricus Regius's claim that the soul and body united *per accidens*): [Johannes de Raey], *Disputatio Philosophica de Mundi Systemate & Elementis. Prima.*; [Adrianus Heereboord], *Disputatio Philosophica de Metaphysicae Constitutione,*; [David Stuart], *Disputatio Eclectica de Unione Animae & Corporis. Pars Prima.*

56   Schlegelmilch, "Andreas Hiltebrands Protokoll."

57   Schlegelmilch, "Andreas Hiltebrands Protokoll," 73.

58   Prögler, *English Students at Leiden University*, 192, 237.

59   Prögler, *English Students at Leiden University*, Plate 14.

students likely stayed and studied longer, as suggested by the careers of the second generation of professors. Petrus Paaw and Otto Heurnius both spent several formative years at Leiden, or even the majority of their period of study.

3   Study Guides for Sharpening the Ingenium (Wit) of the Brain

Medical professors and students spent most of their time reading, listening, talking, and writing (at least, that was the plan). Their ideas and words, as much as we can recover them, are essential and even central to understanding the culture and practices of medical training. But we should not lose sight of their living bodies among the texts and concepts. Students' habits of learning, virtues and vices of study, corporeal experiences in the city, and cultivated "wit" or sharp, agile intelligence all depended on taking seriously the embodied minds of the learners. Strikingly, ideals of learning from books, developing manual skill in anatomy, and gaining operational facility in chymistry all turned on the training and refinement of the *ingenium* or "wit."[60] The medical context made the training of the *ingenium* as the sharpening and altering of the brain explicit. Following Galen, Leiden professors wanted students who naturally had soft, stable parts of their brains to hold memories, and a finer substance for making connections, by noting similarities and differences of things. But they also repeatedly claimed that reading the right books and practicting the art of disputations could sharpen the students' *ingenia*, thus making their brains finer. Book learners needed strong, healthy, manly, and virtuous bodies, while anatomists and chymists learned to be ingenious with their fine manual skills and senses.

Students and professors disciplined their bodies to the work of study and scholarship. We saw this in the disciplined disputation workshops discussed in the previous section. Further, two works by professors of medicine about fifty years apart, from Johannes Heurnius in 1592 and Albert Kyper in 1643, detail the bookish learning necessary for students. These are study guides, with tips for what to read and how to read it. They also portray some of the ideals of medical education, and nod toward some of the other practices in anatomy, medical botany, and clinical instruction.

Leiden University made a name for itself through its humanist scholarship, attracting illustrious humanists such as the Stoic philosopher Justus Lipsius and the "phoenix of all time, the Wonder Man," the renowned philologist

---

60   Ragland, "The Contested *Ingenia* of Early Modern Anatomy." For meanings of *"ingenium"* and related terms, see Marr, Garrod, Marcaida, and Oosterhoof, *Logodaedalus*.

J. J. Scaliger (1540–1609).[61] The young university invested in the humanist academic prestige of research professors such as Scaliger and Carolus Clusius (1526–1609) while it paid young teaching professors and other lecturers to take on the task of education. Scaliger, the most renowned philologist and historian of his time, received a total annual salary of 2,000 guilders and had no teaching duties from the time he arrived in October 1593.[62] In comparison, Scaliger's eminent predecessor, Lipsius, had only worked his way to half that salary. Clusius, appointed prefect of the planned university garden in 1592, brought his wide correspondence network of natural historians and a good part of his extensive collection with him.[63] He likewise had no lecturing duties, though only about a third of Scaliger's salary, but he was supposed to be present in the garden for an hour a day to demonstrate the medicinal plants to interested students.[64]

For all the splendors of the bookish learning displayed by Leiden professors, virtuous medical thought and practice remained embodied. Two attention-grabbing written memorials to Johannes Heurnius adorned the front matter to the 1650 edition of his innovative text on the practice of medicine, the *New Method*. These stories, as we will see shortly, communicated ideals of practice and tales of marvelous curing. The first presented Heurnius as a new, wise Galen who resisted a rush to therapy. The second celebrated his diagnostic skills from the bodily leavings of study. The second is also quite strange to present-day sensibilities: it advertises Heurnius' learning through a scatological warning about the dangers of too much study.

In the 1520s and 1530s, the rediscovery of Galenic texts and wide publication of his works in compendia stimulated a revival of Galenic medicine, re-framing anatomical practice, disease and drug theory, and clinical teaching, at least.[65] The illustrated title page of the Giunta edition of Galen's *Opera omnia* depicted eight scenes from Galen's life, including his famous disagreement with Emperor Marcus Aurelius's three court physicians in 176 AD (Figure 6).[66]

---

61   Grafton, "Civic Humanism," 59–78, 59. Grafton, *Scaliger*.

62   Molhuysen, *Bronnen*, vol. 1, 77.

63   Tjon Sie Fat, "Clusius' Garden." Egmond, *The World of Carolus Clusius*. Ogilvie, *Science of Describing*, 41–44.

64   Prögler, *English Students at Leiden University*, 99–100.

65   Shotwell, "Revival of Vivisection." Bylebyl, "The Manifest and the Hidden." Bylebyl, "The School of Padua." Bylebyl, "Teaching *Methodus Medendi* in the Renaissance."

66   Bylebyl, "The Manifest and the Hidden," 44–45. Bylebyl identifies the emperor only as "Antoninus," but it must have been Marcus Aurelius Antoninus rather than Antoninus Pius, as Galen only served the court of the former. See Mattern, *The Prince of Medicine*, 212–13.

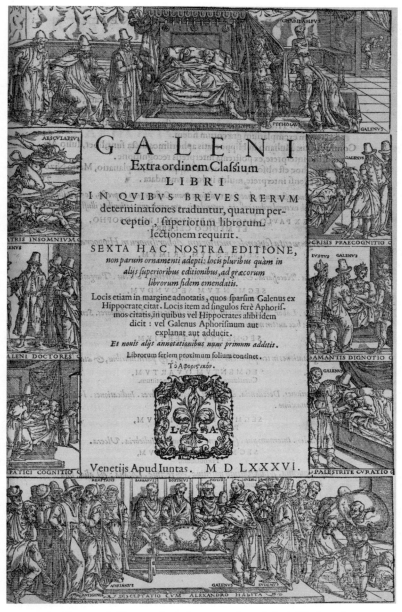

FIGURE 7   Illustrated title page depicting scenes from Galen's life, from the
diagnosis and cure of the emperor Marcus Aurelius Antoninus's disease
at the top to his vivisection of a pig at the bottom. Galen, *Extraordinem
Classium Libri* (Venice, 1556).

(In the bottom scene Galen is vivisecting a trussed pig for a crowd of scholars.) The emperor's three physicians took his pulse and concluded he was suffering a feverish attack. Galen did not yet know the emperor's healthy pulse by long tactile experience, so he resisted taking it, though he later diagnosed the emperor's illness as caused by too much chilling food turned to phlegm. Galen prescribed only wine with a dash of pepper (a hot spice), as well as warming ointment on a wool bandage for the stomach. From then on, the emperor praised him as chief of the physicians and philosophers.[67]

Johannes Heurnius' story was quite similar, though it ended in tragedy for the ruler. A well-rounded scholar of thirty years of age, in 1573 Heurnius returned from medical studies in Italy to a homeland marred by war. The Spanish poisoned the Lord Governor of Noortcarmes, and he fell into a wasting jaundice. The Lord knew the "ambition and envy of physicians," and did not want his fragile health held "under the tyranny of contradiction and disputation," so he summoned all the physicians but invited them in for consultation singly.[68] The older physicians expounded on jaundice and marvelous cures. Youngest of all, Heurnius came last. The Lord Governor, worn out by the earlier questioning, answered nothing to Heurnius. So Heurnius sought "the hidden nature of his disease" by examining all the "symptoms of the injured action, of the changed quality, and of the excrements, and exploring all the internal and external causes." By these "sure indexes" he knew that this jaundice was not customary for the region, but more common in Italy, and there caused by poison. Astonished at the marvelous diagnosis, the Lord Governor sent away all the other physicians. Heurnius alone would care for him, though Heurnius called some physicians back to avoid possible calumnies. Since a cure was not possible, Heurnius used medicines to sooth the Governor's weariness until, wasted by the "inextricable, adamantine disease," he expired.

In the second marvelous occurrence from Heurnius' life as a physician, which his son emphasized in his biography and the editors used to advertise his book, his friend the humanist and Stoic philosopher Justus Lipsius had a morbid scare caused by excessive scholarship:

> For a long time the Very Distinguished Lipsius had been afflicted with a very troublesome disease: he experienced various feverish insults, his stomach and whole body were flaccid and withered. It happened one day that he took a drug to empty his belly: moreover, he felt that when the

---

67   Galen, *On Prognostics*, ch. 11, trans. Clendening, *Source Book*, 50–51.
68   "Something memorable" in Johannes Heurnius, *Nova Ratio* (1650), front matter. Cf. [Otto Heurnius], "Vita Auctoris."

necessity of nature was clear, he began to pour out a huge amount from his belly, and this discharge was continuous and coherent. Inspecting what this thing was, he saw, astonished, that he had poured out a mass that clearly expressed the form and character of the intestines: he was confounded, and called Heurnius over, saying his life was finished since he had poured out all his intestines. Heurnius inspected the discharge of the belly and with a happy face turned to Lipsius, "Look again," he said, "here lies the monument of your disease, the hearth and bilgewater of the whole malady." For there was a tenacious and viscid phlegm, gradually heaped up in the whole intestinal tube, wasted from a sedentary life in study, bearing its figure; which when it had putrefied and communicated its harm to the neighboring parts, propagated the bilgewater of maladies into the whole body. The very Distinguished Man [Heurnius] recreated this from the purged *fomes* of the disease, and Lipsius returned to his former health.[69]

This anecdote likely revealed more than some readers wanted to know. The "bilgewater" metaphor would have been repellently forceful to the Dutch, since this water in the lower holds of ships carried human and rat excrement, decaying food, mold, and other noxious corruption. The story was also intended as a compelling portrait of Heurnius' diagnostic skill, something students and other physicians should emulate. Clearly, this was a world of openly embodied scholarship!

Heurnius frequently included a familiar paean to studying, which could remedy many weaknesses of nature. Through study, students could refine their brains and so sharpen their wits. Untiring study, he advertised to his students, gives "great rewards of learning, lasting fame, and a very happy life." Thus students needed strong, healthy bodies for the hard labor of learning. Ancient wisdom, per Xenophanes, still rang true: "By labors the gods sell to us all good gifts."[70]

He would know. Johannes's biography, written by his son, Otto, described his "peaceful ingenium," which resisted agitation but was also so "slow" that he did not know the alphabet well before the age of eleven, nor grammar before the age of fifteen![71] He had to work his way to success, since his father (also called Otto) had left to live the soldier's life in Hungary when Johannes was young. When his father returned, relatives convinced him that both wife and

---

69   Johannes Heurnius, *Nova Ratio* (1650), front matter. [Otto Heurnius], "Vita Auctoris."
70   Johannes Heurnius, *Nova Ratio*, 566.
71   [Otto Heurnius], "Vita Auctoris."

son had died, and sent father Otto to England so they could eat up Johannes's patrimony. Finally reunited, but with much lessened resources, Johannes's father sent him to study at Leuven. Despite his slow start, Johannes's "diligence" over two years in Leuven with mathematician and philosopher Gemma Frisius allowed him to write a pamphlet on the "terrible" comet of 1577.[72] He never missed a lecture for three years in Paris, and the eminent physician Louis Duret noticed his studies and ability; it pained him that Johannes was not taking part in teaching medicine. With equal diligence, he studied the practical art of cutting for bladder stones with Laurentius Collodaeus; philosophy with Petrus Ramus; and medicine in Italy under Girolamo Capivacca, Girolamo Mercuriale, and Bernardino Paterno, with whom he saw medical practice on patients; while he learned anatomy from Girolamo Fabrizi (Fabricius), and botany, too.[73] He had a few serious fevers in Italy, but reportedly cured himself by bloodletting. Back in the Low Countries, his diagnosis of the Lord Governor of Noortcarmes helped to make his reputation.

After teaching at Leiden for two decades, Johannes's usual health crashed after a university party, and trouble urinating turned to months of fever, then emaciation and a peaceful death on 12 August 1601. His son, Otto, cut up his body and found seven large bladder stones. Johannes's father Otto had died in 1583, and his first son, Johannes, died from measles in Utrecht. Another son, Isaac, a twin, passed soon after birth in 1597. Yet Johannes Senior was spared the massacre of the plague of 1604. His mother Geertruyda died at the beginning, in 1603, and his wife Christina soon after in 1604, at the age of forty-nine. Of his eleven children, six survived. With Christina, daughters Susanna and Margarita died from the plague, at the ages of ten and fifteen, within hours and days of their mother. Abraham had survived his twin Isaac, but died of plague two days after his mother.[74] Fighting the deadly mundanity of disease in early modern Europe demanded serious training.

Pithy descriptions of the proper physician appeared in the study guides for the medical students. These inscribed the ideal traits which the faculty hoped (or at least claimed) to cultivate in students' bodies, and especially their brains. At Leiden, as elsewhere, scholars connected intellectual acumen and bodily dispositions and habits with the concept of the *ingenium*. A companion text added to the *Institutes* detailed Johannes Heurnius' recommendations for the proper "Mode and Rule of Studying, of those who have Dedicated their

---

72   Johannes Heurnius, *De Historie, Natuere ende Beduidenisse der erschrickelicke Comeet* (1577). Jorink, *Reading the Book of Nature*, 125–127.

73   For Capivacca, Mercuriale, and Paterno, see Siraisi, *Avicenna in the Renaissance, passim.*

74   [Otto Heurnius], "Vita Auctoris."

Exertions to Medicine."[75] Calling on his exemplar in medicine, Hippocrates, Heurnius discussed three aids for all arts and sciences: *physis*, *sophin*, and *to chreos*, that is, nature, the study of doctrine, and practice and use. Nature is chief among these three: the student's body should be robust, and the mind possess an "acute *ingenium* for investigating, judging, and teaching."[76]

Most of Heurnius' instructions for the proper study of medicine involved book learning, through which students encountered sharp *ingenia*, and, like iron upon iron, sharpened their own. Heurnius maintained that the true medicine originated with Asclepius, then was elaborated by Hippocrates and passed through Galen. Philosophers helped to give a keen edge to the *ingenium*. Plato, especially his *Timaeus*, "leads us into the deepest parts of our art; more help for physicians is poured out there, than in all the other schools of philosophy, if they were driven together into one."[77] Aristotle, "overcame all before him in order, sharpness, and certitude. But his gold must be vented and sieved from the dust for some time. We will not depart far from him, and we will practice the *ingenium* in him, on account of his sharpness with the highest doctrine. Where he fights against Hippocrates, cast it out."[78] The Aristotelian Julius Caesar Scaliger (1484–1558), the father of J. J. Scaliger, also offered useful exercises through his combative philosophical sharpness.[79] Heurnius' recommendation of Scaliger shows his openness to novelty, since Scaliger was an innovative but partisan Aristotelian who embraced corpuscularian matter theory and small vacua, and was well known as a *novator*.

More recently, Heurnius enthused, another innovator, Jean Fernel (1497?–1558) combined the encyclopedic organization of Arabic works with the philosophical demonstrations of the Greeks.[80] Fernel won fame as a lecturer in philosophy and medicine at the Collège du Cornouailles, and as the official French court physician. Fernel's *Whole of Medicine* (*Universa Medicina*, 1567) synthesized the best of Galenic medicine with Aristotelian and Neoplatonic philosophy to form a comprehensive medical textbook covering *physiologia*, *pathologia*, and *therapeutice*. Paaw lectured from it in 1591, according to the diary of another professor, and cited Fernel frequently in his lectures and

---

75   Johannes Heurnius, *Institutiones*, 557.
76   Johannes Heurnius, *Modus Ratioque* in *Institutiones*, 563–4.
77   Johannes Heurnius, *Modus Ratioque* in *Institutiones*, 576.
78   Johannes Heurnius, *Modus Ratioque* in *Institutiones*, 578.
79   Johannes Heurnius, *Modus Ratioque* in *Institutiones*. On Scaliger, see Lüthy, "An Aristotelian Watchdog as Avant-Garde Physicist." Other leading physicians also turned to Scaliger, especially Daniel Sennert. Andreas Blank, "Sennert and Leibniz on Animate Atoms."
80   On Fernel, see Henry and Forrester, "Introduction," in *The* Physiologia *of Jean Fernel (1567)*, 1–12.

books.[81] Heurnius recommended taking Fernel's book as providing "very lim-pid and firm knowledge," but only insofar as he provided demonstrations and the authority of the ancients, especially Galen. Whatever novelties he brought forward should be accepted, but only if he had reason and utility on his side. Where he departed from the ancients, "demonstration of the ancients breaks the contest." Galen's books ought really to form the "first foundation," along with those of Hippocrates.[82]

The Empirics or "*practici*" offered only more copies of the same remedies, so that if one read one, one read them all. They lacked proper philosophical demonstrations, and did not attend to the crucial variation of individual bod-ies and parts. New remedies proven by use were indeed welcome, but Heur-nius remained sure that physicians would never take up the goal of changing all the remedies. Proven by long experience in use, they fit too well with philo-sophical understanding.[83]

Ancient physicians who adopted philosophical modes of argumentation cultivated medical students' *ingenia*, too. Reading Galen "is not without uses for the cultivation of the *ingenium*."[84] Happily, Galen was the "most faithful expounder" of Hippocrates, used pure, elegant language, and demonstrated everything with strong reasons, refuting contrary positions. Though he "chiefly followed ambition and avarice" in his medical disputes and self-promotion, some sources reported his own medical success: he may have lived a hundred and forty years.[85]

Heurnius closed his guide with advice on reading practices. Hurried reading only resulted in forgetting. Instead, read as you ought to eat: frequently, so that you can digest properly, with the learning softened by much iteration, and the things taken in thus well-concocted. The memory, per the design of the Highest God, has a soft and stable substance so it can receive "characters" and yet retain them. When caught in a tough thicket of a text, mark the place and move on, to return later. Like earlier scholastic teachers, Heurnius advocated attempting to resolve disagreements among authors. Yet he also insisted that students avoid prolix commentaries, which "extinguish the pleasure of learning." Go back to the sources, especially Hippocrates and his expounder Galen. Heurnius pro-vided a list for reading Galen's myriad works in the right order, but he also recommended the ease of his own textbook *Institutes*, instead! To study, make up a list of *loci communes* to aid the memory—use the extra blank pages at

---

81   Bronchorst, *Diarium*, 19.
82   Johannes Heurnius, *Modus Ratioque* in *Institutiones*, 588, 592.
83   Johannes Heurnius, *Modus Ratioque* in *Institutiones*, 598–9.
84   Johannes Heurnius, *Modus Ratioque* in *Institutiones*, 586.
85   Johannes Heurnius, *Modus Ratioque* in *Institutiones*.

the end of this book, he suggested. These *loci*, a common practice used by students throughout the early modern period, followed the order of topics of the *Institutes*, from God and philosophical principles to humors, the non-naturals, diseases, symptoms, medicines, alchemical remedies, and on.

As today, the professor intoned an exhortation to sobriety for his students: excessive drinking dulls the *ingenium* or wit, and utterly washes away the memory.[86] Instead, strengthen your body for the labor of learning. When your mind is tired, get some pleasing exercise. Excessive labors and vexations ruin students' tired *ingenia*. The best times for study are those in the morning, as well as just before dinner. But take caution, Heurnius concluded: studying on a full stomach caused vapors to creep from the stomach to the brain, clouding it with darkness and weakening the *ingenium* into a stupor.

Training students' bodies and minds came about importantly through shaping the anatomical qualities of students' brains. Anatomy was important even for Heurnius' study tips, and teaching anatomy turned on the training of the *ingenium*, too. Professors repeatedly described the purpose of anatomy, academic exercises in medical theory, philosophy, logic, and other disciplines as essential for shaping and sharpening students' *ingenia*. They quite literally wanted to mold students' brains for greater quickness and sharpness. Though this technical term is often translated as "mind" by present-day scholars, the early modern meanings of *ingenium* varied across times and languages.[87] "Wit" is a better present-day and early-modern English synonym. Across the sixteenth century, medical and philosophical sources tended to describe a proper human *ingenium* in terms of faculty psychology, and associate it with the imagination and quick wits.[88]

Among physicians, the primary text for discussions of *ingenium* seems to have been Galen's summary of medical teaching so common in universities, *The Art of Medicine* (*Ars medica*, or *Tegni*, *Techne iatrike*). Galen, ever the advocate for the primacy of the brain over the heart, against Aristotle, began his discussion of the five chief organs with the brain. First on his list of its "commanding activities"—those which arise from the brain alone—is *agchinoia*, which Latin editions translated as *ingenium* or *sollertia*.[89] "*Ingenium* [*agchinoia* in the original Greek] thus indicates a subtle substance of the brain, while slowness of intellect indicates a thick one; facility of learning indicates a substance which easily receives forms, but memory a stable and firm one."[90] Yet, despite Galen's explanation of "cleverness" or "ingenuity" in terms of the speedy working of a finer substance

86   Johannes Heurnius, *Modus Ratioque* in *Institutiones*, 595.

87   Marr, Garrod, Marcaida, and Oosterhoof, *Logodaedalus*.

88   Goodey, *A History of Intelligence and "Intellectual Disability*," 51–58.

89   Laurentius [André Du Laurens], *Historia Anatomica*, 873.

90   Antonius, *Nonnulla opuscula nunc primum in unum collecta*, 72v.

of the brain, anatomists seem to have emphasized training and hard work over inborn aptitude.[91] Like Heurnius, physicians and anatomists across Europe put training the *ingenuim* in a central place in their pedagogical programs.[92]

A later guide to study shows great continuity in the core of Galenic and Aristotelian theory, with increased attention to innovations in philosophy and chymistry. The Prussian Albert Kyper (1614–1655) attended Leiden University as a student in 1638, then worked as a reader in medicine from 1643, and became an ordinary professor of medicine in 1648. His 1643 *Method of Rightly Learning and Training in Medicine* unpacked a vision of the ideal physician for students: "The physician is a Man, pious, good, ingenious [*ingeniosus*], healthy, learned, skilled and powerful in his art, a trustworthy guardian of health and repeller of diseases."[93] Men, after all, are the stronger sex and fit for public life, while women, born from "imperfect seed," can never become men, but need to bear the greater share of care for the home and family.[94]

Kyper detailed sources and guides for training in both experience and reason, often in conjunction. Medicine is an art, and "use and experience dominate in the arts."[95] Thus the students should practice under a teacher the sensible and abstract parts of the "instruments" of medicine: instruments of diet, pharmacy, surgery, nutrition, and medicines. Like nearly all other commentators, Kyper recommended "diligently" contemplating the parts of the body through anatomical dissections (in the refrigerating winter months), alongside "accurate" anatomists at Leiden.

Though a bookish philosopher himself, he warmly recommended chymical books and labor to his students. While his eclectic Aristotelian philosophy happily reduced chymical principles to the Aristotelian four elements, chymistry still demanded attention.[96] Kyper advertised the books of eminent chymists such as Quercetanus (Joseph Du Chesne), Jean Beguin, Johannes Hartmann, and Oswald Croll, as well as the philosophy of Daniel Sennert.

More than books, to learn the art of chymistry one needed to *work*, but also draw on philosophical training to understand the causes of the operations. Kyper recommended finding a "learned man as guide in the labors of the Chymist, who will be able not only to show you the means of manual operations, but even their causes, and to explain thus the dependent changes of the powers

91   For a discussion of Galen, Plato, and Aristotle's uses of the term *agchinoia*, see Goodey, *A History of Intelligence and "Intellectual Disability,"* 49–52.
92   Ragland, "The Contested Ingenia of Early Modern Anatomy."
93   Kyper [Albertus Kyperus], *Methodus*, 25.
94   Kyper, *Methodus*, 26.
95   Kyper, *Methodus*, 249.
96   Kyper, *Transsumpta medica*, 43–161.

of the medicines."[97] Theory mattered, but books alone would not suffice. It was a disgrace that this art took abuse from "learned men who refuse the tedium of Chymical labor."[98] Surely, scholars such as Lipsius and his humanist friend Johannes Heurnius knew about tedium. As we will see in chapter four, Heurnius also knew a great deal about the work and ideas of chymistry, and taught students chymistry in his course on the practice of medicine.

4   Student Life and the Vices of Embodied Learners

Violence, alcohol, poisons, and even too much study threatened students' bodies and minds, at best dulling wits sharpened by the right books, at worst resulting in accidental deaths and murders. The study guides' warnings against inebriation were not unnecessary scolding. Drunkenness wasted professors and students alike, and kindled violence in the city streets. Daniel Heinsius, star student of J. J. Scaliger, was a famed Latin poet, and the leading Greek philologist, began as a student in 1600 and served as professor of Latin, Greek, and politics shortly after, as well as the university librarian (1607–1653). His excessive fondness for the bottle appeared in a celebrated *bon mot* he supposedly penned as a Latin elegiac couplet after walking back one night full of drink: "Stay foot, stay good foot, stay foot, do not slip my foot / Stay foot, or these stones will be my bed."[99] A note once fixed to the door of the Academy Building stated plainly, "Heinsius does not lecture today on account of inebriation yesterday."[100]

Even famed law professor Everard van Bronckhorst (or Bronchorst) had to ask God's forgiveness: he drank so much at a promotion party for a new doctor of law that he vomited, and after suffering for three days from a dinner party with colleagues in 1593 vowed to stay sober and "diligent" for three months.[101] He fell back into his old indulgence until, in December 1607, a celebration for a law student's promotion ended in violence with the city's night watch. In Van Bronckhorst's account, a bloodthirsty night watch attacked boisterous, laughing students, piercing student Assuerius Hornhovius with twenty-one wounds. In the version from the headman of the watch, Jacob Willemsz. van Leeuwen, the students shouted insults at them and drew swords first. Van Bronckhorst swore off dining with students, and the city formed a new night watch with

---

97   Kyper, *Methodus*, 302.
98   Kyper, *Methodus*, 303.
99   Menage, *Menagiana*, Vol. 4, 288.
100   Otterspeer, *Groepsportret*, I, 312.
101   Bronchorst, *Diarium*, 64, 68.

some fifty-four members, under oath to the city and to consult with the city guard but deal politely with students. These students did not take the compromise with city authority over them meekly. Instead, some rioted, smashing windows and destroying symbols of city and university authority; a handful of leaders received punishment.[102]

The great majority of students came from the higher bourgeoisie, and some from the nobility, with a few poor students admitted each year. Most medical students were in their earlier twenties, as were the much more numerous law students, but beginning letters and later philosophy students ranged from an average of about fifteen to about nineteen years old.[103] The university prohibited students from performing manual or trade work while registered, though it did allow booksellers and printers.[104] Paying an annual cost of over 250 guilders each year for room and board, tuition and expenses, many students had the money and social standing to assert themselves, despite the prospect of expulsion for unseemly acts. And, after all, many readily trained with the swords they carried, to embody noble behavior and train to lead soldiers for the Republic.[105] Repeated bans on weapons apparently had limited effects.

The city's street guards and students clashed frequently over the years, but city tax law actually encouraged student drinking in order to attract students. Shortly after it formed, the University pushed for the extension of tax exemptions on beer and wine to students up to the amount of half a liter of wine and four liters of thin beer a day.[106] After receiving the privileged exemptions, but limited to students over twenty years old, the university suddenly enrolled many more students over the age limit.[107] Most of the violent court cases Willem Otterspeer has chronicled spilled out from student drunkenness.[108] This was no surprise, as moralists and professors frequently condemned gluttonous drinking by youth and the hot, irrational violence it enflamed.[109] Further, excessive drinking and student rioting or fighting appears as a theme from early medieval universities, as attested by the longstanding privilege of university students to carry weapons, and cases such as the suspension of lectures at Paris for two years in 1229 after students

---

102   Otterspeer, *Groepsportret*, I, 218–220. Otterspeer, 268, gives the percentage of students
         from the higher backgrounds as 75% in a survey from 1650–1660.
103   Prögler, *English Students at Leiden University*, Plate 7.
104   Otterspeer, *Groepsportret*, I, 257.
105   Otterspeer, *Groepsportret*, I, 267, 270.
106   Roberts, *Sex and Drugs*, 87.
107   Otterspeer, *Groepsportret*, I, 118–119.
108   Otterspeer, *Groepsportret*, I, 130–136.
109   Roberts, *Sex and Drugs*, 76–90.

imbibing "good" wine beat the tavern-keeper and his friends until they were beaten in turn by the prévôt and his men.[110]

Leiden students, many of them from merchant or professional backgrounds and flush with wealth from the expanding Dutch commercial empire, exerted their power and after the 1610s increasingly dressed the part of French military cavaliers to do so.[111] Casting off the traditional Dutch black clothing, they donned bright colors, soft, expensive fabrics, ribbons, and long hair, all topped off with rapiers and pistols. In the heat of June 1608, two students, Anthonius Anselmus and Willem Schade, exchanged heated words and then Anselmus retrieved his sword and ran Schade through the chest. According to Anselmus, they had been friends, but intoxication made them deadly enemies.[112] Other students broke windows, threw stones, fought local Leideners and grappled with swords, even seriously striking local women or assaulting them sexually. In 1647, a drunken student party descended to attacking the landlady with a knife and putting a rope around the maid's neck. Groups of drunken students of different "nations" occasionally fought in the streets—especially, so the Leideners claimed, the largest "nation" of students, those from German lands.[113]

Though the city and university fought over jurisdiction for less-serious disturbances, they also cracked down on public disorder and vice. The university jailed students in the cellar of the academic building for days, banished them from the territory for years for breaking windows, or expelled them for fathering children out of wedlock or other unseemly activities, and the city punished crimes of assault, destruction, and theft with jail time and exile.[114] Thus, the professor's recommendations for proper study, the care and shaping of brains and bodies, were bookish and somewhat idealized, but aimed at cultivating the right bodily, mental, and moral habits among often-unruly students.

5   Conclusions

Learning and teaching at Leiden happened among embodied students and professors, for all of their attention to texts, words, ideas, and ideals. The marriage of reason and experience represented the core ideals of medical learning and

---

110   Haskins, *The Rise of Universities*, 15.

111   Roberts, *Sex and Drugs*, 56.

112   Otterspeer, *Groepsportret*, I, 131.

113   Prögler, *English Students at Leiden University*, Plates 2 and 3, shows that German students made up 22% of the matriculations from 1575 to 1650.

114   Roberts, *Sex and Drugs*, 124–126,

practice. In his lectures and textbooks, Johannes Heurnius crafted a mythic history of medicine which displayed the proper intellectual and moral virtues of true physicians to students. This "Asclepian" medicine flourished with Hippocrates and Galen and demanded sharp and philosophical reasoning combined with personal and collective experience of anatomy, medicines, diseases, poisons, local climates, and the broader cosmos.

Most experience came through the "long experience" of this tradition, which handed on hard-won knowledge about diagnosing and treating diseases with a huge range of medicines. Professors offered study guides that included calls for necessary instruction in object-based learning, such as anatomy and chymistry. But most of the training consisted in sharpening the *ingenium* or wit with books, especially those with keen philosophical edges. Given their Galenic theory of the *ingenium* which grounded it in the fineness or coarseness of the brain, philosophical books, disputations, and exercises literally refined their brains for making better connections. With a fine cerebral substance, students would be better and faster at noting similarities and dissimilarities among things, ideas, and arguments. Disputations, required for promotion to the high social status of "doctor" rather than the practicing "licentiate," forced students to deal with the Hippocratic sources, especially the *Aphorisms*, which formed the wellspring of medicine. Through formal and informal practice in disputations, students trained to be alert, sharp, logical, and bold in their argumentation and responses. In this use of reason to generate knowledge from the appearances of things, students and physicians went beyond the strict empiricism of the Empiric sect, which avoided speculation about causes and hidden states.

For the cultivation of reason, they used the best accounts of the natural world they knew. They prized Aristotle's philosophical works, unless they disagreed with "Hippocrates," as well as books by recent innovative Aristotelians such as the corpuscularian philosopher J. C. Scaliger. Their "Hippocrates" took life through close, humanist scholarship on the best Greek texts, but often read through the system of Galen, whom they thought restored and systematized the tradition of Asclepius and Hippocrates. Students also needed to keep their bodies and brains, the organ of the *ingenium* or wit, in shape, avoiding the drunkenness and masculine violence that impaired the brains and ended the lives of professors and students alike.

Of course, an excess of excellent scholarship posed perils of its own. As we saw earlier, the theology scholarship student Petrus Balen studied too hard and too harshly in the cold. Lipsius, the eminent Stoic philosopher and humanist scholar, could not avoid the morbid effects of sedentary study on his own body. Shaping the brains and disciplining the bodies of the often-unruly students required attention to the embodied life of scholarly practices.

CHAPTER 3

Lecturing about Philosophical Bodies

[T]he substance of a faculty of the individual parts is attributed to the fitting temperament of the individual parts.

–GALEN, *On Prognosis from Pulses* (*Praes.Puls.*) II.9, Kuhn XI, 244.

• • •

On this point many of the philosophers appear to be in some confusion, lacking a clearly articulated notion of 'faculty.' They seem to conceive of faculties as things which inhabit 'substances' in much the same way as we inhabit our houses...

–GALEN, *The Soul's Dependence on the Body* [*QAM*], P. N. Singer trans., *Galen: Selected Works*, 151.

∙ ∙
∙

Sitting in rows on the hard benches of the Academic Building, students heard and transcribed hours of lectures (or they paid a note-taker to sit and write for them). Professors dug intellectual treasures from years of learning in ancient texts, their own university training, and recent works by early modern physicians to write and deliver these lectures. As a philosophical prolegomenon to understanding the practices of experimentation in the garden, anatomy sites, and the hospital, we now join the students for a crash course in medical theory.

To understand their trial-making or experimentation, we must have a clear idea of how they thought about the natures and causal powers of the things they investigated. Understanding living bodies in health and disease took pride of place in medical education, and so in lectures and texts on medical theory, too. Physicians built on the best natural philosophical concepts they had at hand, notably Aristotelian and Galenic theories of matter, qualities, temperaments, and faculties. A close reading of Heurnius' *Institutes of Medicine*, the major textbook for the teaching of medical theory for four or five decades, put in context with other textbooks, provides a map of this complex conceptual landscape. I close this chapter with a new, comprehensive synthesis of medical philosophy, which ran from the Aristotelian primary qualities and elements

© EVAN R. RAGLAND, 2022 | DOI:10.1163/9789004515727_005

through temperaments and organs, and up to the faculties of organs, organ systems, and whole living bodies.

Close readings of the course texts in medical theory (which were based on earlier lectures, and given as lectures) also reveal an important revisionist account of the causal powers of bodies and medicines, or "faculties." I argue against later early modern (and present-day) disdain for faculties as mysterious, immaterial additions inhabiting material bodies, organs, and drugs. After all, this flies in the face of Galen's explicit definitions of faculties, as well as his well-known epistemology grounded in the senses and his preference for material explanations.

Instead, I show that early modern Galenic physicians, like Galen himself, understood faculties as produced by a thing's temperament, or the constitutive mixture of the primary qualities (hot, cold, wet, and dry) of its matter. In order to know these faculties, Galen and his heirs had to follow closely the sensible properties and especially the regular actions of organs and drugs. Dissections revealed the regular actions and states of organs, for instance in Galen's observation of the dissected stomachs of pigs after feeding, which showed the effects of the stomach's power or faculty for concocting food. Faculties were powers or capacities for actions that body parts and medicines, as well as other things, expressed regularly in relation to the same objects.

Over time, this qualitative, material understanding of faculties became more localized in anatomical structures and different types of substances in the body (muscle, heart material, different sorts of contractile fibers, etc.). Increasingly, physicians thought that bodily faculties acted through the types and arrangements of material, anatomical fibers. Even physicians otherwise known for their promotion of innovative non-materialist explanations, such as Jean Fernel, advanced such material explanations of faculties in their medicine. Physicians in early modern Europe distinguished between the concepts and language of philosophers and those of physicians. Of course, physicians trained in philosophy during their arts courses, and used philosophical principles. Speaking as philosophers, physicians described bodily faculties as flowing from and directed by the vital soul or *anima*. Speaking as physicians, though, they emphasized the more material substance and actions of faculties as arising from the qualitative mixture and anatomical structure of body parts.

In the world of physicians, natural faculties or powers produced by the basic material mixture of things linked philosophical principles, anatomy, diagnosis, pathology, and therapy. Drugs, too, worked mostly according to their material temperaments in relation to the different parts of the body. Poisons and purgatives, like magnetic lodestones, worked through occult qualities or, per Galen, their "total substance." Most drugs, though, worked according to their basic qualitative temperament to affect bodily parts in an intelligible—sensible—way.

Material temperament and its qualitative changes and effects thus connected anatomy, disease, diagnosis, and therapy through a shared understanding of what constituted the active powers of different materials. The complexity of these interactions often eluded rigorous analysis and even direct sensation. At least in theory, though, temperaments could be caught by direct bodily sensation disciplined by the proper rational method. Grounding ostensibly successful medical practice in the best natural philosophy available, then, stood as the major task of a properly methodized therapeutics. In sum, professors and students used even their "bookish" philosophy and humanist erudition to understand living bodies in very material, sense-based terms.

To make this case, we will take a seat in the back of the lecture hall and dig out the words and arguments from the lectures and texts Leiden professors used to construct the core of their medical theory books and courses. As usual, we will follow their habit and mine ancient sources for the building blocks of their thinking. Getting early modern physicians' ancient sources right, and then sketching the early modern debates using those sources, once again points to a shared humanist medical culture beyond Leiden.

1   Core Philosophy and Theory

Early modern physicians and patients possessed remarkable confidence in their practices.[1] Although this confidence appears misplaced now, it made the longevity and authority of traditional medicine seem acceptable and respectable. In general, this confidence flowed from two sources: the assumed "long experience" of eminent physicians using similar methods and therapies for roughly two thousand years; and the easy integration of the Hippocratic and Galenic ways of diagnosing and curing with ancient qualitative natural philosophy, especially Aristotelian matter theory. In this section, we will run through a crash course on Leiden medical theory, as presented especially in Heurnius' major textbook and lecture course, the *Institutes of Medicine*. Put in context with early modern and ancient sources, this section and the following two sections present a detailed snapshot of the philosophical medical theory widespread across European academic medicine.

---

1   Stolberg, *Experiencing Illness*, 71–74. Wear, *Knowledge & Practice*, 105.

Broadly Galenic-Hippocratic approaches to medical practices persisted throughout the seventeenth and into the eighteenth centuries, cherished by patients and healers alike, even as persistent critics and new, opposing schools of medicine sprouted with increasing frequency. Despite jarring uncertainty in the face of new diseases such as the French disease (often syphilis), and the prolife-ration of critiques and new theoretical understandings, physicians, especially teaching physicians, often held the pedagogical course.[2] Long experience and shared practices from Hippocrates through the sixteenth century seemed to demonstrate the remarkable persistence and efficacy of core therapeutic prac-tices such as purgation of morbid matter or tempering by contrary qualities.[3]

Of course, physicians could make a distinction between effective practice and true natural philosophy. After all, the debate provoked by the ancient Empiric healers against physicians who claimed to know the hidden causes of health and disease turned on just this difference. Empirics argued that they could avoid the contradictory wrangling over theories and hidden causes by observing and recording only the perceptible phenomena of patients' signs and treatments.[4]

But the everyday intelligibility and traditional scope of thinking in terms of the active qualities hot, cold, dry, and wet, and the faculties produced by mate-rial temperaments of these elemental qualities, fueled a powerful institutional and intellectual inertia. In this, as in much else, the Leiden professors followed Galen. Throughout his works, Galen repeatedly claimed that the "best philoso-phers and doctors" all knew that the hot, cold, wet, and dry qualities were the active principles of things.[5] Of course, he explicitly attributed this doctrine to Hippocrates, rather than Empedocles or Aristotle, but this medical pedigree only helped to establish the doctrine among early modern physicians. Since physicians have to know causes such as these, early modern physicians usu-ally agreed that "the best physician is also a philosopher," as Galen put it in the title of another work (*Opt.med.*).[6] From the eleventh and twelfth centuries on, beginning with the medical school of Salerno, Latinate physicians cham-pioned the use of Aristotle's natural philosophy and the philosophical status

---

2   For stresses on Galenic medicine, see, e.g.: French, *Medicine Before Science*, ch. 6. Cook, "The New Philosophy and Medicine in Seventeenth-Century England." Bertoloni Meli, *Medicine, Experiment, Disease.*

3   Touwaide, "Therapeutic Strategies: Drugs," 261–2.

4   Von Staden, "Experiment and Experience," 187–192. Pomata, "A Word of the Empirics."

5   E.g., Galen, *Mixtures*, trans. Singer, 202. Hankinson, "Philosophy of Nature," 211–217.

6   Galen, *The Best Doctor is Also a Philosopher*, trans. Singer, in *Galen: Selected Works*. Schmitt, "Aristotle Among the Physicians," 2.

of medicine.[7] In the sixteenth century, students first gained a foundation in logic and philosophy for their arts degree, then moved on to medicine.[8] In part drawing on the beginning of Aristotle's *De sensu et sensato*, scholars in the 1500s frequently asserted the commonplace that "where the natural philosopher finishes, there the physician begins."[9]

For the first eight decades after the 1575 founding, Leiden medical professors retained the Aristotelian natural philosophical foundation and the Galenic-Hippocratic structure for their teachings. As we will see in later chapters, they added chymical theory and practice, adopted and defended the circulation of the blood, expanded clinical instruction, and readily practiced anatomical demonstrations and pathological post-mortems, but kept the core vocabulary and concepts. A quick sampling from Heurnius' *Institutes of Medicine* textbook and course should give us a sense of the fundamental principles and language of this natural philosophy.

Heurnius condensed medical theory into a handy topical format, generally following the traditional organization set out in earlier textbooks, such as Leonhart Fuchs's shorter and more intellectually conservative 1555 *Institutes of Medicine*.[10] While Fuchs resisted passing on some of the new findings of the revival in anatomical research, he could still engage with contemporary debates, for instance responding to critics of Galen such as Girolamo Cardano.[11] Both *Institutes* moved from the origins and definition of medicine to considering philosophical topics such as the Aristotelian elements, and the qualities, temperaments, faculties, and humors of living bodies. Of course, they both defined "temperament" as the mixture of the four fundamental qualities, hot, cold, wet, and dry.[12] They also treated basic anatomy, with consideration of the parts and their temperaments, the organs of generation, and then the causes and signs of diseases. Both concentrated on the signs from urine and the pulse for diagnosis and prognosis.

Heurnius also greatly expanded the treatment found in Fuchs's text on most topics, and especially on medical practice. His discussion of the rational method of healing, *methodus medendi*, covers ninety-six pages, over three-and-a-half times longer than the brief account given by Fuchs. As his references make

---

7   Schmitt, "Aristotle Among the Physicians," 3–4. Siraisi, *Taddeo Alderotti and His Pupils*.
8   Schmitt, "Aristotle Among the Physicians," 4–5, 10–12. Maclean, *Logic, Signs, and Nature*, 79–84. Grendler, *Universities*, 316–328. Siraisi, *Avicenna in the Renaissance*, ch. 7.
9   Schmitt, "Aristotle Among the Physicians," 12. Cf. Siraisi, *Avicenna in the Renaissance*, ch. 7.
10   Fuchs, *Institutionum Medicinae*. This approach may have found some roots in Da Monte's work and Avicenna's *Canon*, per Siraisi, *Avicenna in the Renaissance*, 101.
11   Siraisi, *The Clock and the Mirror*, 55–58, 140–141.
12   Fuchs, *Institutionum Medicinae*, 45.

clear, he largely followed Galen's *Method of Medicine* (*Methodus Medendi*).[13] As Jerome Bylebyl suggests, this work had such widespread influence on the craze for "method" in the sixteenth century that it is difficult to find discussions which it did not touch.[14] In his clear and well-organized treatment of the indications of diseases and the method for purging and using other medicines, Heurnius' aim of practical utility comes through clearly, even in the formatting: he frequently made lists set off from the main text and introduced crucial parameters of practice with the typeface in all caps. For example, he moved from the "HUMORES" (humors) in which one often finds the qualitative "antecedent cause of the disease" to the "AFFECTUS" or affect/condition of the disease itself, "WHAT" it is, and then the various steps and cautions for purging or altering the affected part.[15] With these textual markers, students could more easily find and remember the crucial order of the indications they should follow in diagnosis and prognosis.

In brief, the Aristotelian elements of earth, water, air, and fire, with their basic qualities of hot, cold, wet, and dry, mixed to form the simple parts such as flesh, nerve, and bone. These simple parts combined to form the organs and other parts of the body. Since hot and cold are the active basic qualities, as opposed to the passive qualities of wetness and dryness, and the innate heat of the parts vary, they act in part according to their natural heats. Parts perform actions in order to bring about their "work" or "functions," and according to their capacities or "faculties." The vital soul (*anima*) organizes and orchestrates the various functions. The soul acts primarily through innate heat and the natural and animal spirits, which are rarefied, "Aetherial" bodies elaborated from the purest part of the blood, like a thin wind. In all of this, heat, the mixtures or temperaments of the parts, and their anatomical structures are crucial.

Elements are most elementary (at least, for physicians; philosophers started from matter and form). Heurnius and other professors began with the elements. These are the simplest bodies that cannot be divided into different kinds. The world of touch gives us the elemental world. The principal tactile qualities of heat, cold, wetness, and dryness seem to make a thing what it is, and the active qualities heat and cold change the forms of things. The simple pairings of the four qualities constitute the elements and underpin the world of change encountered by the senses. Earth is primarily cold and dry, water cold and wet, air hot and wet, and fire hot and dry. Thus, following Galen and his matter theorist Aristotle, the basic qualitative principles of things made

---

13   Johannes Heurnius, *Institutiones*, 489, 495, 503, 519, 527, 533. 539, 542, 543, 544.
14   Bylebyl, "Teaching *Methodus Medendi* in the Renaissance."
15   Johannes Heurnius, *Institutiones*, 485, 495–555.

up the minimal, basic material elements, though Galen departed from many Aristotelians and argued that dry and wet were active qualities, too.[16] The Aristotelian elements of fire, air, water, and earth are never found pure in the realm of change below the moon. Heurnius invoked Hippocrates again for the claim that fire moves and nutrifies all things, and stressed the power of fire in medicines, making them cook, attenuate, and cut into matter in the body. Rather than simply passing on the simple notion that air is hot and wet, Heurnius put his humanist training to work and resolved apparent disputes among different Hippocratic texts, Stoics, Aristotelians, and Galen over whether air is hot or cold to conclude it is temperate, between them. Hence, medicines with a preponderance of air in them are temperate. Water is clearly very cold and very wet, though of course the water we encounter, like the fire of everyday cooking fires and the earthiness of rocks, is never pure elemental water, but mixed with other elements and mixtures.[17]

Again, Heurnius resolved apparent contradictions between his two main authorities, Galen and Aristotle. Galen had argued that water wets the most, while Aristotle's heirs had argued that air is the wettest element. Heurnius resolved this disagreement by having Galen speak "as a physician": in practice, water wets more because it has a thicker substance, and adheres to things more, thus making them wetter. A nod to Genesis and God's creation of water further established the elemental status of water. Finally, earth is cold and dry, as found by touch. For physicians, per Hippocrates, these four elements can be called hot, cold, wet, and dry.[18]

Mixtures of the elements and primary qualities filled the world. Early modern philosophers, chymists, physicians, and even theologians hotly debated the nature of mixture in early modern Europe.[19] Some, such as the Aristotelian physician, philosopher, and philologist J. C. Scaliger (1484–1558, father of famed Leiden professor J. J. Scaliger), pushed the medieval notion of Aristotelian *minima naturalia* or natural minima to the extreme of endorsing corpuscularism. Scaliger took the *minima*, which were the smallest bits of a substance which could still retain their substantial identity and forms, and conceptually pushed them into little corpuscles or particles. Thus, each living body had a hierarchy of substantial forms, in which one dominant form of the living body organized the forms of the parts, the homoiomerous substances such as flesh, bone, etc.,

---

16   Hankinson, "Philosophy of nature," 212–217.
17   Johannes Heurnius, *Institutiones*, 10–15.
18   Johannes Heurnius, *Institutiones*, 15.
19   Newman, *Atoms and Alchemy*. Lüthy, *David Gorlaeus*. Leijenhorst and Lüthy, "The Erosion of Aristotelianism," 386–400. Siraisi, *Avicenna in the Renaissance*, 296–299.

the humors, and finally the *minima*. True mixture came about through union, but a union that preserved the ingredients' substantial forms. Others, mostly in the Thomist tradition, argued that when substances mixed through division and mutual contact, the "fight" of their opposing elements and qualities resulted in the corruption of the previous substantial form and the emergence of a single new one.

In addition, physicians discussed Galen's *minima* or "little parts" (*particulae*) of things which were too small to sense, which were the elements.[20] They also noted the ancient Methodists' corpuscularianism, especially that of Asclepiades, as well as the atomism of Democritus and Epicurus.[21] In 1546, Girolamo Fracastoro (ca. 1478–1553) precipitated widespread discussion of his atomist theory of contagion. While Galen had discussed "seeds of disease," he emphasized each individual's healthy functioning and impaired states, given each person's natural temperament or mixture of the primary qualities hot, cold, dry, and wet. Thus, what one person might naturally experience as a relatively hot but still healthy brain would be morbidly hot and cause disease impairments for another person with a naturally colder temperament. Fracastoro borrowed atomist seeds from the ancient Roman atomist Lucretius to explain contagion by contact, by material deposits or *fomites*, and by action at a distance. Each occurred through the transfer of material "seedlets of contagion."[22] Heurnius and his colleagues, like physicians across Europe, accepted contagion, of course. After all, they experienced it in their engagement with well-established diseases such as phthisis or consumption, and new diseases such as the French pox.[23] But, as Vivian Nutton has shown, they domesticated Fracastoro's contagion by resisting his atomism and slotting a more robust contagion theory in line with ancient precedents.[24]

Heurnius taught a rather traditional Aristotelian definition of mixture, but resisted the extremes. In short, he thought that in true mixtures the mixed substances divided into minimal parts so their qualities united through mutual contact, but the elements constituting the original ingredients retained their forms and qualities. These elemental forms and qualities, though, remained in potency, under the "command" of the new substantial form of the mixture.[25]

---

20   Galen, quoted in Siraisi, *Avicenna in the Renaissance*, 242, n. 58. Cf. Ragland, "'Making Trials,'" 515–518.

21   Siraisi, *Avicenna in the Renaissance*, 242, 263–5.

22   Nutton, "The Seeds of Disease." Nutton, "The Reception of Fracastoro's Theory of Contagion," 200.

23   Arrizabalaga, Henderson, and French, *The Great Pox*, 121–129.

24   Nutton, "The Reception of Fracastoro's Theory of Contagion."

25   Johannes Heurnius, *Institutiones*, 16–18.

When we eat plants, for example, the form of the plant passes away, but the forms of the elements of the plant remain, even as they are together changed into the form of blood by coction. As Hippocrates taught in *On the Nature of Man*, when we die the elements we drew from our food and drink return to earlier states.[26]

Interestingly, Heurnius maintained that these minimal parts, though Aristotelian unities of matter and form, must exist separately in places and dimensions, with only their qualities mixing. Thus, Heurnius' theory of mixture approached something like a corpuscular understanding of matter. With Fernel, Heurnius rejected the idea of the ancient Neoplatonic philosopher Plotinus that the elemental substances interpenetrated and mixed.[27] Both insisted that the mixing substances divided into very small parts, and their qualities mutually intermingled. But Heurnius endorsed the persistence of the elemental forms in potency in mixtures, something Fernel scorned as a "disgrace," since it asserted there were at least two forms rather than one single, unified substance with one form.[28] Instead, Heurnius taught Leiden students that the elements persisted in mixture and returned to their prior states after the dissolution of the mixture.

This was no mere academic point, however pedantic it might seem to us today. Because our bodies' parts are mixtures of the elements, physicians had to know the proper, healthy temperament for each one. Mixtures of elements formed the parts of the living bodies, and the co-mingling and mutual tempering of the qualities of the elements in these parts produced their temperaments. Moreover, as in the notable case of the contemporaneous Wittenberg medical professor Daniel Sennert, teaching the persistence of elemental forms in mixture, rather than their destruction, also often provided an Aristotelian-Galenic matter theory friendly for chymical theorizing and practice.[29] As we will see in the next chapter, Heurnius inclined toward chymistry, but followed Galen in establishing the qualitative temperament and structure of each part at the center of his physiology, pathology, and therapy.

Historians often describe early modern notions of temperament in terms of each individual's total bodily preponderance of one of the four humors.[30]

---

26   Johannes Heurnius, *Institutiones*, 17.

27   Fernel, *Universa Medicina*, Bk. II, Ch. 8, 63.

28   Fernel, *Universa Medicina*, 64. Johannes Heurnius, *Institutiones*, 16: "Moreover, these elements do not lose their forms in mixtion, but retain them, conquered, under the mutual fight of the qualities."

29   Newman, *Atoms and Alchemy*. Klein, "Daniel Sennert."

30   Maclean, *Logic, Signs, and Nature*, 241, summarizes Renaissance temperament theory in terms of each individual's healthy perfect mixture of the four humors, and a

According to this view, for which there is widespread evidence among non-physicians, people might be said to have sanguine, choleric, melancholic, or phlegmatic temperaments. These humor-based mixtures determined much of the readily-observable human variations in bodily formations, health, disease, and even personality and passions.[31] But there were other definitions and developments. As Michael Stolberg has shown, across Europe in the seventeenth and eighteenth centuries, patients' and physicians' discussions of temperament shifted from more of an emphasis on humors to thinking of "temperament" in terms of bodily strengths and weaknesses, including emotional or mental predispositions.[32] In this later formulation, by the later seventeenth and eighteenth centuries, notions of humoral preponderance or anatomical temperament became considerations alongside many others.

In contrast to both of these views, academic physicians who sought to recover and follow the true Galen published and taught a different theory, one which defined temperaments in terms of the mixtures of the four primary qualities, especially in the principal organs. From organs to drugs, these qualitative mixtures determined the faculties or powers of things, as we will see in greater detail below. For Heurnius and his students, as for Galen and many Galenic physicians, a person's temperament emphatically was *not* due to a natural abundance of one or more of the four humors. Thus, he wrote, we should not call a certain man bilious who has a preponderance of bile. Physicians might attend to the humors, since they were nearer to the senses.[33] But Galen himself defined "temperament" as the form of *each part*, making flesh what flesh is, nerve what nerve is, and so on for each part. Temperament arose from two main sources: the pairs of principal qualities in the elemental matter used in the generation and development of the fetus, and regimen (especially diet), which often reinforced inborn temperament.[34] Thus, Heurnius insisted on the Galenic maxim, "the temperament does not consist in the humors, but in the

---

preponderance of one. For similar accounts, see Wear, *Knowledge & Practice*, 37–38 and Lindemann, *Medicine and Society*, 13, 17–18. In contrast, Siraisi, *Medieval & Early Renaissance*, 101–104, describes temperament or complexion as arising from the mixture of the elements, for the whole body. See also Nance, "Determining the Patient's Temperament." For a more detailed discussion of temperament theory in terms of qualities see Siraisi, *Avicenna in the Renaissance*, 296–315. See also chapter five below.

31   E.g., Nance, "Determining the Patient's Temperament." Stolberg, *Experiencing Illness*, 85–89.

32   Stolberg, *Experiencing Illness*, 88–89.

33   Johannes Heurnius, *Institutiones*, 20.

34   Galen, *The Soul's Dependence* (QAM), Singer trans., *Galen*, 175, K IV 821. Jouanna, "Hippocrates as Galen's Teacher,", 10–11. Kaye, *A History of Balance*, 16

solid parts."[35] Others "err, and do not follow the opinion of Galen, those who consider that he said that this man is melancholic, in whom the melancholic blood abounds; bilious, in whom bile."[36] Rather, the proportions of the humors and qualities in the first formation of the parts in early human development generated the temperaments of the parts.

Reason dictated nine general types of temperament, from the four simple temperaments of one principal quality each, to the four composite (excluding the impossible preponderances of hot and cold or wet and dry), and the one perfect balance in the middle, the *eukrasis*. From these "arise the infinite properties of bodies."[37] In reality the "innumerable varieties of temperaments" fell along a wide latitude, given the nature of each part.[38] Since Heurnius kept his remarks on temperaments of the parts relatively brief in his course and textbook on medical theory, we will save a detailed exposition of his teaching on temperaments and health, disease, and therapy for chapter five.

Other eminent professors across Europe returned to Galen's works to articulate and defend the notion of temperament as the mixture of the four primary qualities, and something which clearly varied from organ to organ and part to part, and *not* the general proportion or mixture of humors in the body. Nancy Siraisi has shown that a series of Italian professors, notably teachers at Padua, defended such a Galenic idea in the sixteenth century.[39] They, in turn, drew on medieval academic medical teaching that also reached back to Galen and Avicenna's systematization of temperament theory.[40] As Linda Deer Richardson demonstrated, this widespread academic teaching sparked resistance and innovation from Jean Fernel, who advanced less-material ideas of diseases based on occult causes, the "total substance" of a thing (a notion also present in Galen's discussions of hidden causation for things like some poisons), and celestial influences.[41] Clearly, knowing the qualitative mixtures of the parts and organs, and their healthy and morbid variations, played a foundational role in medical theory.

---

35   Johannes Heurnius, *Institutiones*, 21. Heurnius followed especially Galen's *The Art of Medicine* and *On Mixtures* for this definition and the foundational concept of temperament for medical diagnosis, pathology, and therapy. For more details and the unanimity of Galen's writings on this point, see chapter five.

36   Johannes Heurnius, *Institutiones*, 20.

37   Johannes Heurnius, *Institutiones*, 25.

38   Johannes Heurnius, *Institutiones*, 20–26, 25.

39   Siraisi, *Avicenna in the Renaissance*, 296–304.

40   Ottoson, *Scholastic Medicine*, 208–212. French, *Canonical Medicine*, ch. 3.

41   Deer Richardson, "The Generation of Disease," 177–179.

How, then, could students know the temperament of a certain part, at least in theory? Touch, disciplined by reason, gives us reliable knowledge of the temperaments of the parts, students learned. But then, budding physicians had to understand the natural temperaments, or non-quantitative calibration, of their bodily instruments for measuring the temperaments of other things. Each part of the body had its own "innate temperament," of course, and from all the parts considered together "we can explore what the temperament of a person is, not from one part alone."[42] Heurnius, like Galen and other Galenists before him, favored the skin, especially the skin on the tips of the fingers for detecting these qualitative temperaments. This spot was "very nervy" and composed of a mixture of nerves and flesh. Of course, all parts of the body seem hot at first touch, but reason together with touch take the judge's seat: one had to touch the different parts of different bodies many times, gaining long experience. Moreover, the human body occupied the middle position among animals, with the median temperament; the healthy "well-fleshed" human held the middle spot among humans, and thus acted as a midpoint for measuring variations of "hotter," "colder," "drier," and "wetter."[43] Galen firmly advocated for the importance of long practice and reported the conclusions of his own "trials" touching "a large number of bodies" and assessing their principal qualities: children have a gentler heat, but larger in quantity; prime-age adults a sharper heat, though less in quantity than children.[44]

Elemental mixture or temperament produced the basic qualitative properties of body parts, but of course the parts interacted and produced "accidental" variations beyond the basic substance. Some parts, such as bone, cartilage, tendon, or even phlegm, might not be hot in themselves, but often draw heat from another source. Careful experience, tutored by Galen's philosophy, shows us that the flowing *spiritus* (a fine vapor, and much like Galen's *pneuma*) is the hottest of all, then the heart, then the liver, followed by the blood, simple flesh produced from blood, the spleen, kidneys, and the skin. Likely for the sake of his beginning students, Heurnius avoided the centuries-old debates over how our own variable and apparently "hot" bodies can act as perfectly temperate measuring instruments.[45] And *whose* body is the most temperate? Instead, Heurnius gave lists, ordering the parts from the hottest *spiritus*, then the heart and liver, to the coldest cartilage, bone, phlegm. Here, he again seems to have embraced

---

42   Johannes Heurnius, *Institutiones*, 31.

43   Galen, *Mixtures*, trans. Singer, in *Galen*, 217, K I 541.

44   Galen, *Mixtures*, trans. Singer, in *Galen*, 241–242, K I 593–594.

45   Ottoson, *Scholastic Medicine*, 208–212. Fernel, *Physiologia*, Bk. 3, Ch. 8. Siraisi, *Avicenna in the Renaissance*, 300–304.

humanist training and his pedagogical vision of making a well-ordered selection of the best teaching. Despite his enthusiasm for chymistry, Heurnius did not adopt instruments to measure heat or other bodily properties such as humidity. In this he was again more in the mainstream of Galenic practice, in contrast with innovators such as the Santorio Santorio, who taught medicine at Padua from 1611 to 1624, and extended Galenic temperament theory tradition far into programs of using new instruments to quantify the changes of human bodies.[46]

For Heurnius, temperament explained many things about each person, but not everything. Though he allowed for a *philosophical* emphasis on *spiritus* and the unitary soul in his discussion of faculties, when he wrote as a *physician* Heurnius rejected Fernel's attempt to minimize temperament and the principal qualities.[47] In fact, Heurnius solidly followed Galen and Avicenna who made qualitative temperament central to matter theory. This made temperament foundational for understanding the faculties or capacities of living bodies and drugs, and thus for diagnosis, prognosis, and therapy. Temperaments unified rational theory with rational practice. Further, Heurnius could add Galen, Avicenna, and more recent natural philosophers to the list of authorities Galen advertised. The "best" and "most distinguished" philosophers and doctors such as Hippocrates and Aristotle, Galen had asserted again and again, defended the theory of the four principal qualities as the basic constituents and fundamental active powers of things; counter-arguments had all failed.[48]

The principal organs of the psychic, vital, and nutritive souls or systems especially determined a person's temperament: "We estimate the temperament of a person most of all from the principal parts...from these parts rightly weighed and estimated separately, and then together, we will apprehend the temperament of a person."[49] An individual's temperament depended most of all on these principal parts—the heart, liver, and brain—and especially the liver.[50] After all, the liver provided the nourishing blood for the whole body, and the temperaments of the heart and whole body "follow the nature of the liver."[51] The heart provides heating, vivifying *spiritus* to the whole body through the arteries, and the liver provides nourishment through the veins. Thus someone with a hotter liver and heart would have wide veins due to temperament, since heat spreads and thins. Usually such

---

46   Siraisi, *Avicenna in the Renaissance*, 237, 304, 314.

47   For Fernel, see Siraisi, *Avicenna in the Renaissance*, 296–299 and Deer Richardson, "The Generation of Disease."

48   Galen, *Mixtures*, trans. Singer, in *Galen*, 202–3, 210–214, K I 510–511, 527–536. Hankinson, "Philosophy of nature," 217–223.

49   Johannes Heurnius, *Institutiones*, 33.

50   Cf. Galen, *The Art of Medicine*.

51   Johannes Heurnius, *Institutiones*, 39.

people would also be thin throughout. But custom and habit could make such a person fat. A fully temperate person, as known by touch and sight, would be moderately warm, with youthful yellow hair turning black in adulthood, but excellently curled. The head should also be nicely rounded. A moderate temperament usually would indicate the proper operation of all the faculties, since those depend on temperament.[52]

Variation in the parts mattered, and students may have attended closely to the longish discussion of different brains. Hot brains showed too much inconstancy of opinions and the *ingenium* (wit), with much quickness of sensation and motion (but little sleep), and a more thoroughly cooked discharge from the eyes and nose. Colder brains showed a similar inconstancy of opinions, and a slowness of the senses and intellect. Dry brains held memories faithfully, sticking them in the desiccated ventricles, and the dryness grew hair quickly. Wet brains, in contrast, learned quickly since they received impressions better, but had slippery memories (physically and experientially). After listing the moderate temperate mixture and the four simple temperaments (more hot, cold, wet, or dry), Heurnius described the mixed temperaments for the chief organs.[53]

In all of this, he followed and cited Galen's mature summary of medical theory and practice, *The Art of Medicine*, and Galen's other works on mixtures or temperaments (Heurnius usually translated Galen's Greek *krasis* as "temperamentum" rather than a Latin term for "mixture").[54] As Per-Gunnar Ottoson put it, "[w]ithin the Aristotelian-Galenic tradition the fundamental mixture in the body is never a mixture of the humors, but of the primary qualities."[55] Ottoson goes on to point out that in Galen's works the four humors "only play a limited role, and are in no ways of any vital importance to his conceptions of health and disease."[56] As we will discuss in greater detail in chapter five, even in their medical practices of diagnosis and treatment Galen and early modern Galenists such as Heurnius prioritized the temperament or qualitative mixture of the body's organs—especially the principal parts—over the qualitative mixtures of the humors.

---

52   Johannes Heurnius, *Institutiones*, 31–34.

53   Johannes Heurnius, *Institutiones*, 30–47.

54   Galen, *The Art of Medicine*, in *Galen: Selected Works*, trans. Singer, esp. pp. 351–364, K I 318–347. Johannes Heurnius, *Institutiones*, 30, 32, 33, 36. Heurnius, pp. 28, 30, 32, 50, also cited Galen's work on mixtures, *De temperamentis* (*Mixtures*). See chapter five below for an extended discussion.

55   Ottoson, *Scholastic Medicine*, 130.

56   Ottoson, *Scholastic Medicine*, 131.

Organs and parts clearly held the primary place in Heurnius' theory of medicine, but he also endorsed the four humors: phlegm, yellow bile, black bile,
and blood. These carried qualities to different places in the body, changed or
corrupted on their own, and often performed vital functions. Each properly
worked for the good of the body, with yellow bile, for example, helping to heat
the body and soften it.[57] Too much of this hot, dry, and bitter-tasting humor,
though, caused burning fevers. Normally, bile entered the intestines via the
gallbladder, but God also arranged it so excess bile naturally went out with
the urine. Too much bile in the intestines would cause dysentery.[58] As we will
see later, Heurnius and many other physicians and patients in early modern
Europe attributed many diseases to anatomically-localized flows or blockages
of morbid humors and matter.

It is important to grasp the tangible reality of the humors (at least, intellectually). Phlegm patently descends from the head all-too-readily in winters in
the Low Countries. Blood, too, flowed from early modern livestock and human
bodies in labor, accident, and war. Yellow bile tinged urine and could be seen
intact at a butcher's shop or among the painters, who used ox bile to thin their
oil paints.[59] Black bile eluded everyday identification, but Heurnius and other
writers in the Galenic-Hippocratic tradition found something to point to in
the dark colors of patients' stools and urine, as well as the frequent practice of
bloodletting. Avicenna described separating out different humoral substances
in his *Canon*, a common resource for medical teaching.[60] Poured into a vessel,
blood drawn from a patient separated into a foamy, ruddy bile, a cloudy dregs
or black bile, a section like the white of an egg, and a watery part. The first
three are the humors bile, black bile, and phlegm.[61] Heurnius, too, urged his
students to trust their senses to pick out the humors from settled blood:

> Inspect the blood that has jumped out from a cut vein, and you will see
> nutritive humors. For while that bloody mass is balled up together, in the
> highest place you will see the bile growing purple: turn over the mass,
> and on the bottom will be black bile: if you inspect the middle, a sticky
> [mass] will be notable, and we call this phlegm: and all these are imbued
> with a certain purple color from the pure blood.[62]

---

57   Johannes Heurnius, *Institutiones*, 117.
58   Johannes Heurnius, *Institutiones*, 311.
59   De Graaf, *Disputatio*, 45.
60   Siraisi, *Avicenna in the Renaissance*.
61   Bertoloni Meli, "The Color of Blood."
62   Johannes Heurnius, *Institutiones*, 123.

With therapeutic bleeding common, and other forms of bleeding even more common, early modern students had ample opportunities for such hands-on learning about the humors. Reasoning from four fundamental qualities to four humors joined with sensory experience to ground the existence and qualities of the humors.

Climate and habit changed bodies, and sex mattered. A birth under a hot Sun and living in heat made bodies harder, darker, redder, thinner, and drier. Too much leisure, especially for women, produced whiter skin. Heurnius agreed with long tradition from Aristotle and Galen that women generally had colder bodies, but he insisted, drawing on longer Hippocratic tradition, that "woman-liness" derived from the presence and activity of the uterus. Thomas Laqueur has broached influential claims that pre-modern physicians thought in terms of a "one-sex model" in which men's and women's genitals were anatomical inversions of each other, and in some cases a person could change sex.[63] But this thesis faces stacks of contrary evidence stretching back to the Hippocratic writings on the diseases of women, misreads key primary evidence, and vastly reduces the rich religious and philosophical cultural worlds which produced thick conceptions of "male" and "female."[64] Even on the question of early modern sexual anatomy, Laqueur's argument is incorrect, as Helen King's close reading of the actual text of Vesalius's *Fabrica* shows: Vesalius did not represent the uterus as the inverse of the male organs, but as the womb itself, its own part with its own actions and use. Early moderns also marked anatomical sexual difference in other parts and characteristics, such as bones, flesh, and temperament.

Like many other anatomists and physicians, Heurnius clearly distinguished the two sexes primarily by the generative organs and their functions. In his lectures and textbooks, which constituted Leiden medical teaching for decades, we find the Hippocratic two-sex model.[65] Heurnius drew on "Hippocrates" to argue that "the foundation of the nature of woman is the uterus, to which the highest maker of things, God, engendered the love of birthing."[66] He also re-told the Hippocratic story of Phaethousa, whose grief over her husband's exile wasted her uterus. Unable to menstruate, become pregnant, or nurse children, Phaethousa became ill and developed a beard and a deep voice.

---

63   Laqueur, *Making Sex*.

64   King, *The One-Sex Body on Trial*. Cadden, *The Meanings of Sex Difference in the Middle Ages*. Crowther, *Adam and Eve in the Protestant Reformation*. Stolberg, "A Woman Down to Her Bones."

65   King, *The One-Sex Body on Trial*.

66   Johannes Heurnius, *Institutiones*, 165–166.

Therefore, Heurnius argued, the uterus, "the cause of the menses, is the *he gunaikeie physis kai chroie*, that is, the nature and color/complexion of the woman." Different organs made real differences, since they performed different actions and displayed different faculties.

In sum, our crash course in medical theory from the first section of Heurnius' textbook, given as lectures and used by other professors for decades, reveals a very Galenic medicine that used the best natural philosophy of the time to explain the matter and basic operations of bodies. The qualities hot, cold, dry, and wet mixed to form the temperaments of things, from organs to food and drugs. In these courses, at least, Heurnius avoided most of the contentious debates over the nature of the elements and qualities, or the metaphysics of mixture. Still, he accepted innovations such as pluralism about forms and the preservation of the forms of ingredients in mixtures and a domesticated contagion theory. For the most part, though, Galen's approach to the healthy and morbid temperaments of organs, and their subsequent faculties, grounded the theory students learned.

2   Basic Principles vs. Hope for Certainty

These basic principles persisted in Leiden pedagogy, though they appeared less robust after decades of attacks from chymists and mechanists.[67] Even as late as 1654, Albert Kyper, a Prussian philosopher and physician who taught natural philosophy and medical theory at Leiden, argued for maintaining the established precepts of healing, even after taking on board disruptive doctrines such as the circulation of the blood. Writing to beginning students of medicine in his *Transsumpta*, Kyper insisted that "what ought to be done in Medicine should not be changed, although the reason according to which it ought to be done is disputed."[68] If the principles of natural philosophy which undergirded the theoretical or rational part of medicine really lacked integrity, perhaps students and physicians could fall back on historical or *to hoti*, "the that," knowledge. But beginning students in medicine could not possibly have enough experience of all the particulars they needed for learning all the "thats" of medicine: medicinal plants, diseases, constitutions, therapies, etc. This sort of experience "comes from use through a series of years, thus it is necessary that one draws it from good and proven Authors, among which by the judgment of all Hippocrates

---

67   Klerk, "Galen Reconsidered."
68   Kyper, *Transsumpta Medica*, unpag. preface.

and Galen are eminent."[69] Books handed on past experience for students of medicine, supplied the rational principles for thinking in terms of universals rather than just particulars, and trained students' wits. Thus the two central principles of medicine—"experience and reason"—stood on the teaching of "skilled men" of the past and present.[70]

Yet the point of the *Transsumpta* was to give students the Aristotelian philosophical prolegomena supposedly necessary for medicine: detailed theories of the elements and mixed bodies.[71] Kyper's philosophy represents the increasingly eclectic Aristotelian pedagogy of natural philosophy of the middle of the 1600s.[72] Pedagogical inertia accounts for some of this constancy. Like others, Kyper held on to Aristotelian core concepts such as the immobility of the Earth—largely on the testimony of scripture—as well as the four elements and four elemental qualities, and conceptual schemes which retained pairs of agents and patients, as well as the four causes (formal, final, material, and efficient).[73] Yet Kyper's confidence in the Galenic-Aristotelian natural philosophy of the principal qualities (hot, cold, dry, and wet) perhaps had waned enough that, by the 1650s, he no longer described the faculties and actions of drugs in those terms. Instead, he provided a methodical doctrine of drugs by organizing them by their effects for removing morbid matter: purgation, salivation, sweating, and urination.[74]

Despite growing problems in matter theory or the basic principles of natural philosophy, the old philosophies offered ready lecture material. The Aristotelian system ordered the world of knowledge and experience, and did so in a way that provided a shared vocabulary and way of thinking so necessary for students. All things under the Moon are composed of a mixture of the four elements earth, water, air, and fire, which acted and could be perceived by their sensible qualities of hot, cold, wet, and dry. Hot and cold, especially, seemed to be the most active qualities in sublunar nature, from the change of the seasons to cooking, fevers, the inflammatory or cooling powers of drugs, and patients' own sensations of their states of health and disease. Teaching philosophers such as Kyper, and others across Europe, often expressed a reluctance to give up such a useful pedagogical system when they did not have a unified, comprehensive philosophy to replace it. Even with errors such as claiming the

---

69   Kyper, *Transsumpta Medica*, unpag. preface.

70   Kyper, *Transsumpta Medica*, 8.

71   *Pace* French, *Harvey's Natural Philosophy*, 346–348.

72   Ruestow, *Physics*, 39–43. Martin, "With Aristotelians Like These, Who Needs Anti-Aristotelians?"

73   Lüthy and Thijssen, "The Tradition of Aristotelian Natural Philosophy," 6.

74   Kyper, *Institutiones Medicae*, 305–307, 317–332. Cf. Klerk, "Galen Reconsidered," 155–6.

heart as the chief organ of sensation, rather than the brain, Aristotle remained the "Prince of the Philosophers" who still stood close beside Hippocrates and Galen.[75]

With so many different philosophical voices making new and contradictory declarations, Kyper hoped for a reconciling synthesis. He accepted opposing innovations such as the unity of the heavens and the earth and the mutability of the heavens. Yet he had no rival physics to the geocentric order of elemental place, and so endorsed Tycho Brahe's model of a stationary Earth around which the Sun revolves, and the planets revolve around the Sun. He also attempted a theory of the elements and mixed bodies which reconciled the teachings of Aristotle, Galen, Avicenna, and even recent chymical writers. In short, chymical theory reduced to Aristotelian natural philosophy with the Aristotelian elements of earth, water, air, and fire forming the chymical principles.[76] Aristotle, for Kyper, still held the unchallenged title of "the Philosopher," and his quotations, principles, and vocabulary dot Kyper's pages.

A decade earlier, just beginning his lecturing at Leiden in 1643, Kyper had explicitly hoped Descartes might settle the disputes by providing real, mathematical certainty to natural philosophy.[77] Given the profusion of different philosophies and claims about phenomena—chymical, Aristotelian, Platonic, atomistic, skeptical, etc.—Kyper hoped for someone to distinguish "the certain from the uncertain, demonstrations and true histories from opinions and tales, so that nothing would be held as true and recognized as such except what is either deduced from first principles directly by necessary consequence, or was so congruous with experience, that the observations of all times attest to its truth; the rest, however, he may take up as more or less probable."[78] These would render "true and solid foundations" for constructing Medicine with the least danger of ruin. Here, Kyper likely echoed the rhetoric of Descartes's 1637 *Discourse*, in which the French mathematician and philosopher claimed to begin with the indubitable truths of the existence of God and of the thinking mind, and to deduce chains of reasoning "more certain than

---

75   Kyper, *Institutiones*, Dedication, ††.

76   Kyper, *Transsumpta Medica*, 43–50.

77   Kyper, *Methodus*, 274: "Descartes, a man of sharp judgment, gives us hope for the elaboration of his work, which does not yield place to Mathematics with regard to the certitude of demonstrations, and unfolds clearly and solidly the causes of all natural effects, and even of marvels, commonly referred to occult qualities. O our happy time, if he might render back effects equal to the promises and darings! But I wish for that more than I trust in it, and I do not want, yet, my judgment to jump ahead of the outcome. Meanwhile we are nourished by hope, we will judge of our work, to learn further in Physica what we can."

78   Kyper, *Methodus*, 276.

the demonstrations of the geometers."[79] Descartes even claimed the "force of mathematical demonstrations" for his account of the action of the heart.[80]

What is more, Kyper agreed with Descartes that philosophers and physicians needed more diligent labor to increase the stock of "new findings" alongside those things well-found by the Ancients. Descartes wound down his *Discourse* by reiterating the need for a renewed, "practical philosophy" versus the "speculative philosophy" of the universities, to make us "lords and masters of nature," especially in medicine.[81] Since "even the mind depends so much on the temperament and disposition of the bodily organs," medicine was uniquely necessary for making humans wiser and more skillful.[82]

Descartes's evaluation of the state of medical knowledge, and his ambitions for its expansion, contrasted sharply with the more piecemeal programs of reform advocated at Leiden and elsewhere. Deprived of Cartesian philosophy, Descartes claimed, what physicians knew about the body, "is almost nothing in comparison with what remains to be known."[83] Descartes himself needed time (and patronage) to make the *expériences* (experiences or experiments) necessary for knowing bodies better, given his metaphysics. The last passage of his *Discourse* announced his promise to "devote the rest of my life to nothing other than trying to acquire some knowledge of nature from which we may derive rules in medicine which are more reliable than those we have had up till now."[84]

Despite the bold promises of Cartesian certainty, Kyper later critiqued Cartesianism and re-asserted Aristotelian natural philosophy in the 1650s. It seems quite likely that after his early enthusiasm he found Descartes's contributions to be a sad disappointment, especially given the Frenchman's extravagant anatomical and philosophical claims.[85] Among Leiden physicians and students, sharply unfavorable views of Cartesian anatomy became common by the middle of the 1600s.[86] By then, experimentalist medical investigators sought to locate the active principles of the body in chymicals such as acids and alkalis. But from 1575 through the 1640s, by far the most common explanatory principles of organs and drugs were capacities, powers, or "faculties" (*facultates, dunameis*).

---

79   Descartes, *Discourse*, in *The Philosophical Writings of Descartes*, translated by Cottingham, Stoothoff, and Murdoch [*CSM*] I, 131; AT VI, 41.
80   Descartes, *Discourse*, CSM I, 136; AT VI, 50.
81   Descartes, *Discourse*, CSM I, 142–3 AT VI, 62–3.
82   Descartes, *Discourse*, CSM I, 142–3 AT VI, 63.
83   Descartes, *Discourse*, CSM I, 142–143; AT VI 62–63.
84   Descartes, *Discourse*, CSM 1, 151; AT VI, 78.
85   Molhuysen, *Bronnen*, III, 107.
86   Ragland, "Mechanism."

3 Galen on Faculties, Matter, and Souls

But what were these "faculties"? Despite modern historians' interpretations, ancient and early modern Galenic faculties did not allow physicians an easy escape from anatomy, matter theory, or philosophical explanation.[87] In the standard view, faculties are mysterious or "immaterial" or "nonmaterial" entities added to the matter, structure, and elemental qualities of body parts.[88] It is certainly easier for us, from our present-day vantage point, to think of pre-modern physicians as hastily slapping an immaterial "faculty" on any activity of the body which they could not easily explain by sensory phenomena or rational theorizing. We might also join some of Galen's early modern critics such as John Locke and suspect that "faculties" are obviously superfluous, immaterial nonsense blocking real thought about how bodies act.[89] But such dismissive thinking is rash on our part. After all, this immaterialist interpretation of Galenic faculties flies in the face of Galen's lifelong commitment to grounding his claims in the phenomena of the senses, and in his emphasis on material explanation.

Faculties, in Galen's view, and the views of his early modern physician followers, were not strange, immaterial, or mystical things added to living bodies.[90] In short, they were powers or capacities for action. They were real powers or dispositions arising from the qualitative temperament of a part or parts (or drug), in relation to an object. They also worked through the structure of a part or organ, especially through the different types of basic contractile fibers. Thus, faculties were powers of a thing to act on a given object, produced by the relation of the thing's material substance and structure and the substance of the object. Magnets attract iron and aloe cleanses eyes.

To understand later Renaissance ideas of faculties, we must join the throng of humanist scholars and head back to their sources, especially Galen's works. Recovering a more faithful reading of Galenic faculty theory, and putting it in philosophical context, will also show that the Leiden physicians taught a doctrine faithful to the ancient ideas, especially many of Galen's ideas, a doctrine embraced across Europe. The ancient texts surveyed here found wide and frequent use in early modern medical education.

---

87   *Pace* French, *Dissection and Vivisection*, 1–2; Cunningham, *Anatomist Anatomis'd*, 197. For a more nuanced view, see Bertoloni Meli, *Mechanism, Experiment*, 14–15.

88   *Pace*, e.g., Cook, "Medicine," 426; Bertoloni Meli, *Mechanism*, 11.

89   Locke, *An Essay concerning Humane Understanding* II, Ch. 21, sec. 20, 130.

90   For a view of Galen's concept of faculties or powers across his works, which harmonizes with many of my claims here and which I discovered after composing this chapter, see Hankinson, "Galen and the Ontology of Powers."

In this and the following section, I will argue for four interrelated theses. First, that Galen and his physician followers did not call for a "faculty" every time they observed something happen, but only for the regularly-observed actions of different substances. Second, that temperaments or mixtures of the four qualities constituted the "true essence" or "*ousia*" of faculties Galen invoked more cautiously in his work *On the Natural Faculties*. In this way, Galenic physicians used the best matter theory at hand to make regular actions of substances intelligible, and to connect physiology, pathology, and therapy. Yet, as Galen claimed, it was almost impossible to know precisely *which* temperaments produced all the cascades of effects, especially in living bodies. Third, that Galen and his early modern heirs self-consciously compared facultative explanations with simplistic material speculative explanations, such as those of atomists and other corpuscularians. Fourth, that the "faculty" concept was called a relative one in logic, indicating a cause-effect relation between a given substance and an object.

First, physicians from Galen on invoked faculties based on phenomenal regularities of anatomical actions and substances. Hearts, muscles, livers, bladders, and other organs across animal kinds all displayed perceptibly different anatomical substances—anyone who thought the heart was a muscle should eat both and note the clear differences in taste—and so organs of each kind performed the same actions.[91] Similarly, mobile organs performed faculties of attraction, retention, and expulsion by means of fibers observable in dissection: specifically, straight, oblique, and circular fibers.

Second, across his writings, Galen described the substance of the faculties in material terms, as consisting in the qualitative mixture or temperament of the given part or parts, yet balanced this with his commitment to the wisdom and foresight of Nature or the Craftsman shown in the construction of living things. The lodestone appears in his work as the model of a material substance showing the action of a natural faculty, namely, the capacity to attract iron. When describing substances and faculties, Galen frequently explained the causal powers of nonliving and even living bodies in terms of their material substance and powers, in which elemental mixtures, temperaments, and anatomical structures determine higher-level actions, without much recourse to thinking in terms of forms: "All philosophers and physicians who are experts in natural science [*physis*] agree that activities accord with the peculiarities of substance."[92]

---

91   Galen, *On Anatomical Procedures*, trans. C. Singer, 182–183, K I 610–612. Galen calls taste "a most important indication of a difference of nature."

92   Galen, *On Anatomical Procedures*, trans. C. Singer, 182, K I 611. Singer, "Levels of Explanation in Galen."

Here, Galen used "substance" to mean the physical make-up or type of "stuff" constituting a bodily part, medicinal ingredient, lodestone, or other thing. As R. J. Hankinson has pointed out, Galen often used the term "substance" to refer to material things, or material substrates, while at other times giving a more Aristotelian expression of a compound of form and matter.[93] For Galen, as opposed to his Stoic opponents, the four elemental qualities of hot and cold, wet and dry, are not bodies themselves. But they are always embodied, properties of matter that make up substances, especially substances in Galen's more material way of speaking.

Galen stuck doggedly to his realism about the senses. Against Sophists and Pyrrhonists, as well as atomists, Galen followed Aristotle and, he claimed, Hippocrates, in concluding that there were four primary qualities making up all things, and that we can be confident that the senses reliably perceive the true qualities of things. Our senses and the intervening medium between us and objects all interact in reliable causal chains since they are like one another, and all ancient philosophers seemed to agree that like affects like.[94] Thus, the senses perceive the primary qualities of hot, cold, dry, and wet, and that hot and dry are most active in living things. They also reliably pick out the simple parts of our bodies in which all their bits are alike (in philosophical terms, they are homoiomerous): the liver, spleen, kidneys, lungs, heart, brain, etc.[95] Usually, anatomists relied on sight and touch to distinguish the parts—a finger placed in the heart reveals it is the hottest part—but cooking and eating the "substance" of the heart shows most clearly that it differs from muscles in its "variety of fibers" and its "taste, a most important indication of difference in nature."[96] Anyone who thought the heart a muscle was only "blundering where they could have learned by the senses." Throughout his works on mixtures, temperaments, and some later discussions of the soul, Galen emphasized materiality, bottom-up causation, and the elemental mixtures of the parts as the substance of the faculties, which mixtures and structures determined higher-level faculties and actions.[97]

Yet, Galen rejected explanations for natural complexities based on matter and chance *alone*. The atomists advanced such absurd stories about the origins of natural things, but the complex, wise construction of living bodies had to come from a rational plan, not chance. Even in his treatise on mixtures or temperaments, Galen objected to claims that differing amounts of the primary

---

93   Hankinson, "Substance, Element, Quality, Mixture."
94   Lehoux, "Observers, Objects, and the Embedded Eye."
95   Galen, *On the Natural Faculties*, trans. Brock, 1.6, 15, 23, K II 8, 13–14.
96   Galen, *On Anatomical Procedures*, trans. Singer. 7.8, 183, K I 612.
97   Singer, "Levels of Explanation in Galen." Von Staden, "Teleology and Mechanism," 197, 204.

qualities caused and explained the construction of passages and structures in bodies. These sorts of theories foolishly failed "to regard the natural cause of our construction as a craftsmanlike power, whereby the parts are formed in a way suited to the characters of our souls." Matter alone cannot dispose itself properly to form such complex and fitting anatomical structures, thus the fundamental material qualities are "only instruments, whereas the cause responsible for construction is something different from them."[98]

Galen celebrated the foresight and wisdom of the Craftsman or Demiurge or Nature (the activity of the Demiurge) throughout his works, especially his youthful *On the Usefulness of the Parts*.[99] Only such divine intelligence and power could arrange the "construction" (*diaplasis*) of living bodies out of matter so artistically, with perfect fit of form to function, no superfluities, and precious few monsters.[100] In his late work *The Construction of the Embryo*, Galen affirmed a well-earned nescience about the role of the soul—whether individual souls or a Platonic world soul—in the formation of living bodies. Citing his more physicalist late work *The Dependence of the Soul on the Mixtures of the Body* (*Quod animi mores*), he claimed only that the "faculties of the soul are brought to perfection of function *along with* their organs."[101]

In the face of contradictory arguments about the nature of the soul, Galen kept to a middle course. He considered different explanations for the construction of embryos one-by-one, and then rejected each as unpersuasive given the anatomical evidence and philosophical argumentation. Positing a formative soul transmitted from parents to offspring seems a good way to explain hereditary resemblance. Further, young animals seem to act as if their souls know how to use parts before they are fully formed; puppies bite without formed teeth and birds try to fly with incipient wings. But then, we voluntarily move our limbs and muscles without *knowing* the dozens or hundreds of muscles involved. Similarly, the alleged soul which constructs the embryo in its early stages seems to be the nutritive soul, but that soul is seemingly present in plants, too, and obviously lacks the "divine" reason and intelligence necessary to construct complex functional bodies.[102] In other works, such as *On the Natural Faculties*, Galen would restrict the soul to animals, who display the faculties

---

98   Galen, *Mixtures*, trans. Singer, in *Galen*, 261, K I 636.
99   Singer, "Levels of Explanation in Galen." Hankinson, "Philosophy of Nature," 233–236.
100   Singer, "Levels of Explanation in Galen," 537–9.
101   Galen, *The Construction of the Embryo*, trans. Singer, in *Galen*, 187, K IV 674. Italics added.
102   Galen, *Construction*, trans. Singer, in *Galen*, 200, K IV 700.

or capacities of sensation and voluntary motion, while plants show only the faculties of nutrition and growth, which are effects of nature, not soul.[103]

To craft a functioning body, Galen reasoned, one would have to know thousands of parts and functions. Anatomists counted the more than three hundred muscles and more than two hundred bones of the human body, each with ten or more functions. Adding in the organs summed to tens of thousands of purposes for "the whole apparatus," and each one "perfectly completed."[104] A Platonic World Soul would possess this superhuman skill and power, but the consequence that this Soul also constructed spiders, mice, mosquitoes, and worms seemed to verge on blasphemy. In the end, Galen concluded only that Epicurus and other materialists were clearly wrong to hold that "everything happens without design." Complex bodies without any useless parts, and tens of thousands of functions, could only result from "an extraordinarily intelligent and powerful craftsman."[105] After its construction, three causes of motion "managed" the living body: "that from the brain through the nerves and muscles; that from the heart through the arteries; and that from the liver through the veins."[106] Thus, in polemical attacks on the crude or simplistic materialism of rivals such as the atomists Epicurus and Asclepiades, or his polemical depiction of Erasistratus, Galen stressed the necessity of invoking the artistry and foresight of Nature or a Craftsman. Matter alone could never generate the wise and beneficial complexity revealed in anatomical dissections.

Other polemical contexts pushed him away from these repeated emphases on the external teleology of the Craftsman. Galen famously leaned in the opposite direction in his arguments against Platonists about the nature of the soul and its relation to the body. These Platonists possibly followed Plato's *Charmides*, which allowed for *no* influence of the body on the soul in the generation of diseases (instead, Plato argued there that all diseases originated in the soul).[107] In contrast, Galen's therapeutic practice blended bottom-up and top-down views of bodily causation. Diseases of the mind or soul had to be expelled by the application of reasoned discourse, yet most of his therapies for diseases of perceptible body parts aimed at restoring the proper action of a

---

103   Galen, *On the Natural Faculties*, trans. Brock, 1.1, 3, K II, 1–2.
104   Galen, *Construction*, trans. Singer, in *Galen*, 198, K IV 695.
105   Galen, *Construction*, trans. Singer, in *Galen*, 194, 198, 201; K IV 688, 695, 701.
106   Galen, *Construction*, trans. Singer, in *Galen*, 201, K IV 701.
107   Singer, "Levels of Explanation in Galen," 536, n. 47, referring to the Platonist targets of QAM. "All diseases are born from the soul," Plato, *Charmides*, trans. Lamb, 21.

part or parts by restoring the proper qualitative or elemental temperament, or purging morbid matter.[108]

Material explanation and external teleology came together through the formative wisdom and power of Nature or the Craftsman. Galen focused on the material powers and changes of bodies, whose construction always displayed the greatest intelligence and wisdom, with no part or structure crafted in vain. Thus, while materialist bottom-up accounts seem incompatible with Galen's external teleology, a rough harmonization remained possible by invoking an external cause or agent acting wisely to arrange the materials to bring about the best construction, then allowing the material powers to operate.[109]

Third, Galen and early modern Galenic physicians weighed facultative explanations against competing material explanations such as those of the atomists, and they rejected *crude* or simplistic explanations that did not fit the phenomena while accepting other material or mechanical explanations. As Sylvia Berryman has argued, Galen happily invoked comparisons to mechanical devices to explain bodily structures and actions.[110] After all, the Craftsman was divinely skilled and intelligent as a technician—Nature was the best architect. Only Nature could make *truly* self-moving, growing things. The observed actions of living bodies also demanded other powers beyond those apparently present in human art or nonliving objects, especially faculties of growth, nutrition, and generation.

Finally, faculties, at least those attributed most often by Galen and Galenic physicians to medicines and body parts, were usually relative concepts, meant to indicate that a given medicine or body part had a capacity for a certain kind of action, given the right object. Most simply and generally, then, a "faculty" is a logical relation, standing in for the actual cause, the *specific* substance or nature of which was yet unknown.

4 Galen among Ancient Sources on "Powers" or Faculties

The above sketch is already more complicated than the standard story among present-day histories of medicine and philosophy. So how should we refine our understanding from here? In this section, I will set a broader historical foundation for early modern debates and defend the revisionist view of faculties

---

108   Hankinson, "Actions and Passions." Garcia Ballester, "Soul and Body."
109   Von Staden, "Teology and Mechanism," 204. Singer, "Levels of Explanation in Galen," 538–9, 542.
110   Berryman, "Galen and the Mechanical Philosophy."

through a more detailed study of the ancient debates over faculties, with special attention to Galen's influential work, *On the Natural Faculties*.

First, like good humanists, we should attend to the words. Galen and other ancient Greek philosophers such as Plato and Aristotle used the term *dunamis* as the noun derived from the verb *dunasthai*, and especially from the form *dunamai*, "I am able to."[111] Thus "faculties" in ancient Greek medical and philosophical works denoted powers or capacities for action.

Next, we should recover a historical sense of the ancient debate, beginning with Hippocratic sources. *On Ancient Medicine* offers a likely source for Plato's notion of a faculty or power in the *Phaedrus*, and was widely read deep into the middle of the 1600s. In the Hippocratic text, the author described the origin of medicine in the common practice of observing and reflecting on the bodily effects of different foods on different people. Raw foods such as those eaten by animals made people sick, and so humans developed cooking. Cheese nourished some people but made others diseased. Next, people noticed that the foods that benefitted the sick, such as very thin gruel, did not necessarily benefit the healthy.[112] Then people began to note general patterns, namely that a person with a weak nature (*physis*) could not overcome the unblended powers or faculties (*dunameis*) of stronger foods.[113] An individual's sense of taste can pick out the overpowering faculty (*dunamis*) of a perilous food by taste, perceiving too much unblended saltiness, sweetness, etc. Similarly, the powers or faculties in human bodies are indexed by these flavors: "there is in the human being the salty and bitter and sweet and acid and astringent and insipid and myriad other things having powers of all kinds in quantity and strength."[114]

Using this new notion of powers or faculties, the author of *On Ancient Medicine* took aim at other Hippocratic writers whose works came to form the core of medical thinking after Galen. He attacked and rejected the rival Hippocratic hypothesis that food, bodies, and other things are composed of the hot, cold, wet, and dry, and so changes and proportions of these qualities are the true causes disease and health. He set up an alternate system based on powers or faculties in food and bodies revealed by taste and by an individual's experience of the effects of different food. The author closed by calling for greater understanding of the anatomical structures of the body which might attract or convey poorly-concocted or otherwise pathologically powerful food throughout the body, as well as greater understanding of the effects of the humoral powers

---

111   Corcilius, "Faculties in Ancient Philosophy," 19–58.
112   *On Ancient Medicine*, in Schiefsky, *Hippocrates*, trans. Schiefsky, 81.
113   *On Ancient Medicine*, in Schiefsky, *Hippocrates*, trans. Schiefsky, 88, 92.
114   *On Ancient Medicine*, in Schiefsky, *Hippocrates*, trans. Schiefsky, 92–93.

individually and in relation to each other. A sweet humor would likely change first into an acid humor on its own (as sweet wine into vinegar), so if sweet humors are best for patients then acid humors are second best. It would be best, the author concludes, to investigate these powers and changes "outside the body," perhaps in a sort of kitchen chemistry.[115]

Plato borrowed from Hippocratic writings on nature and drug action to articulate his concept of faculties and how to know them. In his *Phaedrus*, Plato took a Hippocratic discussion of "nature" (*physis*) as a model. Socrates argues, per Hippocrates and "true reason," that when we want to become learned about a given thing and teach others about it, we must investigate "what power [*dunamis*] of acting it possesses, or of being acted upon, and by what, and if it has many forms, number them."[116] Then, we should see how it acts and is acted upon, according to each form. Despite Plato's reference to "Hippocrates" here, there is no clear source among extant Hippocratic writings for this concise description of learning and teaching about the nature of a thing by knowing its powers, and learning about its powers by seeing how a thing acts and is acted upon in various ways. But this approach matches the method and language of Hippocratic discussions of drug action, and especially the early methodological sections of *On Ancient Medicine*.[117]

Plato's discussions of faculties tied his faculties closely to his account of the soul. As is well-known, Plato developed an influential conception of a tripartite soul, defining three major types of faculties, seated in different locations: the thinking, spirited, and desiderative parts, based in the head, chest, and belly, respectively.[118] The soul possesses, and is the subject of, the faculties (*dunameis*), which are capacities or powers relative to their objects. The faculty of knowledge has for its object *mathêma* (learning or systematic knowledge), the desiderative faculty desires food, pleasure, and other objects common to humans and beasts. Faculties were not just relatives, but really existed for Plato, and he thought of the soul as distinct from them (especially the rational soul), such that the soul is the self-moved mover which causally moves the body.

With Plato's student Aristotle, there were notable differences, with more emphasis on the living body. For Aristotle, the soul is not distinct from the faculties since it is the set of all faculties of a living body, but the *living body* is

---

115   *On Ancient Medicine*, in Schiefsky, *Hippocrates*, trans. Schiefsky, 109.
116   Plato, *Phaedrus*, trans. Fowler, 548–9. Cf. Corcilius, "Faculties in Ancient Philosophy," 22.
117   Johansen, *The Powers of Aristotle's Soul*, 1, n. 2. Schiefsky, *Hippocrates*.
118   For this and the following paragraph, I rely mostly on Corcilius, "Faculties in Ancient Philosophy."

the bearer of the faculties, not the soul.[119] Rather, the soul just is the inseparable form of the living body, as a wax seal is inseparably both the impression
and the wax. Better, the soul as the actualization of capacities is to the body as
sight is to the eye.[120] Aside from the thinking or rational faculty, which seems
separable, incorporeal, and unitary in a way that vexed commentators for centuries, the faculties of Aristotelian bodies are not things in their own right,
existing independently of a living body.

Aristotle's method for *identifying* faculties appears very similar to Galen's,
centuries later. Faculties are causal powers of the living body which we bun-
dle together and ascribe to a unitary soul as the form of the body, due to our
observation of regular activities which are characteristic of living things. For
instance, Aristotle identifies the material cause of anger as the boiling of the
blood or some hot substance around the heart.[121] Thinking in terms of the faculties' relations, and what they are *for*, he argues that the lower faculties are
potentially contained in the higher faculties, in a way similar to the potential
containment of triangles in squares, pentagons or other geometric shapes. Thus
animals' perceptual faculties contain nutritive faculties, which exist for the sake
of perception and other higher faculties. They are also united by their primary
seat, in the heart of animals. For Aristotle, the heart is the primary organ of the
sensitive soul, on which imagination, pleasure, pain, memory and "reasoning"
(*dianoeisthai*) depend, and which serves as the common organ of all the senses.[122]

Centuries later, Galen followed Plato in categorizing the concept "faculty"
(*dunamis*) as a "relative," indicating that it is only attributable relative to some
action (as the cause) or some effect of an action or function (*energeia*).[123] Galen
constrained his faculties by anatomical and clinical evidence for bodily actions
and structures, and used them as placeholders for complete explanations: "so
long as we are ignorant of the true essence of the cause which is operating,
we call it a faculty."[124] In other words, "faculty" is a word we use as a marker of

---

119 Corcilius, "Faculties in Ancient Philosophy," 44–45. Of course, Aristotle famously applied
     the philosophical terms of faculty or capacity (*dunamis*) and activity or action (*energeia*)
     to being, such that things come to be and act on each other in terms of actuality (*ener-
     geia*) acting on potentiality (*dunamis*).
120 Aristotle, *De anima*, 412b17–413a3.
121 Aristotle, *De anima*, 403a25.
122 Aristotle, *De anima*, 408b1–19. Tracy, "Heart and Soul in Aristotle." Vesalius, *Fabrica*, Bk. VI,
     Ch. XV.
123 Galen, *On the Natural Faculties*, trans. Brock, 17, K II 9–10. Corcilius, "Faculties in Ancient
     Philosophy."
124 Galen, *On the Natural Faculties*, 1.4, trans. Brock, 17, K II 9–10. Cf. Galen, *The Soul's Depen-
     dence on the Body*, trans. Singer, in *Galen*, 151 K IV 769–770.

ignorance about the *essence of* the specific cause or causes of a known phenomenal relation. But we can know these causes must be of a certain type,
without knowing their specific constitution.

In many places across his works Galen insisted that the *substance* of most
bodily faculties must be the qualitative mixtures or temperaments of the
part(s). In *On the Natural Faculties*, he expressed this view, tempered by the
caution just noted. Early in the work, he stated that "it appears to me, then,
that the vein, as well as each of the other parts, performs an activity [*energein*]
in such and such a way according to the manner in which the four qualities
are mixed."[125] He reiterated this point later on: "every part functions in its own
special way because of the manner in which the four qualities are compounded."[126] In this way, parts lacking the right mixture of their qualities did not act
rightly, and so were diseased. Thus, even in his more cautious work on faculties, Galen favored the idea that the efficient causes of actions—which causes
he called "faculties" (*dunameis*)—arose from or just were the material mixtures of each part.

Other works repeat this point. In *On Prognosis from Pulses*, Galen explained
how careful attention to all the variations of a patient's pulse revealed signs
and indications of an important vital faculty, the pulsative faculty of the heart
and arteries. The mixture or temperament of the heart was the substance of
this faculty, as with other faculties and other parts: "the substance of a faculty
of the individual parts is attributed to the fitting temperament of the individual parts" and "the substance [*ousia*] of a faculty [*dunamis*] is nothing other
than a certain mixture."[127] The elemental or primary qualitative variations of
each body part altered the faculty or capacity to act healthily: when an individual part is very temperate, it performs vigorously; when it is intemperate (too
hot, cold, wet, dry, etc.), it performs its faculty badly.

Emphatically, Galen's faculties were not strange or immaterial additions
to things. Galen clarified his position on faculties explicitly in his late work,
The Dependence of the Soul on the Mixtures of the Body: "On this point many of
the philosophers appear to be in some confusion, lacking a clearly articulated
notion of 'faculty.' They seem to conceive of faculties as things which inhabit
'substances' in much the same way as we inhabit our houses, and not to realize

---

125   Galen, *On the Natural Faculties*, 1.3, trans. Brock, 13, K II 7, slightly amended.
126   Galen, *On the Natural Faculties*, 2.8, trans. Brock, 185, K II 118–119. Cf. 189, K II 121: "[I]f dis-
       proportion of heat belongs to the primary diseases, it cannot but be that a proportionate
       blending [*eucrasia*] of the qualities produces the normal activity [*energeia*]."
127   Galen, *Praes. Puls.* 11.9, 244, 305–6, trans. Singer, "Galen."

that the effective cause of every event is conceived of in relational terms; there is a way of talking of this cause as of a specific object, but the faculty arises *in relation to* the event caused."[128] Aloe, relative to body parts, is able to cleanse, so we say it has a cleansing faculty. Given Galen's matter theory, the primary qualities of hot, cold, dry, and wet must have been the main causal powers, but it was vexingly unclear just *how* those produced so many different phenomena in the parts of living bodies.

Galen also distinguished between *natural* faculties found throughout living and non-living things, and the faculties found only in animate things. As he put it in his major work on the natural faculties, sensation and voluntary motion are characteristic of animals, while they share growth and nutrition with plants. So sensation and voluntary motion are faculties which can been seen as effects of the soul, growth and nutrition as effects of nature.[129] Living things, made artistically by Nature, showed clear capacities for generation, growth, and nutrition which non-living things obviously lacked. Animals demonstrated capacities for feeling and voluntary motion, both effects of the soul, while they shared with plants generation, growth, and nutrition. These general capacities, and especially the faculties of attraction, retention, and expulsion on which they depend, Galen termed "natural" faculties.

Throughout his treatise, Galen presented the lodestone's attraction of iron as the model of natural facultative action. Vessels of the body attract nutriment in the same way the lodestone attracts iron, seed or semen attracts blood, and likewise drugs draw out poisons.[130] These all work by similarity of qualities, rather than drawing a lighter substance as the bellows draw air.[131] He also spent several pages working through rival, non-facultative accounts of the lodestone's action. The atomistic explanations of Asclepiades did not work, since he denied even the facts of attraction. Epicurus accepted the attractions of the lodestone and amber, but his scheme of rebounding hooked atoms faced obvious rebuttals.[132] As Galen pointed out, this scheme requires the atoms to hook together and to rebound. But if they get hooked together, how do they rebound? And how can atoms which penetrate one, two, three, or more pieces of iron in sequence then hook onto and rebound from the fourth or

---

128   Galen, *The Soul's Dependence on the Body* [*QAM*], trans. Singer, in *Galen*, 151, K IV 769–770. Italics in original.

129   Galen, *On the Natural Faculties*, 1.1, K II 1.

130   Galen, *On the Natural Faculties*, 2.7, 1.14, 2.3; 165, 83, 133, K II 105, 53–54, 84–85.

131   Galen, *On the Natural Faculties*, 3.15, 319, K II 206–207.

132   Galen, *On the On the Natural Faculties*, 1.14, K II 45–52.

fifth pieces? Galen himself had seen five iron writing styli attached to a single lodestone. For Galen, these crudely materialist, atomistic explanations failed: living bodies performed selective attraction and elimination as they changed qualitatively and continuously in their parts.

Unlike most inanimate objects, living bodies develop and grow, transforming qualitatively different substances into their own parts. Only Nature, acting with the natural faculty of growth, could make living parts grow by adding matter in all dimensions at once. Galen's rival Erasistratus claimed that animals grew like ropes, sacks, or baskets, with additional weaving added to the ends or margins.[133] Yet this is not growth but the coming-to-be of the artifacts. Children in Ionia might fill pigs' bladders with air and then rub them in the ashes of a fire, so the bladders get larger, but this is not growth but stretching.[134]

Nature works through faculties of generation, growth, and nutrition. In growth and nutrition, especially, living bodies are selective, attracting and assimilating what is good for growth and health and eliminating waste. "Nature does everything artistically [technikôs] and equitably, possessing certain faculties [dunameis] by virtue of which each of the parts attracts to itself its appropriate fluid, and having done so attaches it to every part of itself and completely assimilates it."[135] This attraction and assimilation without the action of fibers happened due to the similarity or "affinity" (suggeneia) of the nutriment's qualities to those of the bodily substance.[136] Those parts of nutriment not assimilated are rejected by an expulsive faculty. Galen argued that this selectivity of the body, especially shown in the process of nutrition, distinguished living bodies from things like rocks and cadavers.

To explain the selective action of bodies in taking up nutriment and eliminating waste, Galen and Galenic physicians postulated attractive and retentive faculties responsible for these sorts of actions. Galen ascribed this view of nature, working by attractive and eliminative faculties, to Hippocrates.[137] All parts had the natural faculties of attracting appropriate nutriment—material substance friendly to or like their own—and rejecting opposing substances.[138] The types and structures of fibers or filaments, detectable by dissection, determined the faculties of the mobile organs. As Galen put it, in On the Natural

---

133   Galen, On the Natural Faculties, 2.3, 136–137, K II 87.

134   Galen, On the Natural Faculties, 27, K II 16–17.

135   Galen, On the Natural Faculties, K II, 29–30, trans. Hankinson, "Philosophy of nature," 223.

136   Galen, On the Natural Faculties, 1.10, 32–3, K II 20.

137   Galen, On the Natural Faculties, 1.13, 49, 61, K II 30, 38.

138   Galen, On the Natural Faculties, 1.13, 49, K II 38–39.

Faculties, "the movements of each of the mobile organs of the body depends on the setting of the fibers."[139]

The activity of fibers as basic facultative structures comes through in dissections. They are most obvious in the case of muscles, which show clearly the dependence of the action of the muscles on the direction of the fibers. Other parts mix fibers to have faculties for performing different actions. The stomach has two coats: one for drawing substances along by straight or longitudinal fibers, the other for peristaltic motion by the contraction of transverse fibers. Importantly, it also possesses a retentive faculty, retaining the food until it is properly concocted and changed qualitatively to be more like the parts to which it is then assimilated. The pylorus opens at just the right time to allow the expulsive faculty, acting through the specific structure of the stomach's fibers, to push the nutriment along. The longitudinal fibers contract and elongate, dragging their contents along their lengths. The intestines, too, have transverse, circular fibers, which narrow the passages, generating peristaltic motions.

Crucially, *simple* or *crude* mechanical or material explanations failed to account for the selectivity of facultative actions. For Galen the gallbladder possessed faculties for attracting bile, retaining it, and expelling it at different times. Galen could infer the existence of these faculties from the actions observed or inferred from dissections. His method for articulating "faculties" explicitly traveled back along causal chains, from the observed effect (*ergon*) to the discovery of how this results from a specific bodily activity (*energeia*), to the efficient cause of the activity, the faculty (*dunamis*).[140] In dissections, one sometimes found the gallbladder very full of bile, sometimes empty, sometimes moderately full. For Galen, this indicated that the gallbladder drew in bile, held it for different periods of time, and expelled it. These actions indicated that the gallbladder possessed attractive, retentive, and expulsive faculties. Galen's ancient rival, Erasistratus, could not account for this well-ordered, selective process in terms of the material contractions of the stomach alone.[141]

Another rival, the atomist Asclepiades, denied the presence of selective faculties in the body. Instead, he favored crude material explanations. For instance, he treated the bladder in material terms, as like a cloth or sponge that soaked up and condensed the vapors from what a person drank.[142] But *these* sorts of explanations, at least in such simplistic terms, could not explain

---

139   Galen, *On the Natural Faculties*, 3.8, Brock trans., 263, K II 169.
140   Hankinson, "Philosophy of nature," 224.
141   Galen, *On the Natural Faculties*, 3.4 and 3.5 K II 152–159.
142   Galen, *On the Natural Faculties*, 1.13, K II 32.

the specific selective attraction of bile from the blood, since the serum in the blood was even thinner and finer. Any channels or pores small enough to select for the tiny particles or thin substance of the bile would also allow serum to pass through. Pores-and-particles contrivances for filtering, of the sort atomists such as Asclepiades favored, could not explain *this* selective action in the gallbladder.

Interestingly, Galen used dissections and vivisections to eliminate rival explanations. The brash Asclepiades had described the bladder merely as a sponge or piece of wool, passively letting vapors pass through its coats, which then condensed into urine. Galen countered with an anatomical demonstration of the ureters, which carried urine from the kidneys to the bladder. Yet one rival even challenged Galen by pointing to the common knowledge that a bladder filled and tied at the neck or urethra did not let anything escape—surely any connecting channels would let fluids in and out? Once again, Galen chastised his opponents for estimating Nature's artistic skill by their own. In dead and living animals, he demonstrated by dissection and ligature of vessels that urine flowed from the kidneys through the ureters, into the bladder, and out the urethra, but not back from the bladder into the ureters.[143] The insertion of the vessels prevented this backflow, as in mechanical one-way flow valves.

Similarly, vivisection experiments made against Erasistratus and his followers showed that swallowing did not happen merely passively, due to the pushing of the ingested stuff, but due to the attractive action of the elongating fibers of the inner coat and peristaltic, propulsive action of the outer coat of the esophagus. The throat of a dead man still dilated and contracted outwards and inwards when force-fed water passed through, but it did not contract along its length. And systematic cutting of organ coats in live animals eliminated their characteristic actions and faculties.[144]

Having ruled out competing explanations, Galen argued, we should invoke a "faculty" whenever we observe some regular action the nature or "substance" (*ousia*) of which we do not *yet* fully understand, and which is not *yet* explained otherwise. Thus, lodestones, drugs which draw out poisons, ointments which attract thorns when manual extraction failed, kidneys, gallbladders, and other parts of living bodies all exhibit attractive faculties. Given the phenomenal actions we consistently observe, we must use talk of "faculties" to think in an orderly way about otherwise inexplicable regularities.

Yet Galen and early modern physicians working in the Galenic tradition did not invoke faculties in a knee-jerk fashion. Anatomical studies and clinical

---

143   Galen, *On the Natural Faculties*, 1.13, K II 36–37.
144   Galen, *On the Natural Faculties*, 3.8, K II 171, 175–177.

experience had to indicate the existence of an action, such as the fact that the gallbladder collects bile and not serum, and the kidneys pass on urine. Further, even fine anatomical structure still mattered: the kidneys selected out urine through a combination of an attractive faculty which drew the blood to them and a seemingly porous structure which filtered the attracted matter. Galen needed to postulate an attractive capacity or "faculty" since mere mechanical pressure from weight of the blood in the vena cava and descending aorta would drive most of the blood right past the kidneys, placed on either side of these major vessels. But Galen also argued that attracting organs could filter out thinner, finer fluid from the thicker parts of the blood by means of tiny outlets, so that the kidneys filtered out urine "as if through a strainer."[145] While the kidneys attract the watery substance of the blood and then filter it, at least in part, through a material structure, the bladder does not attract urine, but only receives it due to the action of the kidneys. Thus, as Michael McVaugh argues, Galen "appears to think mechanically up to the point where he has to conclude that mechanical explanation will no longer work, at which point he turns to attraction as an explanatory principle."[146]

Clearly, Galenic faculties were not "mechanical" in the sense of operating *only* as human-made machines do, nor in the sense that they are explained *only* in terms of matter undergoing local motion. But the matter and machine-like actions still played important roles. More important still, though, was the material qualitative mixture of each part, which produced the faculty of a part in relation to an object. Later philosophers who worked explicitly to develop some sort of "mechanical philosophy" differed on many points, many endorsing active principles, some not, but, as Domenico Bertoloni Meli has argued well, what they shared foremost of all was the rejection of souls and faculties as explanations for the actions of living things.[147]

Further, despite Galen's programmatic search for the anatomical specification of bodily actions and diseases, his acceptance of analogies from ancient machines to living things, and his use of fibers and channels to explain some key actions, Galen also tended to conceive of organs and parts as continuous, undergoing continuous *qualitative* changes. Like Aristotle, Galen distinguished his view of continuous matter undergoing continuous, qualitative changes and acting throughout its substance from the atomist view of tiny, discrete,

---

145 Galen, *On the Natural Faculties*, with amended translation from McVaugh, "Losing Ground," 107.

146 McVaugh, "Losing Ground," 109–110.

147 Bertoloni Meli, *Mechanism, Experiment, Disease*, 12–16.

discontinuous parts of matter undergoing rearrangements.[148] Nature, after all, is much more artful than even the best sculptor or engineer, even those who made mobile puppets, such as the apparently self-moving cart of Hero.

Yet Galenic faculties were not obviously "vitalist," either. After all, the lodestone attracting iron remained his model for natural faculties, and he always attributed the substance and cause of faculties to the temperament or qualitative makeup of the objects under consideration. While Galen insisted on the intelligence and power of the creator demonstrated in the things created, especially the heavens and developed bodies, he did not rely on a cosmic vitalism of a universal spirit or a local vitalism of a principle of life distinct from but added to matter.[149] Galen consistently tried to show that the substance of the faculties just was the elemental or qualitative mixture of the parts involved, and most often expressed a cautious agnosticism about the soul.

For the operation of animal and rational faculties beyond the vegetative ones of nutrition, growth, and generation, Galen also had recourse to a directing soul. At least, to the "mortal part of the soul," which according to a late work, just *was* material, namely "the mixture of the body."[150] Galen claimed to know from anatomical or philosophical demonstrations a few things about the soul: that there were three kinds or forms of the soul, that each had its seat in a different location, and that the rational part was "divine" and seated in the brain, the spirited part in the heart, and the desiderative part in the liver.[151] He ascribed to Plato the claim that the rational part of the soul was immortal, but could not himself decide whether it was or not. Despite occasional Stoic claims that the soul was just psychic *pneuma*, he remained explicitly agnostic about its nature or substance.[152] After all, in systematic dissections of the brains of a range of living animals, incising the brain's ventricles must have allowed the fine, active *pneuma* to escape, and thus, according to the theory of the Stoics, should have caused death, yet produced only a variation in the animals' responses, depending on the location and extent of the cut.[153] For Galen, the activity of each part depended on its elemental temperament and the action of a material *pneuma* flowing to the part through channels in the body. Innate heat, especially distributed by *pneuma*, orchestrated the faculties. Galen had identified *pneuma* as the finest, lightest matter of the body, finer than vapor,

---

148   Berryman, "Galen and the Mechanical Philosophy," 238–244.
149   For a concise discussion of Renaissance vitalisms, see Chang, "Alchemy as Studies of Life and Matter."
150   Galen, *The Soul's Dependence on the Body*, trans. Singer, 157, K IV 782. Donini, "Psychology."
151   Galen, *PHP* V 793, in Hankinson, "Partitioning the Soul," 87, 92, 97.
152   Donini, "Psychology," 184–5.
153   Donini, "Psychology," 250–251.

carried through the veins, arteries, and nerves. He distinguished three kinds, natural, vital, and psychic.[154] But his writings, and those of early modern physicians and philosophers, remained shaped by Plato and Aristotle's ascription of the particular capacities of animals to move and sense to a soul (*psuche*).

Of course, Galen's long experience in dissections drove him to advertise the anatomical errors of Aristotle. As Galen and his followers relished pointing out, Aristotle's description of the heart as the seat of perception badly missed the entire nervous system. Anatomical dissections, especially the systematic dissections Galen performed, showed clearly that voluntary motion and sensation in the body depended on the nerves, which had the brain as their center and chief organ. Cutting or tying off the intercostal nerves of a live pig, for example, dramatically proved that these nerves controlled phonation—the pig's screams stopped with the nerves tied, then rent the air when Galen loosed the ties.[155] He explicitly followed Plato, and, he claimed, Hippocrates, in arguing for three chief anatomical seats of different parts of the soul, as noted above. Again and again, Galen followed his anatomical experiments, reasoning, and matter theory as far as he could to identify the faculties and nature of the mortal soul.

In sum, across his works Galen emphatically denied that his faculties or powers were immaterial additions "inhabiting" material parts of bodies, medicines, or magnetic lodestones. Except for the marvelous order and craftsmanship displayed in nature, and especially in the anatomy of bodies, Galen argued for grounding the entities of his world in matter. The temperament of a given sort of matter (flesh, fire, lodestone, heating drug) produced or just was the substance of its faculties. Explanations in terms of the soul did not play much of a role, especially in his later works in which he argued for a more materialist reading of the soul itself in terms of the mixtures or temperaments of the body. While early modern physicians took care to keep more theological space for the soul, they followed the main lines of Galen's accounts and uses of faculties.

5   Early Modern Medical Discussions of Faculties

Leiden professors and students worked with an eclectic but very Galenic understanding of faculties. After all, they studied, quoted, and systematized many of the same texts we have just surveyed in the previous section. Galen's

---

154   Brock, "Introduction," in Galen, *On the Natural Faculties*, xxxv.
155   Galen, *On Anatomical Procedures*, trans. Singer, 217. Galen, *On Anatomical Procedures*, trans. Duckworth, 210–212, K I 672–675.

On the Natural Faculties, his major focused discussion of faculties, which we reviewed in the previous section, appeared in at least ten editions from 1537 to 1596.[156] This work also informed medical education across Europe, with frequent citations in textbooks such as Fuchs's *Institutes*, Fernel's *Whole of Medicine* (*Universa Medicina*), and Johannes Heurnius' *Institutes*.[157] These physicians, and many others, embraced a Galenic eclecticism, with various Aristotelian, Platonic, and Paracelsian inflections. Their discussions of the faculties, though, in emulation and critique, engaged most of all with Galen's works. In this section, we will survey some select moments in this broad engagement and debate.

Throughout the 1500s, physicians debated definitions of natural and bodily faculties, often alternating or combining the more localized, reductive accounts found in Galen with definitions referring faculties to the power or activity of the soul. In the middle of the 1550s, Leonhart Fuchs, for example, argued in his textbook that physicians should follow Galen's arguments for reducing faculties to local temperaments of organs and parts. They should leave philosophical ways of speaking about faculties coming forth from the soul to the philosophers.[158] Other professors and physicians maintained a similar distinction, and emphasized Galen's more material notion.

Giambattista da Monte, teaching at Padua in the 1540s until his death in 1551, discussed faculties at length in his lectures, which students published after his death. Commenting on the second fen of Avicenna's *Canon*, Da Monte suggested that Galen and Aristotle actually taught the same *method* for identifying faculties: specify the object, then the operation acting on it, and then trace back to the faculty of the acting subject. But Da Monte instructed his students to follow Galen's more material definition. Faculties are the immediate causes of actions, and the acts of a given "organic body," but "not as you know from Aristotle."[159] The operation of a faculty is not from the simple form of the single soul, but from the composite form of the organic body and its parts. As Da Monte noted, Galen taught clearly in his *Dependence of the Soul on the Mixtures of the Body* (QAM) that the actions and faculties depended on the mixture or complexion of the acting parts. According to the grade or degree of the qualitative or quantitative fault in the complexion of the part or parts, different

---

156   Durling, "Chronological Census," 259, 263, 264, 265, 267, 269, 274, 278, 279.

157   Fuchs, *Institutiones*, 19, 74, 93, 175, 185, 369. Fernel, *Universa Medicina*, 85, 101, 102, 130, 134, 138, 145. Johannes Heurnius, *Institutiones*, 13, 72, 73, 78, 80, 84, 170.

158   Fuchs, *Institutiones*, 165–166: "According to Galen, it is nothing other than the natural constitution, or the native temperament of things."

159   Da Monte, *Lectiones...In secundam Fen primi Canonis Avicennae*, 23–24. Here Da Monte may have reflected the naturalism about the soul learned from his teacher Pomponazzi. See Siraisi, *Avicenna in the Renaissance*, 290.

sicknesses resulted. All sicknesses came from either a bad complexion of the simple parts (flesh, nerves, etc.), or a fault in the composition of many simple parts into a complex part (e.g., a hand), or the dissolution of natural continuity. Thus, for Da Monte, anatomical faults impaired facultative actions, which constituted diseases.[160]

On the soul, Da Monte went even further, insisting that Galen, Hippocrates, and Aristotle all taught that a thing's substantial form and temperament were identical. Revelation and theology, as well as "the Arabs and more recent Latin writers," taught the opposite, that the body's substantial form (the soul, *anima*) and its temperament were distinct.[161] Yet philosophers and physicians, speaking as such, had to follow the force of proper reasoning, concluding that the organic soul (the *anima*, or principle of life), not the rational soul, was the proper temperament of the living body and thus was mortal. Divine theology might teach otherwise, that the substantial form of the living body was immortal, but Da Monte judged that there was "nothing worse than to mix philosophy with theology."[162]

In contrast to Fuchs and Da Monte, the influential French physician and medical philosopher Jean Fernel entertained Galen's obvious materialism about faculties, then firmly rejected this materialist explanation as the complete story.[163] He propounded a Christian and Platonic interpretation of Galen's texts, for instance emphasizing ideas of the soul and other entities shaping matter. Fernel tried to reduce materialistic interpretations, emphasizing the activities of an intelligent, wise, and powerful Creator, foresighted Nature, or a "crafting faculty," rather than the mixture of the elements, as the makers of the heavens, earth, and living bodies.[164]

In his *Physiologia*, Fernel insisted on an immortal, immaterial, incorporeal Platonic intellectual soul, and attacked the "philosophers" who argued that even the soul as the form of the body was divided and not unitary.[165] Here he may have had in mind an influential tradition, defended by Averroes, Avicenna, and Thomas Aquinas, of ascribing independent powers to the soul's faculties, rather than thinking of them as the soul itself acting.[166] Although he only explicitly attacked the "Averroists" for their over-reliance on material

---

160 Much further discussion on this point appears in chapter five.

161 Da Monte, quoted in Siraisi, *Avicenna in the Renaissance*, 290.

162 Da Monte, quoted in Siraisi, *Avicenna in the Renaissance*, 292, n. 108, my trans.

163 Fuchs, *Institutiones*, 165. Fernel, *Universa Medina*, 96.

164 Hirai, *Medical Humanism*, 53.

165 Fernel, *Physiologia*, trans. Forrester, 393.

166 After Fernel, Suarez and Zabarella would defend some notion of independent powers as well. William of Auvergne, William of Ockham, and others attacked it and defended some version of the alternative. See Perler, "Faculties in Medieval Philosophy."

explanation, he may also have had in mind the surge of Aristotelian philoso-phy in the 1500s which explored systems of pluralities and hierarchies of sub-stantial forms, often allied with corpuscular explanations. Pluralists rejected the Thomist idea that substances had only one, single form, while the forms of the elements became corrupted. They held that the parts of bodies and other complex things retained their own forms, but subordinated to the substantial form of the whole. This often included corpuscularian explanations, as in the case of J. C. Scaliger discussed above, since corpuscles or atoms with their own forms made good sense of chymical phenomena.[167]

Against pluralists such as J. C. Scaliger, Fernel proclaimed that each living thing had only one sort of soul, either natural (plants), sentient (animals), or intelligent (humans).[168] This soul was the living thing's single substantial form, given by the heavens or World Soul, and responsible for the construction and faculties of living bodies. Following Plato and Aristotle, it still made sense to talk of natural, sentient, and intelligent "parts" of a single soul, uniting in "har-mony." Fernel contradicted physicians and naturalists of Aristotelian leaning, such as Fuchs, and instead argued that a faculty really was a power the soul brings out, as it were, from its pocket or "bosom" (*sinus*), as a property of the soul or as if part of the soul itself.[169]

For Fernel, humans possess only one soul, immortal, immaterial, and simple. This one soul itself is the "principle and cause of the functions of the living body."[170] Though the soul is one in essence, we can distinguish "parts" by their actions. Our mind or intelligence is the "ruler and queen" of all the other so-called parts of the animate soul, and clearly knows things that are incor-poreal and immaterial, the "universal concepts and forms of things," "unlim-ited knowledge of innumerable things," and things hidden and distinct from every sense and the body.[171] Thus, we recognize immediately that "its essence is simple, individual, abstracted from all matter and body," and does not need a bodily instrument to act.

The external senses transfer the qualities of external things to internal senses, which receive "images" of these, which are presented to the mind.[172] The common sense or internal faculty of distinguishing, comparing, and judging

---

167   Newman, *Atoms and Alchemy*, 36–43, 108–115. Blank, *Biomedical Ontology*.
168   Fernel, *Physiologia*, trans. Forrester., 306.
169   Fernel, *Physiologia*, trans. Forrester, 309.
170   Fernel, *Physiologia*, 304, my trans. For more discussion of Fernel in relation to longer Aris-totelian and Galenic traditions, as well as to Descartes, see Sloan, "Galenizing Descartes," *forthcoming*.
171   Fernel, *Physiologia*, trans. Forrester, 357, 395.
172   Fernel, *Physiologia*, trans. Forrester, 359.

these images, "like a ruling governor, occupies a permanent sure place in the body of the brain, which it uses like a platform for surveying the images."[173] These images are "branded and carved on the brain"; if they are imprinted more deeply, they are retained longer in the memory.[174] While the sensitive part of the soul is spread throughout the whole of the brain, the single unified soul needs no brain for higher-order abstract thinking about particular and universal forms.[175] It acts on the images and fashions concepts, ultimately reaching universal, eternal, necessary, and divine concepts, and thus enacting a life of wisdom.[176] On its own, independently of the body, the "independent free mind thinks, reasons, and remembers," distinguishing of what sort things are "purely and clearly." These actions of the mind the soul performed on its own. For other faculties and actions, though, the soul needed "the help of the bodily faculties [*corporearum facultatum*]."[177]

Even for Fernel, anatomy and material qualities and causes mattered. Neither the elements nor the temperaments of the parts were the essence or the causes of the faculties.[178] Yet the bodily faculties operated through the parts of the body according to their elemental temperaments and structures, as coordinated by the innate heat carried by the *spiritus*, and as instruments which flowed from the soul.[179] Even the initial stages of mentally "distinguishing, and fashioning in thought, and remembering" used the services of the brain, which is fit for these activities in its temperament, size, shape, and *spiritus* contained in its vessels.[180] All natural, animal, and vital faculties worked this way, from attraction of materially similar substances to sensation and nutrition. Like Galen, Fernel still employed natural faculties to explain the action of lodestones turning toward the Earth's poles, and the action of some drugs. These natural faculties or powers were common to living and non-living things.

Anatomical fibers played central roles in Fernel's vision of bodily faculties, and those of other physicians.[181] Fernel even went so far as to argue that dissection allows one to enumerate the fibers and faculties: "the number of faculties residing in each part can be discovered from the variety of its functions, and

---

173   Fernel, *Physiologia*, trans. Forrester, 337.
174   Fernel, *Physiologia*, trans. Forrester, 339.
175   Fernel, *Physiologia*, trans. Forrester, 361. Here Fernel terms this the "active intelligence," following Aristotelian terminology.
176   Fernel, *Physiologia*, trans. Forrester, 497–499.
177   Fernel, *Physiologia*, trans. Forrester, 395.
178   Fernel, *Physiologia*, trans. Forrester, 523.
179   Hirai, *Medical Humanism*, 57–74.
180   Fernel, *Physiologia*, 350, my trans.
181   Siraisi, *Avicenna in the Renaissance*, 329. Cheung, "Omnis Fibra Ex Fibra," 70–74.

accounts for the different sorts of its filaments. And conversely, the variety of filaments determined by dissection declares the number of faculties of any part."[182] Like Galen, Vesalius, and other physicians such as Johannes Heurnius at Leiden, Fernel often explained the attractive, retentive, and expulsive faculties of organs, especially digestive organs, by the structure and action of their straight, oblique, and circular fibers. Similarity of nutriment and the substance of a bodily part could explain passive attraction, and, for Vesalius, all parts could attract, retain, and expel by a force or power seated in each part.[183] Other anatomists, such as Falloppio, used their new dissection-based knowledge to disagree, for instance rejecting the idea that the gallbladder attracted, retained, and expelled bile by faculties. Instead, he argued, the gentle pressure of the liver in upright creatures, or the stomach in "beasts" pressed out the bile into the intestines.[184]

Writing around the same time as Heurnius, the philosopher Rudolph Goclenius of Marburg sketched the broader semantic field for the meanings of "faculty" in his *Philosophical Dictionary*.[185] Most properly, a "faculty" is a quality by which whatever is capable to be affected in a certain way, is affected. In good Aristotelian terms, it can be an active or passive potency, as an aptitude for acting or receiving action. Some defined it as an efficient cause, drawing on Galen's discussions we have just seen from *On the Natural Faculties* and *Quod Animi Mores*. Active faculties likely derived from or were part of the form, since actions proceeded from the form. Per Aristotle, there are faculties of the human arts: the orator has the faculty of persuasion, the physician the faculty of healing or spoiling health. Art itself is a faculty, since it is turned toward an object in our power, which determines whether or not something comes about. In machines, levers, pulleys, wedges, and screws are all faculties, since "by them great weights and loads can be moved and raised up."[186] Just as with Galen, early modern physicians and philosophers thought of faculties as relational concepts, and they did not need to seek them in immaterial powers— even a block wedge could provide a faculty for moving or raising objects.

At Leiden, Heurnius and his students drew on Fernel's Christian Platonic reading of Galen, and their own strong emphasis on the temperaments of the parts, to frame an eclectic Leiden doctrine of faculties. Following Galen, Heurnius taught students to define "faculty" as "the efficient cause of all actions,

---

182   Fernel, *Physiologia*, trans. Forrester, 329.
183   Vesalius, *Fabrica* (1543), 258.
184   Falloppio, *Observationes Anatomicae* (1561), 177v. Siraisi, *Avicenna in the Renaissance*, 307–9.
185   Goclenius, *Lexicon Philosophicum*, 565–566.
186   Goclenius, *Lexicon Philosophicum*, 566.

seated in the proper temperament of each thing."[187] He also noted Galen's insistence that the essence or substance of a faculty consisted from the hot, cold, wet, and dry principal qualities. As in Fernel's work, for Heurnius a special innate heat was the substance of the faculties of the body, or at least their primary and necessary instrument.

It is important to note that Heurnius moved from a fascinating discussion of *spiritus* in the cosmos and living bodies to the faculties. This was only natural since the three sorts of *spiritus* act as "the vehicles of the powers of the soul."[188] As in Galen, the natural spirit formed principally in the liver pervades all the parts, while the hot vital spirit carried by the heart and arteries heats and vivifies the parts, and the animal spirit generated in the ventricles of the brain flows through the nerves to provide motion and sensation. But Heurnius added alchemical and Stoic ideas, too. All *spiritus* or spirits are airy or aetherial bodies, "elaborated" (as in alchemical distillation) from the purest part of the blood, and changed into a hot, very thin, windy substance. As the Stoic philosophers argued, there is a spirit of the whole cosmos, poured out from the heavens, and especially the Sun, from which all things draw life. Even metals and gems vegetate and grow deep in the "viscera" of the earth due to the vivifying heat of the Sun.[189] Aristotle and Avicenna both attested to this vivifying spirit's closeness to a celestial nature, and its active power in the generation of living things: Aristotle's *Generation of Animals* 2.3 taught that this spirit is contained in the seed or semen and a "foam-like body," and the spirit is "analogous to the element of the stars."[190]

For Heurnius, physicians used the term *faculty* rightly, in the sense of the efficient cause of a bodily action or function, when they expressed "the various aptitudes of the soul."[191] Siding with Aristotle, Heurnius insisted on thinking of a unitary soul which makes something the sort of thing that it is, and is the efficient cause of the various works or functions (*functiones*) of the body. Thus, Galen's frequent reduction of the substance of bodily faculties to the proper temperaments of the parts absurdly overlooked the faculties as powers of the unitary soul. Speaking *philosophically*, Fernel had it better when he described the faculties as coming forth from the "bosom" of the soul.

---

187   Johannes Heurnius, *Institutiones*, 66. Here Heurnius quoted from Galen's work on simple drugs: Galen, *De simplicium medicamentorum facultatibus libri XI*, 2–3. Kühn XI, 381. He also referred to Galen's *On the Natural Faculties*.

188   Johannes Heurnius, *Institutiones*, 66.

189   Johannes Heurnius, *Institutiones*, 62.

190   Aristotle, quoted in Hiro Hirai, *Medical Humanism and Natural Philosophy*, 25–6.

191   Johannes Heurnius, *Institutiones*, 70.

Yet anatomy and matter remained essential objects of study, since the variety of bodily actions and functions comes from the differences of the "structure and temperament" of the various parts of the body.[192] Of course, Heurnius agreed with Galen and other philosophers that non-living things also displayed faculties, so, speaking philosophically, faculties in general are the most proximate and chief causes bringing forth actions, or, in short, they are the forms of things. The soul or *anima*, as Aristotle showed, just was the power of the living body, and the first cause of actions. Soul or form had unity and causal priority; diversity of action followed from the diversity of the matter. While the soul was unitary, as the one form of the living thing, it acted through the organs ("instruments") of the body, as the author of sense and motion in the brain and nerves, of the pulse in the heart, and of blood in the liver. Each of these organs and parts, in turn, had the proper "structure and temperament" for bringing about their proper facultative actions.[193] The specific matter, especially the innate or native heat, of each part determined how the soul used each part as an instrument for its proper action. Different faculties are powers of a single form or soul of the body, just as Aristotle said the figures of the triangle and quadrilateral are in potentiality in the pentagon.[194]

Most philosophically, Heurnius argued, a given faculty should be defined as the most proximate and chief cause bringing forth an action characteristic of a thing—a faculty is thus the form of the thing.[195] Parts of living bodies have forms constituted by their distinct temperaments (qualitative mixtures) and anatomical structures. At least, this is how to understand forms, and hence, faculties, as "accidental." Taken as "essential," the form and faculties of a living body are defined in terms of the soul and its operations. This is not the immortal, rational soul of course, but the *anima* as the potency of the living body, the chief cause of the actions of the living body.[196]

Despite his philosophical definition of a faculty as essentially part of or an action of the organic soul, like other physicians Heurnius hewed closely to material accounts of faculties in his medicine, and emphasized material-qualitative interventions to restore their proper actions. He particularly prized Galen's explanations of the anatomical bases of these facultative actions, constructing an easy scheme for his students: the attractive faculty uses right fibers, the expulsive transverse, and the retentive oblique. Thus the gallbladder,

---

192   Johannes Heurnius, *Institutiones*, 69.
193   Johannes Heurnius, *Institutiones*, 69.
194   Aristotle, *De anima*, II.3, trans. W. S. Hett, 83.
195   Johannes Heurnius, *Institutiones*, 67, cf. 59–69.
196   Johannes Heurnius, *Institutiones*, 68.

uterus, veins, stomach, and intestines, all attract, retain, and expel by means of anatomical fibers with specific structural orientations.[197]

Variations in the actions of faculties depended on the materials and qualities of the body. Like most other Galenic physicians, Heurnius taught that a "pulsific faculty" caused the motions of the heart and arteries—systole (contraction) and diastole (expansion)—and the periods of rest after each one.[198] By "necessity," when the temperament of the heart changes due to causes such as the heat of wrath, hot food, or exercise, the faculty of the pulse changes, becoming more violent in its action.[199] All the dozens of different pulses Galen took pains to taxonomize—violent, languid, hard, great, small, intermittent, undulating, worming, hectic, turbulent, etc.—follow from the causal effects of the qualitative changes of the temperament of the heart.

Later, Gilbertus Jacchaeus (Gilbert Jack, ca. 1585–1628) a Scottish teaching philosopher and physician at Leiden, also distinguished between the physician's purview of bodily parts and their faculties and actions, and the philosopher's disputation about the nature of the living soul. He commended Aristotle for exceeding the industriousness of all philosophers in explaining the soul (*anima*), and recommended his account of the soul as the form of the body and the efficient cause of all its operations. The body's actions come about by faculties, inherent to different body parts, which must be disposed in the proper way for them to function, in structure and temperament. Thus, faculties mediate between the soul and the actions. Philosophers or logicians might dispute about the nature of the soul and discourse about the rational faculty of the soul, but the physician did not since the rational faculty does not inform a part of the body. But even the rational faculty "depends antecedently on an organ," the brain, whose impaired structure or temperament remained part of the physician's purview to diagnose and treat.[200]

Across the renaissance of anatomical practice beyond Leiden, anatomy mattered for the operation of faculties. In the early sixteenth century, the anatomist and surgeon Berengario performed experimental tests of kidney filtration. Attempting to weigh in on ancient and medieval debates, he wanted to know whether the kidneys filtered passively, due to their material structure alone.[201] As mentioned above, anatomical fibers and structures remained important to

---

197   Johannes Heurnius, *Institutiones*, 85.
198   Johannes Heurnius, *Institutiones*, 339. Bylebyl, "Disputation and Description."
199   Johannes Heurnius, *Institutiones*, 342, 348.
200   Jacchaeus, *Institutiones medicae*, 40.
201   McVaugh, "Losing Ground."

Vesalius's explanations of many facultative actions, though he also noted the importance of powers or faculties implanted in all the parts, apart from fibers.

In the seventeenth century, structural explanations continued to work hand-in-hand with facultative thinking. The leading Galenic anatomist Jean Riolan (1580–1657) advanced even more localized structural explanations of the action of faculties, which he tested by experiment. Riolan used his dissections of kidneys to argue that the selective facultative action occurred in their small eight to eighteen glandular structures.[202]

In sum, it is clear that later critiques of faculties as unquestioned covers for ignorance or in opposition to anatomical or rigorous philosophical thinking cannot be sustained as historically accurate. Galen's notion of "faculty" reveals his sophisticated logical thinking, his close attention to anatomical phenomena, his philosophical caution about identifying the substance of a poorly-known relation, and his frequent critical use of material and even mechanical explanations. True, Galen and his critical followers often rejected crude or simplistic material explanations, such as fanciful pores-and-particles speculations to explain bodily selectivity. But they followed material anatomical phenomena to generate and revise their facultative explanations, and reached for what seemed to them the best-established matter theories and philosophies of the soul, and action and passion.

Scholastic philosophers developed a lively critique of the various philosophical explanations for such capacities or powers for centuries in the medieval and early modern periods. Early modern Galenic physicians followed them in taking the soul as philosophically primary in causal or substantial accounts of the faculties. But they also sharply distinguished their own emphasis on material, qualitative, and anatomical thinking, which served the art of medicine. Even Heurnius' philosophical defense of the soul or even the World Soul in schemes of facultative action and bodily powers, inspired by Fernel, bowed to a much more mundane and perceptible medical practice of body parts, sensible qualities, and perceptible phenomena in his teaching and practice, as we will see in the following sections.

Renaissance Galenists' understandings of faculties remain misunderstood by historians, in a way that reflects the superficial critiques of their rivals. In the early modern period, with the rise of anatomical dissection, Aristotelian naturalism, Platonic natural philosophy, and chymistry, physicians and philosophers articulated compelling accounts of faculties which attempted to do justice to the epistemic demands of anatomy, theology, matter theory, logic,

---

202   McVaugh, "Losing Ground," 123.

and a range of ancient sources. John Locke and other seventeenth-century critics of appeals to faculties dismissed such thinking, but aimed at a caricature. According to Locke, "faculties" were circular pseudo-explanations which stopped inquiry: "For it being asked, what it was that digested the Meat in our Stomachs? It was a ready, and very satisfactory Answer, to say: That it was the *digestive Faculty*."[203]

Locke's polemical critique badly misses the mark. Digestion, like other bodily faculties, worked through the best anatomical and philosophical causes physicians could find. For Galen, as for Heurnius and countless other physicians before Locke, digestion in the stomach works necessarily through the shortening of the fibers in two coats around the stomach. One sort, the longitudinal fibers, pull food in; the other, transverse fibers, extend and contract and move it along. During digestion, the pylorus closes tightly and the stomach contracts around the food, squeezing and cooking it through its heat and temperament to help transform it into nutriment through qualitative changes. This takes time. Pigs dissected a few hours after a big meal of wheat flour and water still show food in their stomachs, a procedure Galen often carried out.[204] Like other organs, the stomach worked through its anatomical structure and temperament, as revealed through dissections. As Aristotle showed in his works on generation and corruption and meteorology, which academic Galenists knew well, digestion by gentle cooking and qualitative changes happened due to the four primary qualities and anatomical structures, as did most bodily changes.[205] In addition to its temperament of the four primary qualities, the stomach may have had a special power of changing different sorts of food into the same sort of nutrifying chyle, a power that escaped direct sensation or reasoning, but digestion was not a black box, with the word "faculty" covering sheer ignorance.[206]

Locke certainly rejected the real primary qualities of Aristotle, Galen, and many of his predecessors, but that does not mean they did not use them in sophisticated, sensory-based accounts of the body's action and its faculties. His objection does not do justice to rich notions of late Renaissance Galenic faculties, grounded in anatomical observation and a range of natural philosophical concepts and commitments, and gradually developing into better anatomical and philosophical accounts of their substance and action.

---

203   Locke, *An Essay concerning Humane Understanding*, 130.
204   Galen, *On the Natural Faculties*, III.4 and III.8. Johannes Heurnius, *Institutiones*, 78–86, follows Galen closely.
205   Galen, *On the Natural Faculties*, III.8.
206   Johannes Heurnius, *Institutiones*, 80. Fernel, *Physiologia*, trans. Forrester., 404–405.

6   Conclusions

Leiden University medical theory over its first five decades was more and less than historians have thought. It was more substantive, for one thing. Professors readily extended theory beyond description or historical accounts.[207] Extensive theory, harvested from ancient, medieval, and early modern sources, but above all Galenic works, had a foundational place. It was far less "vitalist," mysterious, or credulous since the key dispositive properties for action, faculties, derived from material structures and qualitative temperaments in relation to some other object (which received action according to its own temperament). Clearly, describing faculties as "immaterial" or "nonmaterial" is not accurate, and stands at odds with the persistent material thinking and tendency toward materialization of the medical professors.[208] While philosophers could follow Aristotle in speaking of faculties of the soul, physicians self-consciously turned the other way, and emphasized material structures and bodily qualities. Physicians' faculties were not immaterial additions to the substance or stuff of bodily parts, magnets, or drugs, but relative causal powers that always worked through and from the material structure and qualitative temperament of the acting thing.

Temperaments, too, had a different definition than is often advertised. Despite persistent claims by historians, early modern Galenic physicians did not describe temperaments in terms of whole-body mixtures of the humors.[209] Physicians emphasized the temperaments of individual parts and organs, and always in terms of their fundamental mixture of the four qualities. After all, these were the basic principles of the world, and the grounds for faculties.

The fact that this account closely followed Galen's own teaching strongly suggests that thinking of faculties as extra, immaterial entities inhabiting material objects was widely rejected in other medical schools, too. As Linda Deer Richardson noted some time ago, in the middle of the 1500s eminent teaching professors Da Monte in Padua and Jacobus Sylvius (Jacques Dubois) in Paris both identified the essence of a faculty with the temperament of the relevant part.[210]

There were frequent puzzles and objections to temperament theory in the sixteenth century. For example, that the different temperaments of the organs

207   *Pace* Cook, *Matters of Exchange*, 111.
208   *Pace* Cook, "Medicine," 426; Bertoloni Meli, *Mechanism*, 11.
209   Cf. Stolberg, "Post-mortems," 75. Siraisi, *Avicenna in the Renaissance*, 24–27, 296–305. *Pace* Maclean, *Logic, Signs, and Nature*, 241.
210   Deer Richardson, "The Generation of Disease," 177–178.

could not really be felt, that recourse to faculties should be restricted in favor of *spiritus* and occult causes, as Fernel argued, or that Hippocrates had not really used the concept. But, as Nancy Siraisi has mentioned in her study of commentaries on the first *fen* of Avicenna's *Canon*, nearly every academic physician commenting on the subject adopted some sort of Galenic temperament theory to link drugs, diseases, diagnosis, and treatment through their sense-based realism about the primary qualities.[211] Temperament was central to Galenic physicians' causal thinking, and grounded on their sensory realism about primary qualities as the primary causes of natural changes.

It is worth flagging the relation between temperaments as qualitative mixtures and the seats of faculties, and concepts and practices of pathology and therapy. We will discuss these relations much further in the context of early modern teaching and practice of diagnosis, pathology, and therapy in chapters five and six. For now, it is worth repeating that when Galen, Heurnius, and other early modern Galenists mentioned temperaments or mixtures of the body, they almost always meant the basic qualitative mixtures making up the principal parts, simple parts (such as flesh, bone, sinew, etc.), organs, and humors. Galen frequently mentioned health as "balance" and disease as "imbalance," but he almost always defined these in terms of relations of the four *qualities* hot, cold, dry, and wet, especially of various organs, and *never* as a simple description of the four humors in general.[212] Sensible and localizable qualitative and structural changes could impair or restore organ function, and they concentrated their senses—sight and touch, especially—on identifying these.

Depending on how we understand the term, medical theory at Leiden was either more or less "empirical" than we and early modern proponents of the new science have assumed. As was the case with their theories of drugs, discussed in the next chapter, from our point of view this approach seems *too* "empirical"—they took the most prominent sensory qualities as important agents of physical changes. The four qualities of hot, cold, wet, and dry stood out as the fundamental and everyday principles of change, according to venerable tradition and daily experience. Ancient authorities such as the Hippocratic author of *The Nature of Man*, the philosophers Empedocles and especially Aristotle, and most influential, for physicians, Galen himself, founded their theories of natural changes on these four qualities.

From our present-day view, we might easily overlook the power and ubiquity of this way of thinking, and perhaps favor the attacks of ancient and early

---

211   Siraisi, *Avicenna in the Renaissance*, 296–300.
212   Kaye, *A History of Balance*, 168. For further discussion, see chapter five.

modern critics. We could join with the ancient Empirics in rejecting these writers' jump from repeated sensation of hot, cold, dry, and wet to assuming these are the philosophical causes of things. With them, we could stick to phenomenal descriptions and avoid speculations about causes. Or we could celebrate the emergence of mechanical or corpuscular philosophies, which dismissed the four qualities and faculties as explanatory or ontological principles.

To generate some historical sympathy for our Galenic actors, we should remember that it is not obvious that the speculative subvisible mechanisms of Descartes and Boyle, and the different empiricism of Locke, were great improvements. As Margaret Wilson sharply argued some time ago, we probably should not sign on to the qualitative theories of Descartes, Boyle, or Locke, over those of their more traditionalist opponents.[213] Despite strict mechanists' heroic (or quixotic) efforts to rid matter of qualities or modes beyond size, shape, and motion, other powers persisted and proliferated. Active powers, qualities, and forces only multiplied in new and productive forms from chymical affinity theory to Newtonian physics.[214]

Even the noted mechanical philosopher and chymist Robert Boyle developed a view of chymical powers and properties as non-reducible to the strictly "mechanical" qualities such as size, shape, motion, and arrangement. As Marina Paola Banchetti-Robini concludes in a very recent study, Boyle argued for chymical properties, such as solubility or salinity, as "dispositional, relational, and emergent properties."[215] Building on work by Boyle scholars such as Peter Anstey and William Newman, Banchetti-Robini shows that Boyle held to a fundamental ontology of particles characterized only by size, shape, and mobility, which formed corpuscular concretions, which Boyle called "texture."[216] But the chymical properties could not be reduced to this austere ontology. Instead, they are emergent dispositions or powers inclining a body to affect or to be affected by other bodies in certain ways. They are also relational: they emerge only in the interactions between bodies or chymical substances in the proper settings.[217] Unlike the speculative, hasty Cartesians, Boyle refrained from establishing direct links between chymical qualities and his fundamental mechanical ontology.

---

213   Wilson, "History of Philosophy in Philosophy Today."

214   E.g.: Henry, "Occult Qualities and the Experimental Philosophy." Newman, "Elective Affinity."

215   Banchetti-Robino, *The Chemical Philosophy of Robert Boyle*, ch. 4.

216   Banchetti-Robino, *The Chemical Philosophy of Robert Boyle*, 112–113. Newman, *Atoms*, 182–192. Anstey, *Philosophy of Robert Boyle*, 47–49, 68–69, 80–88, 90–99.

217   Banchetti-Robino, *The Chemical Philosophy of Robert Boyle*, 167.

Boyle's view of chymical powers was remarkably similar to the Galenic notion of faculties. Both distinguished the causal effects and properties of material things as dispositions or powers, as relational properties between things, and as emergent rather than reducible to their fundamental ontologies. Of course, their ontologies differed starkly, with Galenists committed to the "best" natural philosophy of hot, cold, wet, and dry mixtures and Boyle holding to his universal basic matter possessing size, shape, and motion. But thinking through the baffling diversity of the powers of things in terms of dispositional, relational, and emergent properties was a productive and powerful use of reason for Galenists and Boyleans alike. Both camps' accounts counted as rational explanations, whatever the tensions in their open-ended programs, and despite Locke's sneering.

Since temperament theory based on the primary qualities was so foundational to Galenic medicine, it was a vulnerable soft spot for attacks using different, rival philosophical principles. Polemical, philosophical assaults from Paracelsus began in the 1520s, and revived with the increasing popularity of his works in the 1560s. Jean Fernel mounted an attack closer to home in the middle of the 1500s, writing an influential medical textbook which demoted temperament in favor of *spiritus*, the soul, and occult causes. As is well known, celebrated champions of the new science wrote works weaponized in campaigns against the Aristotelian-Galenic theories of qualities, temperaments, and forms: Francis Bacon (1620), Galileo (1623), Descartes (1637), and Van Helmont (1648). By the middle of the 1600s, cumulative assaults on this foundational Aristotelian-Galenic natural philosophical system broke into open war. Our own historical understanding of how these ideas worked in medical education seems to be a casualty of this intellectual and social warfare. I hope to have helped remedy our historical understanding by identifying some of the major intellectual casualties.

Inevitably, early modern medical theory traveled back to bodies, with perceptions of bodies shaped by the senses and books. Joining a chorus of others, Leiden teachers certainly rejected the idea that there was only one sex with different, inverted anatomical arrangements. Yet their medicine was not egalitarian. They maintained that only men could be learned physicians, and that women's distinguishing function was child-bearing. Through ideals of learning, exercises and hazards for embodied learners, curricula of books and lectures, and theory from elements to faculties, professors led students to understand healthy and diseased bodies in material, sense-based terms. There was a marked trend toward teaching more recent, innovative works in anatomy and philosophy, as well the professor's own texts, ideas, and experiences. Most notably, a clear rise in emphasis on the local and material nature of diseases developed in concert with a far greater emphasis on localized therapy in the courses on the practice of medicine, as we will see in later chapters. Increasingly, too, professors and students followed ancient methods and checked their teachings with the sensory phenomena displayed in drugs, the ingredients of drugs, and the operations used to make them. We will see this and more as we turn to the materials, methods, and faculties of medicines in the next chapter. After all, the university garden is just out the back door, its hundreds of plants growing in neat rows and its gallery building stocked with the essential books, and animal and mineral specimens, of the new humanist discipline of natural history.

CHAPTER 4

Learning to Make Medicines: Reading, Viewing, Tasting, and Testing

> For by experience the faculty of a simple remedy is known. With these cautions for this work: Let the remedy examined not be mixed, and be given to a healthy human, or one occupied by a simple disease. Let it be a pure remedy, not imbued with any other quality than its own: and discern what is exerted by its own power, and what by another. If you bring judgment to this matter, experience will be more steadfast. However, many things escape judgment, such as those which follow from substance or essence, and are to be explored by use alone.
>
> –JOHANNES HEURNIUS, *Institutiones Medicinae*, 482

∙ ∙ ∙

> If God had not been present, and poured powers into plants, / What, I ask, would dittany, would panaceas help?
>
> –JOHANNES HEURNIUS, *Institutiones Medicinae*, 554

∙∙
∙

Learning about medicines joined the lecture hall and the garden, since practices of knowing and experiencing medicinal ingredients and compound drugs developed in close spatial and intellectual proximity. For medical students, the most obvious places for first-hand practical instruction were the garden (founded 1590), the anatomy theater (founded 1593), and especially bedside teaching in the hospital (begun at least by 1636, and likely earlier). The garden grew just behind the Academic Building, and the theater lay just across the canal in front. Since the anatomical and clinical practices drew together many of the forms and methods of knowledge cultivated across the curriculum, we will look at those in the following chapters.

Now we have the chance to learn about the primary form of medical intervention: medicines. Historians have noted some of the sophisticated

© EVAN R. RAGLAND, 2022 | DOI:10.1163/9789004515727_006

combinations of theory and practice, and the debates over the ancient sources, which characterized Leiden teachings on pharmacology.[1] Here, we will add important pieces of theory and practice, notably previously-unknown early chymical teaching, the foundational importance of Galen's writings on drugs, professor's methodologies for making trials or tests of medicinal ingredients, and professors' discussions of drug temperaments and faculties in the context of fifteenth-century debates over these topics.

First, we will stay in the lecture hall to hear about the essential importance of chymistry for medicine and even daily life, a message emphasized by the courses on practical medicine taught at Leiden for several decades. Deeply Galenic physicians at Leiden embraced practices and ideas from this new, often rival, discipline. Historians of alchemy and chymistry have also omitted its important place in even the earliest period of medical instruction at Leiden.[2] By 1587, and very likely earlier, medical students received instruction about basic chymical operations and recipes for making chymical medicines. It is quite possible they could learn more of the theory and secrets of the art, even as part of the curriculum. Their professor Johannes Heurnius had published an enthusiastic history and summary of Paracelsian-flavored alchemy as a preface to three ostensibly medieval treatises on alchemical transmutation.[3] He even included some personal, attested witnessing of marvelous transmutations. By 1587, he taught about chymical procedures, substance, and some theory in his course on medical practice, his lectures mirroring his book on the subject published in the same year, the *New Method of the Practice of Medicine*. The great size, complexity, and erudition of the book strongly suggests he developed its contents in lectures earlier.

Through chymical apparatus and procedures, such as distillation, physicians could extract and refine the effective materials and powers from minerals or the plants they studied in the garden. Johannes Heurnius' course and textbook on the practice of medicine, the core of Leiden medical teaching for decades, included extensive presentations of chymical operations and medicines. Heurnius expressed public enthusiasm for chymical transmutation and

---

1   The best work is by Saskia Klerk, too little of which has seen formal publication. Klerk, "Galen Reconsidered," chapters 1 and 2, though still only parts of a fine dissertation, provide helpful overviews of the teaching of the garden teaching and some of the theories of Dodonaeus and Johannes Heurnius on drug properties and philosophy. See also Klerk, "The Trouble with Opium."

2   Powers, *Inventing Chemistry*, 47–48, puts the beginning of Leiden chymical instruction in 1642. Spronsen, "The Beginning," 333, notes only in passing that Johannes Heurnius endorsed medicines produced by distillation.

3   Johannes Heurnius, "Praefatio" in *Secreta Alchimiae*, ed. Brouchuisius (1579).

philosophy in early publications, and insisted to students that chymistry was "not just *very useful*, but rather *necessary*" for medicine and for life.[4] Students likely did not practice hands-on chymistry, let alone real experiments, as a formal part of their education (though they probably tried remedies out on themselves and members of their close social circles). But chymical substances and procedures were matters of public interest and teaching in the lecture hall and garden.

Learning about medicines in the garden is worth a long visit. Textbooks and lectures presented exemplary ancient authors such as Dioscorides and Galen as models, especially for their catalogues of drugs' faculties. But professors also celebrated the ancients' sense-based epistemology, especially their reliance on their own sensory perceptions of plants and other medicinal ingredients, as well as their methods of making trials to discover or test drugs. Echoing Galen, Leiden physicians proclaimed that knowing the properties of drugs and the right, effective method of healing were deeply connected, so that you could not understand one without knowing the other. In the program Galen described in his works on mixtures and simple or compound drugs, one had to make trials of substances to determine their capacities for altering living bodies, or their "faculties." Rules or conditions for making trials appear throughout Galen's pharmacological works, as well as narrative descriptions of his actual performance of a few trials, on patients or his own person. Only methodical, rational trial-making could avoid confounding or accidental interactions, and reveal the cause-effect relations between a medicine's temperament and the range of changes in living bodies. In part following Galenic and Arabic discussions of testing poison antidotes, Renaissance physicians set up parallel trials, in which the physician divided test subjects (usually unfortunate dogs or, occasionally, condemned criminals) into two or more sets, and administered the test substance to only one or some of the subjects.[5]

Yet the very sophisticated persuasiveness of Galen's pharmacological works, combined with early modern physicians' confidence in the long experience of Hippocratic and Galenic medicines, subdued motivations to carry on systematic testing. There are occasional records of physicians and students carrying out their own trials of drugs or other remedies, but these are usually incidental, and not part of the systematic programs Galen advocated. Of course, even he did not have the time or energy for the labor-intensive, exhaustive tests of the hundreds of simple ingredients and hundreds more compound medicines available in the second century A.D. In the sixteenth century, a flow of new substances from the Americas joined a wave of local discoveries and medicines

---

4   Johannes Heurnius, *Nova Ratio*, 67.
5   Rankin, "Of Antidote and Anecdote." Rankin, *Poison Trials*.

from the east and south. How should physicians come to know their properties and faculties? One could, as Galen argued at length, rely at first on taste,
since the flavors supposedly acted as pointers or indexes to the faculties. After
all, both flowed from the same material mixture of the medicine, its temperament. But this was less reliable, and, for the physician, potentially more perilous than making careful tests of small doses in patients, and perhaps animals.

Students, professors, and natural historians of many stripes flocked to the
university garden, set up their own verdant plots, and made happy herborizing
trips to the windy coasts or inland meadows and forests. Learning to identify
plants required long practice with living specimens, preserved samples, and
visual representations available when the plants were not at hand, due either
to the distance of seasons or geography. Apothecaries such as Dirck Cluyt, who
with the scholar Carolus Clusius organized and ran the early university garden,
gained expertise and recognition for their collected *naturalia* and knowledge.
For naturalists such as Clusius and his friend, the Stoic philosopher Justus
Lipsius, years of collecting, corresponding, reading, and writing all cultivated
the delights of appreciating and knowing beautiful, new, and rare plants. For
physicians and physicians-in-training, discerning the differences among plants
could divide life from death. Different varieties of the purgative hellebore had
different strengths, some too violent for weak or severely ill patients. Other
ingredients, such as "doronicum," a type of sunflower in a large family of similar flowers, might be deadly or a reputed curative. Such skills of identification
and memory came only through practice, even for professors who had to study
hard to get ready to teach in the new garden.

Temperament theory, discussed in the previous chapter, linked theory and
practice across domains of academic medicine, with drugs as a key node. As
we will see over this and the next two chapters, knowledge about drugs, diseases, faculties, and post-mortem appearances all joined together through the
causal nexus of ideas about qualitative temperament as the source of most
of the powers of drugs and changes in the body. Anatomical dissection and
even medical theory served medical practice, too. Professors viewed, touched,
and smelled healthy and diseased living bodies, and cut deep into dead ones
to sense the phenomena of disease changes. They tasted, smelled, touched,
and viewed plants, minerals, animal products, and some chymicals in order to
know their qualities and faculties, too.

In these practices and pedagogical programs, ancient, medieval and early
modern texts and practices supplied models, language, and concepts for
experimentation. Except in the case of learning the properties of drugs, this
usually fell far short of experimentalism. Even Galen's explicitly experimentalist method of testing for drug faculties was overshadowed by the optimism

of healers about their medicinal stores, stocked over centuries with medicines supposedly proven effective by "long experience" in their uses. Galenic texts and theory became the common language and conceptual lenses for studying the properties of drugs, as well as the framework and tools for understanding living bodies and diseases.

1   Fire and Transmutation

In 1579, six years after his return to Utrecht from his medical studies abroad, Johannes Heurnius published a lengthy preface extolling the secrets of alchemy.[6] The rest of the book reprinted medieval treatises on alchemical transmutation by pseudo-Thomas Aquinas, John of Rupescissa, and pseudo-Raymond Llull. Yet recent works, including those claiming to be comprehensive histories of Leiden chymistry teaching, do not mention Heurnius' interest in alchemy or chymistry.[7] This book and preface enjoyed sustained readership, appearing in three editions, with printings in Cologne and Leiden. At least two Leiden editions appeared in Heurnius' lifetime, including one printed in 1598 while he was still the most visible professor of medicine at the university.[8] Hence his enthusiasm for transmutation could hardly have been a secret.

Heurnius and the editor, Danielis Brouchuisius (Daniel van Broekhuizen), intended the book as a clear, even introductory exposition of alchemical practice and theory. As the prefatory poem announced, each one of the treatises used clear language to describe operations for different stages of alchemical work. Other writers twist riddles; a few pages here demonstrate "everything nature sets up by the secret Stone, which has been revealed by art to ingenious men." To make the operations even clearer, the printer included detailed illustrations of the proper "physical furnace" to use, as well as the "egg" of the alchemists: a divided metal sphere to enclose the ingredients (Figure 8).[9] As did other Paracelsians at the time, though, Heurnius sought to elevate and establish the academic status of alchemy as natural philosophy by narrating an ancient pedigree for the theory and practice of the art. He may well have

---

6 J. Banga, *Geschiedenis van de geneeskunde*, 163. Johannes Heurnius, "Praefatio." Brüning, *Bibliographie der alchemistischen Literatur*, Vol. 1, 80, 115, 176.

7 *Pace* Powers, *Inventing Chemistry*. See also Lindeboom, *Dutch Medical Biography*, col. 858. Huisman, *Finger of God*. Otterspeer, *Groepsportret*. Kroon, *Bijdragen*, does not discuss this work or Heurnius' later practice of chymistry, but he does list the preface, 93.

8 Brouchuisius, ed. *Secreta Alchimiae* (1598).

9 Brouchuisius, ed. *Secreta Alchimiae* (1579), 47–48. Subsequent references are to the 1579 edition.

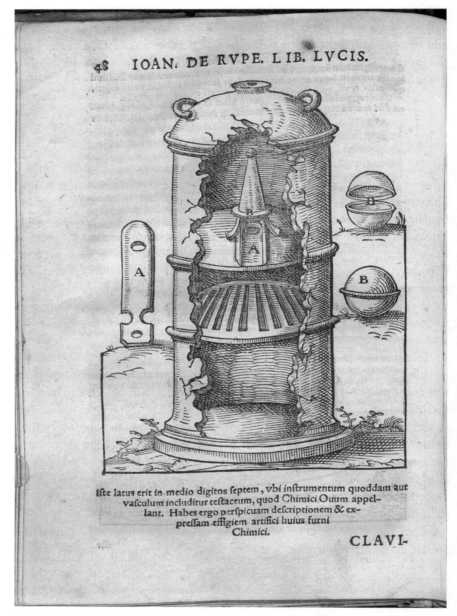

ₐ48   IOAN. DE RVPE. LIB. LVCIS.

iſte latus erit in medio digitos ſeptem, vbi inſtrumentum quoddam aut
vaſculum includitur teſtaceum, quod Chimici Ouum appel-
lant. Habes ergo perſpicuam deſcriptionem & ex-
preſſam effigiem artifici huius furni
Chimici.

CLAVI-

FIGURE 8   Chymical furnace for transmutation, with the metal "philosophical egg" for
enclosing the ingredients to the right. *Liber Lucis* in *Secreta Alchimiae* (1579), 48.
COURTESY, BAYERISCHE STAATSBIBLIOTHEK MÜNCHEN, ESLG/4 ALCH. 90,
P. 48, URN:NBN:DE:BVB:12-BSB00014904-4.

followed Petrus Severinus here, as he did in other parts of his account of chymical theory, as we will see.[10] Reading through Heurnius' approach, in which he tried to construct a legitimating history of chymistry from approved ancient sources, allows us to see his humanist scholarly practices at work.

Although recent histories of chymical teaching at Leiden assert that it only began six decades later, in 1642, and then as a very marginal practice, I argue in the following that chymical operations, theory, and medicine had a place in Leiden medical learning from near the very beginning of the university.[11] Even in his university lectures on the theory of practice, which began at least by 1587, Heurnius praised "the art of distillation" as "not just *very useful,* but rather *necessary*...without which indeed no life can be led commodiously enough. Medicine certainly now stumbles without *this art.*"[12] As we will see, he spent serious time and effort in learning and communicating chymical medicine.

Heurnius' enthusiasm for chymical philosophy and history, as well as his strong belief in processes of transmutation, shines through in his first publication. In his 1579 preface to the medieval alchemical treatises, Heurnius wove together a history of ancient knowledge, Paracelsian chymical theory, and his own experiences of marvelous transformations. Heurnius articulated an ancient and medieval history in which alchemical learning and skill is a golden thread of power, an art wielded by Egyptian priests and Greek philosophers, suppressed by Roman bellicosity, and then recovered by medieval writers and, most of all, by Paracelsus.

The art of alchemy, Heurnius declared, came "as from a very rich flood" out of ancient Egypt.[13] As in the early modern period, the Egyptians' development of alchemy demanded hard work. Even with their more excellent wits (*ingenia*) and more capacious minds, the Egyptians and their heirs won discoveries by "much dampness of sweat and force of the philosophical mind." Alchemy has long demanded hard labor, even from ancient sages. For the benefit of future generations, the Egyptians inscribed some of the secrets of their art on their tombs and columns. The people of Colchis emerged from the Egyptians,

---

10   Shackelford, *A Philosophical Path for Paracelsian Medicine,* 154.

11   Powers asserts that "for the first sixty years after its founding in 1575, the University of Leiden did not offer chemical instruction as part of its curriculum," and begins the institutionalization of chemistry there with the 1642 hiring of Niclaes Chimaer, an apothecary, to demonstrate the fabrication of medicines and general instruction as part of the *collegium medico-practicum.* Powers, *Inventing Chemistry,* 47.

12   Johannes Heurnius, *Nova Ratio,* 67. Molhuysen, *Bronnen,* 1, 157*.

13   Johannes Heurnius, "Praefatio," 3.

bearing fleeces or vellum hides marked with these secrets. Through alchemy the learned of Egypt and Colchis enriched and ennobled their kingdoms. With such an art, "even a very weak kingdom was formidable to the most powerful Monarchs of the whole world."[14]

Heurnius used his humanist textual skills to present the best ancient philosophers and sages as alchemists. Repeatedly, he interpreted striking references to "gold" in ancient myths and histories as markers of an ancient group's mastery of alchemical processes. He cited the Greek historian Herodotus for the origin of the Colchians in Egypt, and he interpreted the story of Jason and the golden fleece in alchemical terms.[15] The golden fleece Jason stole bore the secrets of alchemical art, written for the king. Outstanding Greek thinkers also sought out secrets through travel. Democritus of Abdera, Heurnius averred, through the force of his "more excellent mind," traveled throughout India, Scythia, and Egypt, recovering texts from Egyptians such as the "magus Dardanus." With this harvest of bookish learning, Democritus enriched every discipline, and wrote "spagyric books, which even today I know remain in a certain place."[16] In using the term "spagyric" for "chymical," Heurnius followed Paracelsian practice, which humanists supported with a Greek etymology (*"span"* or "to separate" plus *"ageirein"* or "to collect together").[17] Heurnius also participated in a widespread humanist construction of various *personae* for Democritus as an anatomist, an atomist, a laughing philosopher, and an alchemist. References to Democritus's supposed travels appeared in ancient works by Pliny, Petronius, Seneca, and others, and his contested status as an alchemist, practitioner of natural magic, and atomist spread in the second half of the sixteenth century.[18]

Heurnius draped Pythagoras in alchemical gold, too—at least, his leg. He turned longstanding claims that Pythagoras had a golden leg (an ancient sign of divinity) into a mark of alchemical wisdom. In Heurnius' historical defense of the ancient wisdom of alchemy, Pythagoras sailed to Egypt to learn the art, and with such knowledge (*scientia*) he "covered his whole leg with gold so thickly that the whole thing was judged to be gold." Similarly, Heurnius interpreted Plato and other philosophers scoffing at offers of wealth as evidence for their status as adepts: true alchemical philosophers ordered gold about, not the other way around. Only Roman warlike practicality ended the flow of alchemical knowledge and gold from Egypt. Diocletian, fearing threats

---

14   Johannes Heurnius, "Praefatio," 4.

15   Herodotus, *The Persian Wars*, trans. Godley, 104, 391.

16   Johannes Heurnius, "Praefatio," 4.

17   Newman, "From Alchemy to 'Chymistry,'" 509.

18   Lüthy, "The Fourfold Democritus."

to the empire, occupied Alexandria and ordered "all Chemical writing" put to the fire. Yet "men gifted with divine *ingenia*" in Alexandria suffered many labors and dangers, preserving the divine alchemical art and other parts of ancient knowledge.

Like others in his time, Heurnius read Paracelsian natural philosophy back into ancient texts. In this view, the active, seminal cores of material things occupied the center of this ancient knowledge. Greek philosophers Timaeus, Pythagoras, and Plato learned from "Orpheus" that "nature spread into all things certain hidden and seminal reasons." These active, seminal reasons produced marvelous effects if freed from their "elemental chains" or stirred up by "a spiritual or sidereal agitation."[19] Heurnius also adopted the language of illumination, writing that "a more perfect light" between "friendly seeds" could gently attract sympathetic objects, drawing quicksilver or *argentum vivum* out of gold just as the magnet attracts iron. Discord between seeds or natures also produced marvelous actions, such as Pliny's classic example of the warlike lion's fear at the gaze of the rooster.[20]

Heurnius described these seeds as "divine" in at least three senses. First, earthly seeds often moved toward the heavens. Certain flowers followed the Sun, the stone selenite grew and decreased with the Moon, and other gems had Classical warrants for their sympathetic actions with stars and celestial spirits. Second, in Paracelsian or Neoplatonic fashion, Heurnius argued that these seeds acted best when freed from their material "chains" or corporeal "bridles." Finally, in each "divine seed there is something of their proper intelligence [*intelligentia*]."[21] This divinity and intelligence came from God's initial creation via rational seeds, as well as the influence of celestial or heavenly bodies. Thus the alchemical practitioner sought to practice "the spagyric art" or the "heavenly star" by which one could entice seminal forms free of bodies, acting purely by sympathy, in a way that echoed the "great fermentation" of God's first mixture of Creation. Adepts needed some knowledge of astrology, too, such as Pythagoras developed in his high tower in Babylon.

In sum, Heurnius constructed a history in which the true art of alchemy (and some allied astrology) began with Adam, then poured out from Egyptian priests and even, in side remarks, from "Hermes Trismegistus," next passed to the Colchians and Greek philosophers, and was then carried off by the Romans. He also claimed these arts received cultivation after their "long exile" at the hands of the Goths and Vandals. Among Arabic alchemists he identified

---

19   Johannes Heurnius, "Praefatio," 5.
20   Copenhaver, "Natural Magic, Hermetism, and Occultism," 277.
21   Johannes Heurnius, "Praefatio," 6.

especially "Geber" and Rhazes. Among more recent Latin writers, he praised the incongruous companions Thomas Aquinas and Paracelsus. (Pseudo-) Thomas Aquinas surveyed the whole of "Chymistry" and found it supported by nature but reaching even the deeper "recess" of nature, and began a "trial of the matter [*experimentum rei*] with great detriment to his body, as he himself testifies."[22] Only through sacrifice and bodily engagement could anyone hope to advance this "laborious work." Paracelsus, in turn, "a very sharp fighter for this art," praised (pseudo-)Thomas Aquinas. While other alchemists deliberately obscure the ingredients and practical steps of the art, and some even write pseudonymous treatises "under the names of great men," Heurnius wrote, the *Treatise on the Philosophical Stone* by "Thomas Aquinas" is free of all suspicion! Pseudonymous authorship was common in later medieval and early modern alchemical texts, and Heurnius knew it.[23] While he expressed justified skepticism about many pseudonymous alchemical treatises, he declared this one to be true gold.

But how is one to learn this art? In his preface and in his collaborative act of putting out the book, Heurnius was clearly advocating for Latinate scholars reading books as a first step. The act of writing down the secrets of the art and then the preservation or recovery of those writings is the main thread of his history of alchemy, from the Egyptians to the Greeks, Romans, Arabic writers, and beyond. But Heurnius also emphasized personal labor and bodily practice. In Heurnius' own sad age, the "very idle" think they can manufacture the philosophers' stone from "little receptacles of paper," especially those obscurantist and deceptive books of the "unlearned" (*idiotae*). The true adept needs clean hands to enter into the sacred art, and must see with the mind as well as the corporeal eyes, in order to follow the footprints of brilliant men through the "labyrinth of nature."[24] Only with God's favor, study, and personal labor could the reader follow the proper path of the art. Done rightly, this would allow the adept to produce great wonders or "*magnalia*" drawn out from gross matter.

Heurnius recounted his own and others' stories of these marvelous transformations and transmutations. As he said, nothing prohibited art, the imitator of nature, from producing natural effects. Common experience grounded some of his claims. Daily experience (*experimentum*) taught that living things came from inanimate sources, and in very specific relations. Toads generated out of bits of a duck boiled and then covered against the sky; bees came from

---

22   Johannes Heurnius, "Praefatio," 7
23   Long, *Openness, Secrecy, Authorship*, 144–148.
24   Johannes Heurnius, "Praefatio," 8.

a dead calf; wasps from donkey flesh; scarab beetles from horseflesh; locusts from mules' flesh. Nature "transmutes" flax into farner, dead wood into mint, and different kinds of wheat into one another.

But Heurnius also accorded strong epistemic weight for marvelous changes to individual scholars' testimonies. As he declared, "At Paris Petrus Ramus showed us a stone thrown down by thunder and lightning."[25] Likely, this marvel appeared as part of Ramus's philosophical instruction in Paris, and Johannes's son Otto reported that his father was "very familiar" with Ramus.[26] His personal witness secured an even more marvelous transmutation than the traditional "thunderstones." Heurnius went on, after citing a report of a fountain which turned immersed objects into copper: "In Padua I saw the breast of a woman turned into stone by the power of a water." These marvelous events of natural transmutations—witnessed by credible persons such as Petrus Ramus, Heurnius, and his colleagues—made the case for alchemy: "Why therefore would it be wholly irrational for crude metal to be guided so that it matures, as here our Thomas Aquinas demonstrates?" Thus, the ancient wisdom and art of the Egyptian alchemists, preserved and cultivated in text and practice, found immediate warrant in Heurnius' personal testimony on behalf of singular, historical instances of transmutations by nature.

In its theory, Heurnius' vision of alchemy plainly articulated a moral and epistemological program of clear language and practical work. Though he mentioned "Hermes Trismegistus" in passing, there are no clear allusions to the identified Hermetic works of the period, such as the *Pimander* or the alchemical *Emerald Tablet*.[27] Instead of exploring the nature of Soul and Mind, and the relations between divine Mind and things in the world, Heurnius' alchemy is mostly a formalized Paracelsian theory of divine, active seeds in matter which interact at a distance and which can work marvelous practical transmutations when freed from their material bodies or elements. He likely drew from Petrus Severinus's 1571 philosophical articulation of Paracelsian medicine, the *Idea of Philosophical Medicine* (*Idea medicinae philosophicae*). Both texts share an emphasis on natural causation by seeds or *semina*, sympathetic action, and astral influences.[28] Unlike Severinus, though, Heurnius does not attack Galen for perverting medicine in a search for geometric method and certainty.[29]

---

25   Johannes Heurnius, "Praefatio," 8.
26   [Otto Heurnius], "Vita Auctoris."
27   Copenhaver, "Natural Magic, Hermetism, and Occultism." Robichaud, "Ficino on Force, Magic, and Prayers."
28   Shackelford, *A Philosophical Path for Paracelsian Medicine.*
29   Severinus, *Idea medicinae philosophicae,* 2–3.

Instead, Heurnius seems to have constructed his history of alchemy by stitching together histories from antiquity with selective readings from ancient philosophical and natural-historical sources. A 1589 publication of letters by a German physician, Johannes Lange, gives a similar history, citing sources such as Exodus for the flood of Egyptian gold, the early Christian historians Eusebius and Orosius, and the Greek lexicographer Suidas.[30] Heurnius' explicit sources for seminal reasons and alchemical and astrological sympathy, though, were Neoplatonic and magical texts. He emphasized especially "Orpheus," as well as Timaeus, Pythagoras, Plato, Theophrastus, and Proclus. He almost certainly had in mind the long Greek poem on stones and their magical properties, the *Lithica* (Λιθικα) of pseudo-Orpheus.[31] This "Orpheus" is Heurnius' explicit source for the central claim that stones have magical sympathetic powers, and perhaps for the notions that alchemy required hard labor, as well as his report that the Egyptians hid the secrets of their art in recesses in the earth.[32]

Thus Heurnius' first publication—prefixed to medieval treatises on alchemical chrysopoiea—endorsed a broadly Paracelsian, Neoplatonic philosophy of the hidden *semina* of natural things. He put his humanist historical and linguistic training to use to stitch together a legitimating history for chymistry, drawing passages from Herodotus, Pliny, Suetonius, Seneca, pseudo-Orpheus, and other ancient and supposedly ancient authorities. In his vision, Democritus handed on true medicine and philosophy when he taught alchemy, Pythagoras transmuted his golden thigh with alchemical skill, Plato and his heirs recommended the art, and Paracelsus had recently revived it. Yet he still adopted a somewhat conciliatory stance toward Galen, unlike other Paracelsian writers such as Severinus. He also sought epistemic credibility not only from ancient and medieval texts, but his own witnessing, and that of other named figures, of marvelous transmutations.

2   Chymical Teaching in the Lecture Hall

In his lectures, Heurnius taught students how to *do* things with chymistry, especially how to make medicines. Eight years after printing his transmutational preface, Heurnius published a new textbook of practical medicine which included some thirty-seven detailed pages on chymical operations, recipes, and some theory. He used this very text for his regular courses in the practice

---

30   Lange, *Epistolarum medicinalium volumen tripartitum*, 270–271.

31   Ps.-Orpheus, *Musaei opusculum de Herone et Leandro*.

32   Johannes Heurnius, "Praefatio," 5–6.

of medicine, at least from 1587. The first official *series lectionum* from October 1587 records him teaching "the practice of the art composed by himself," and Heurnius' dedication of the *New Method* praised the university Curators for allowing him to teach his "interpretation of Medicine" in their Academy.[33] Since the extensive book appeared in early 1587 in print, he must have been teaching from similar lectures developed over the previous six years, since his appointment in 1581. Like his textbook on medical theory, Heurnius' textbook for practical medicine enjoyed popularity into the middle of the 1600s, with six editions published in Leiden and Rotterdam.[34]

As a whole, Heurnius' major medical project aimed to bring the rational theory of therapeutics into closer, and more methodical, engagement with head-to-toe practice. His project received accolades. In February of 1587, the Curators of Leiden University awarded Johannes Heurnius a silver dish worth 10 great Flemish pounds for the dedication of his *New Method of the Practice of Medicine* (*Praxis Medicinae Nova Ratio*).[35] Extending over seven hundred pages, Heurnius' synthesis of ancient, medieval, and early modern learning on medicines, their production, and use joined very practical instructions for making medicines to an exhaustive method for diagnosing and treating diseases of the body from head to toe. This very practical textbook deeply informed his more philosophical *Institutes* book and courses, which were the mainstay of Leiden medical teaching into the 1640s.

In the *New Method*, his first published treatise, Heurnius presented a new, rational method for healing predicated on the precise measurement of drug ingredients, with remedies carefully calibrated and specified to the location and qualitative intensity of each disease. Given his strong emphasis on the book's rational method, we might translate *ratio* here as "method," following Cicero's influential rendering of the Greek *methodos* as *via et ratio*, and earlier modern equations of "*methodus*" and "*ratio*."[36] In short, his program aimed to bridge teaching students how to make medicines with traditional theories of diseases and therapies.

Importantly, Heurnius also reached beyond Galen and adopted chymical apparatus and techniques as part of his project of therapeutic reform in the

---

33   Molhuysen, *Bronnen*, 1, 157*. Johannes Heurnius, *Nova Ratio* (1609). *2v.

34   Kroon, *Bijdragen*, 93. The text remained substantially the same since at least the 1590 edition, and apparently exactly the same from the 1609 amended edition on. Unless otherwise noted, my references are to the 1650 edition: Johannes Heurnius, *Praxis Medicinae Nova Ratio* (1650).

35   Resolutie Curatoren Feb. 9 1587, in Molhuysen, *Bronnen*, 1, 51. Johannes Heurnius, *Praxis Medicinae Nova Ratio* (1587).

36   Wightman, "*Quid sit Methodus?*" 361, 366.

New Method. His therapeutic approach remained largely Galenic-Hippocratic, though with a remarkably fine specificity in the match of the qualitative grades of diseases seated in individual parts of the body to the powers and doses of the remedies. He described chymical apparatus, operations, and recipes in detail. Woodcut illustrations of basic chymical apparatus made his teachings clearer to students. Heurnius' sources, too, drew from a wide range, including Hippocrates, pseudo-Llull, Gesner's *Euonymus*, Avicenna, Albertus Magnus, Aristotle, Galen, Michele Savonarola, Dioscorides, and Pietro Mattioli, and thus made for an eclectic chymical practice. He also repeated his praise for Paracelsus, who strove to bring "the highest majesty to this art."[37] In Paracelsus's age, chymistry, "this *ingenious invention*" rose up to it greatest vigor, as never before. Medical students and physicians needed this art. As he insisted at the beginning of the long section on distillation and other things chymical, distillation is "not just *very useful*, but rather *necessary*" for life and medicine.[38]

Heurnius put into practice his humanist training, and displayed humanist values to the students, especially in his laudatory history of chymistry. Most often, he described chymistry in terms of distillation and alchemy. In his *New Method* he insisted that Hippocrates knew and approved of chymistry.[39] He informed his students, "if we are to believe Raymond Llull, Hippocrates wholly burned for this art, *and he knew the modes by which one could fix the stars from metals* ... Let them be silent, therefore, who think that this art was unknown to *Hippocrates and the ancients*."[40] Here, he referenced the pseudo-Llullian alchemical text, *On the Secrets of Nature, or On the Fifth Essence*.[41] With this attribution Heurnius shouted his own approval of alchemy ("Alchimia"), since for him Hippocrates "showed the true Medicine of the Gods to men."[42]

According to Heurnius, Hippocrates "the Great" learned philosophy from Democritus and could trace his lineage back seventeen generations to the mythical founder of Greek medicine, Asclepius himself. Once again, Heurnius flashed his humanist reading skills to follow the ancient Greek poet Pindar, and subsequent mythic histories, and report that Asclepius learned his art from Chiron, trained by Apollo, and that Hippocrates counted himself a twentieth-generation descendent from Hercules.[43] Echoing his earlier

---

37   Johannes Heurnius, *Nova Ratio*, 69. Here as elsewhere, Heurnius used italics in the original to emphasize points for his students and readers.

38   Johannes Heurnius, *Nova Ratio*, 67. Italics in original.

39   Johannes Heurnius, *Nova Ratio*, 68.

40   Johannes Heurnius, *Nova Ratio*, 68. Italics in original.

41   [Pseudo-]Llull, *De secretis naturae*, 22.

42   From his oration on the origin of medicine of 1589, reprinted in Johannes Heurnius, *Institutiones* (1638), *3r-*5r. Kroon, *Bijdragen*, 94, gives a first edition of 1589 and a second of 1608.

43   Johannes Heurnius, *Nova Ratio*, *3r-*4r. Edelstein and Edelstein, *Asclepius*, 22–24.

enthusiastic history of alchemy, Heurnius followed the historian Suidas to trace alchemy to the ancient Egyptians. So long as he had ancient Greek or Latin sources to cite—Pindar, Ovid, Soranus, Pliny—in loose corroboration of each other, Heurnius remained as confident in his epic history of the true medicine as he was in his earlier history of alchemy. Careful reading of Pliny's ancient *Natural History* revealed that the emperor "Caius" (Caligula) ordered a large amount of auripigment (yellow arsenic sulphide) melted, and clearly made excellent gold, but of a very small amount.[44]

Chymistry helped the physician fine-tune the faculties or powers of his remedies. For Heurnius' larger project of carefully calculating and compounding the powers of different medicinal simples to produce medicines calibrated for specific affects in specific parts, chymistry provided real help. "*This art* by the power of *fire* draws out liquors from all the parts *of plants* and *animals*, which bear the *flavor, color, odor,* and *power* of those parts from whence they flow out."[45] In general, chymistry worked through processes of separation: "This art is certainly of the greatest *use* in Medicine, for it separates the heterogeneous and adds nobility to things, while it entirely rescues them from *fetidness,* and harmful corruption."[46] Distillation rarified and thinned substances, enhancing their ability to penetrate and remove humoral blockages without violence. Heurnius himself proved this in experiences treating colic pains and difficulty in urination.[47]

He also added personal suggestions for better practice, likely indicating his own experience. For instance, he suggested that students use spirit of wine to draw away the vaporous parts of distillates, based on his own estimation.[48] For successful distillations, he specified precise dimensions of the apparatus and ingredients.[49] Again, his own experience in sickness and health further warranted the use of distillation. He had good results with using distilled almond and chamomile oil as a liniment, and especially with the ingestion of oil of vitriol: "frequently, the oil of vitriol calls out to me."[50] As in his earlier witnessing for marvelous natural transmutations, Heurnius added his own testimony to establish the credibility of the effects of chymical practice.

Students needed to know about apparatus, operations, and materials in order to *do* chymistry. Most of thirty-seven-page discussion of chymistry focused on operations and apparatus for making medicines, including

44   Pliny, *Historia mundi naturalis,* Bk. 33, Ch. 4, 464, l. 50.
45   Johannes Heurnius, *Nova Ratio* (1650), 67.
46   Johannes Heurnius, *Nova Ratio,* 69.
47   Johannes Heurnius, *Nova Ratio,* 70–71.
48   Johannes Heurnius, *Nova Ratio,* 93.
49   Johannes Heurnius, *Nova Ratio,* 102.
50   Johannes Heurnius, *Nova Ratio,* 104, 98.

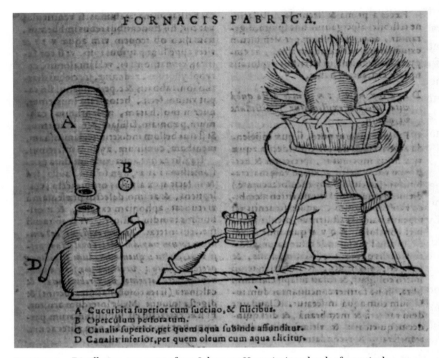

FORNACIS FABRICA.

A Cucurbita superior cum succiao, & filicibus.
B Operculum perforatum.
C Canalis superior, per quem aqua subinde affunditur.
D Canalis inferior, per quem oleum cum aqua elicitur.

FIGURE 9   Distillation apparatus from Johannes Heurnius' textbook of practical
            medicine, *Nova Ratio* (1609 [orig. 1587]), 49. The same illustration appears on
            p. 52 of the 1587 edition.
            COURTESY, STAATLICHE BIBLIOTHEK REGENSBURG, 999/MED.491, P. 49,
            URN:NBN:DE:BVB:12-BSB11106351-6.

diagrams of crucibles, retorts, cooling apparatus for distillates, etc. Heurnius'
pedagogical aims come through in the sequences: general procedures (e.g., distillation), then specific procedures and uses (e.g., distillation in a sand bath),
and then illustrative examples (e.g., distilling oil of antimony in a sand bath).
He cautioned his students that the grades of heat are important, and different
authors used different grades.[51] The grades of heat ranged from the gentlest
warmth of water vapor, horse dung, and the Sun to fermentation by a kind
of ebullition, to digestion, and finally a consuming heat.[52] Gentle distillations
changed substances in ways analogous to cooking or coction in the body; from
food into chyle, or chyle into blood, etc.

   Theory was never far from Heurnius' thoughts, though. He followed precedent to argue that one never produced pure Aristotelian elements, not even

51   Johannes Heurnius, *Nova Ratio*, 81–82.
52   Gesner gives three grades of heat: gentle, moderate, and violent. Gesner, *Euonymus*, 27.

through distillation. Many substances, Heurnius argued, work "most power-fully by reason of their form" or by some hidden power.[53] For example, fresh opium and raw garlic, distilled together, produced a narcotic drink. The garlic worked by a hidden power to bring out the power of the opium. Similarly, three spoonfuls of distilled water of garden nightshade extinguished internal inflammations of the guts.

In medical theory, the proper sensible qualities of things—especially flavors, odors, and colors—provided indexes for reasoning back to their fundamental elements and qualities, and perhaps their faculties.[54] But neither flavors nor colors stayed consistent through distillation. Flavors varied with the movements of the earthy parts, and colors did not seem to depend on elemental temperament. The important philosophical question of colors in chymistry provoked Heurnius to enter a longish discussion of the origin of colors. Did they arise from the temperament or the substantial form? Could one say, following *some* of Galen's contradictory writings, that the substantial form *is* the temperament? Perhaps for the benefit of students, Heurnius worked through accounts from Galen and Aristotle, then seemed to favor Plato, whose *Timaeus* argues that varying color follows from different kinds of fire.[55]

In short, Heurnius mostly borrowed what he found valuable in chymical writers and practice, while holding to an Aristotelian-Galenic natural philosophy in which "all *corporeal things* by *nature*, depend on the *form*, which consists from the *sure tempering* of the four elements."[56] Putrefaction produces real changes, as a result of "the death of the substantial form of the mixt."[57] Yet he also made passing remarks to some key components of the chymical philosophy he celebrated in his earlier preface. As we have seen, Heurnius followed (pseudo-)Llull in ascribing to Hippocrates the apparent ability of physicians to direct the astral powers of metals. He also explained the attractive power of distilled liquors by a reference to a sympathetic "mutual similitude."[58] While Heurnius did not design a curriculum for the purpose of advocating the experimentalist investigation of nature via chymistry, his chymical medicine certainly combined making and knowing across a range of operations and substances.

This approach comes through clearly in the final long section on *aqua vitae* (in our terms, primarily ethanol). Like his alchemical predecessors

---

53   Johannes Heurnius, *Nova Ratio*, 70.
54   Klerk, "Galen Reconsidered," 106.
55   Johannes Heurnius, *Nova Ratio*, 73–5. Plato, *Timaeus*, 175–177.
56   Johannes Heurnius, *Nova Ratio*, 100. Italics in original.
57   Thus Heurnius adopted a fairly standard Scholastic view of mixture, per Newman, *Atoms and Alchemy*.
58   Johannes Heurnius, *Nova Ratio*, 71.

pseudo-Llull and Rupescissa, Heurnius extolled the powers of the thin, distilled part of wine, *aqua vitae*, to preserve all things from corruption, guard the human body from putridity, excite the body's heat, renew its spirits, and even prolong life.[59] Heurnius also insisted that it excited the brain and renewed memory (at least when taken in the proper amounts), and cited two cases of prominent physicians who lived well into their eighties through the use of this "distilled liquor of wine."[60] Those hotter by nature, age, or disease ought to abstain from *aqua vitae*, but for others it fed vital heat through its "celestial heat." Acting by a tempered heat like that of the celestial bodies, *aqua vitae* acts through its own form, the form of fire. Repeated distillations of *aqua vitae* make it more fragrant and even thinner—"Llull turned [distilled] this water for a whole year"—so it seems acceptable to call very pure *aqua vitae* the "quintessence."[61] Yet, in his lecture course and textbook, Heurnius still resisted the earlier Paracelsian-Severinian matter theory of active, astral *semina* interacting from within coarse matter. He denied that distillation could draw out a distinct fifth essence, since all corporeal things by nature depend on form, "which consists in a *certain tempering* of the four elements."[62] Anything perceptible to the senses must result from a mixture of the four elements and qualities.

In his course and textbook on practical medicine, then, Heurnius domesticated the alchemical enthusiasm of his earlier 1579 preface. He skipped over the central philosophical theory of rational, astral *semina* found in the preface, and instead oriented chymical practice and concepts toward a fine-tuned rational method of compounding medicinal ingredients according to broadly Hippocratic and Galenic schemes of qualities. He retained the core of the earlier legitimating history of alchemy, arguing that Hippocrates approved of the art of distillation and that he learned it from Democritus, who had it from the Egyptians. Strikingly, in his discussions of theory and the grand claims for the necessity and power of chymistry, Heurnius frequently referenced works on transmutation, especially books attributed to Llull. There are bright glimmers of his earlier alchemical interests scattered across the more Galenic-Hippocratic system and remedies of his daily courses and major textbooks.

This domestication likely followed from the official requirements of the students' exams and disputations. As we saw earlier in chapter two, university rules

---

59   Johannes Heurnius, *Nova Ratio*, 92–97. DeVun, *Prophecy, Alchemy, and the End of Time*, 70, 93, 105.
60   Johannes Heurnius, *Nova Ratio*, 94. The fifteenth-century Paduan physician Michele Savonarola is his source for one such anecdote.
61   Johannes Heurnius, *Nova Ratio*, 97.
62   Johannes Heurnius, *Nova Ratio*, 100.

demanded that students explain an aphorism of Hippocrates and a particular disease from Hippocrates or Galen, and then move on to a public disputation. A great majority of the disputations over the first five decades discussed a single disease of a certain kind (angina, pleurisy, putrid fever, phthisis, etc.), and in a Galenic-Hippocratic framework.[63] So Heurnius bent the conventions as he could, especially in his legitimating history of distillation, which presented Hippocrates as a chymist who learned the art from Democritus. In sum, chymical apparatus, practice, and some theory occupied a prominent place in early Leiden education in practical medicine.

Of course, the broader roots of university instruction in chymical theory and practices burrow back further and wider than Heurnius. Heurnius had studied in Paris, Padua, and Pavia in the later 1560s and early 1570s.[64] Gabriele Falloppio (or Falloppia) had passed away already in 1562 but had established instruction on distillation and analysis of the components and medicinal powers of waters, as well as of metals and minerals.[65] Heurnius included chymical recipes from Padua in his discussion of chymistry, such as the oil of balsam of Falloppio.[66] Earlier than Falloppio, of course, Luca Ghini's 1543 appointment to teach pharmacy at the University of Pisa had included instruction in the garden and laboratory.[67] Italian universities established some regular teaching in chymistry in the early 1600s, but set up professorships a century later.[68] Thus Heurnius' own course points to the much older adoption and development of chymistry in more traditional Galenic and Aristotelian medical settings.

Heurnius very likely moved in the vanguard of chymical teaching when he included chymistry in his core medical practice courses and textbook before 1587. In contrast, Leonhart Fuchs's popular medical textbooks, which introduced the "Institutes" form into medical teaching, only mentioned distillation in the context of excessive mucus draining from the brain, or catarrh.[69] The most popular textbook of medicinal ingredients, or medical "simples," Pietro Mattioli's lengthy *Commentaries* on the ancient herbal of Dioscorides, included a very short discussion of distillation procedures in just a few pages appended to the main text, and only from a later 1565 edition.[70] But, as Allen

---

63   Lists are incomplete, but over eighty percent of the disputations listed from 1593 through
      1625 discuss one disease in the title. See Harskamp, *Dissertatio medica inauguralis*, 21–35.
64   "Heurnius (van Heurne, van Horne), Johannes," *Dutch Medical Biography*, col. 857.
65   Ragland, "'Making Trials,'" 515–518.
66   Johannes Heurnius, *Nova Ratio*, 79.
67   Frietsch, "Alchemy and the Early Modern University," 127.
68   Kahn, "First Private," 259–260.
69   Fuchs, *Institutionum medicinae* (1555), 414; Fuchs, *Institutionum medicinae* (1605), 601.
70   Mattioli, *Commentarii*.

Debus argued some time ago, chymical teaching in universities was no doubt more widespread than official course listings and chairs in chymistry suggest.[71]

Including chymistry in European medical teaching seems to have been increasingly common around 1600, despite violent attempts to suppress it by some physicians' associations, such as the Paris faculty of medicine. By the later 1500s, the University of Basel produced many students interested in chymistry, as suggested by their disputations and later publications.[72] Dedicated courses for chymistry likely appeared first in German lands, especially those taught by Johannes Hartmann at Marburg and Daniel Sennert at Wittenberg, and embraced far more detailed and expansive chymical theory and practice. At Marburg, students pushed for practical instruction in chymistry, and this pressured administrators to include the topic in the curriculum from 1608–1620.[73] There, Johannes Hartmann offered a blend of Hippocratic and Paracelsian medical teaching. Professors at Jena such as Andreas Libavius and Zacharias Brendel the Elder may have been teaching some chymistry by the 1590s, judging by a few student disputations on metals.[74] At Wittenberg, Sennert even included a long discussion of chymistry in his medical textbook of 1611, and later editions. Sennert also likely taught more detailed, hands-on "private" chymistry courses in his own home, which was also a possibility for Heurnius.[75] Famously, Sennert used sophisticated laboratory methods to argue for chymical atoms and the chymicalization of ancient medicine and philosophy, a program that inspired Robert Boyle, G. W. Leibniz, and other innovators.[76] Didier Kahn has very recently clarified the early situation in Paris.[77] Joseph Du Chesne, Theodore Turquet de Mayerne, Ribit de la Revière, and Pierre Paulmier likely lectured on chymistry in Paris around 1597. Jean Beguin, famous as the founder of the didactic French chymical tradition, borrowed from Libavius and probably began lecturing around the end of 1607 or 1608.

Leiden formal instruction in chymistry, as part of the standard *practica* course, began earlier and enjoyed a more open embrace. Practical goals and possibilities enlivened interest in chymical medicine at Leiden, although Heurnius stayed mostly well within the well-ordered fields of Galenic theory

---

71   Debus, "Chemistry and the Universities in the Seventeenth Century."

72   Debus, "Chemistry and the Universities in the Seventeenth Century," 181. Frietsch, "Alchemy and the Early Modern University."

73   Krafft, "The Magic Word Chymiatria." Moran, *Chemical Pharmacy Enters the University.* Moran, *Andreas Libavius.*

74   Principe, "Changing Visions," 182.

75   Klein, "Alchemical Histories." Klein, "Daniel Sennert." Newman, *Atoms and Alchemy.*

76   Newman, *Atoms and Alchemy.* Blank, "Sennert."

77   Kahn, "First Private."

and practice. Like Sennert, he hoped for a reconciliation between chymistry and Galenic medicine, but, in contrast, one that mostly tamed the wild new speculations of chymists and brought them more clearly into the fold of "Asclepian" medicine. From the time of "Asclepius," plants had filled the lists of ingredients for most medicines, as detailed in the next section.

3   Cultivating Knowledge and Medicinal Simples in the Garden

Now is the time for a stroll in the university garden, where students could learn about medicinal plants in person, and begin thinking about how to use their powers to treat specific diseases. As much as possible in a brief discussion, we will attempt to recover the types of plants encountered, their origins and arrangement in the garden, and the teaching tools and practices which constituted Leiden education in medicinal substances. The verdant abundance of the garden mirrored the variety of practices for knowing plants. As always, academic practices combined humanist scholarship with first-hand sensory experience. Professors and students collected plants on herborizing field trips, received them as gifts in local or global exchange networks, appropriated plants as the fruit of empire, followed and critiqued ancient sources, wrote and read newer textbooks, consulted herbals, examined watercolors of plants in the winters, visited apothecaries' shops, viewed, touched, smelled, and tasted samples, and tried out remedies on themselves, their relations, and patients. Like the anatomy theater, as we will later see, the university garden flourished as a node for the exercise of these different practices. As Petrus Paaw and Johannes Heurnius discovered when faced with the task of instruction in the garden, even professors had to endure long practice to learn how to identify plants and their properties.

Founded in 1590, then developed quickly through 1594, the university garden nestled next to the main academic building on the Rapenburg canal.[78] Like the garden site itself, the plantings fit together in rectangular blocks, with four main quadrants of twelve or sixteen rectangular beds. The Ambulacrum, an enclosed, covered gallery on the south side built in 1601, provided lecture space in rainy or cold weather, housed medical books for reference, and displayed natural historical specimens such as shells and preserved animals, as well as minerals and plants brought in for the winter. A Latin inscription on the Ambulacrum stipulated visitation only under supervision: students were

---

78   Tjon Sie Fat, "Clusius' Garden."

permitted only to see and smell the plants, and not harm them. They could not pull on the tender or growing parts, or pluck off branches, flowers, or seeds, or dig up bulbs or roots. Nor should they jump over or trample the "pillows" of earth in which the plants grew.[79] Despite these restrictions, students apparently remained eager for their hour in the garden.

Accounts from the professors and the students detail similar practices and interests. Petrus Paaw began teaching botany and anatomy in 1592, and by 1599 he was prefect of the garden and living in the adjoining university house.[80] His 1601 garden work-book for students announced his teaching, and provided an index of plants, but consisted mainly of 175 pages with fill-in-the-blank boxes, one for each "pillow" in the garden. He advertised some 900 plants, and taught the students the plants' "names, etymologies, powers, and faculties," explaining how strong each is, and when it should be used in medicine.[81] One copy of his book, apparently used by a student in 1601, is mostly completed (Figure 10). Names of plants and their origins appear in most boxes, but absent are frequent mentions of their powers or medicinal uses.[82]

Later, while defending his teaching and expertise against critics, Paaw reiterated that he taught the plants in person over the summers, noting their "nature, powers, and affections." He taught from the Latin expanded editions of the ancient Greek herbal of Dioscorides daily, "so those things which the spectators had seen in the garden, those the listeners could hear in the lecture and learn, and so by the twin senses they would make their way to our discipline."[83] He also took the students on herborizing trips, excursions popular in other European medical schools: "as the occasion arose (moreover it arose three or four times a year), I furnished to the students the not-inglorious work of medicine in fields, in hills, in woods and forests, and in marshy places."[84]

Students prized these activities and the expertise they cultivated. In 1598, after the early death of the apothecary and naturalist Dirck Cluyt (1546–1598) who helped found and direct the garden, seventeen students submitted a detailed petition to the university Curators asking for the appointment of

---

79   Paaw, *Hortus Publicus*, front matter.

80   Molhuysen, *Bronnen*, I, 122.

81   Paaw, *Hortus Publicus*, *4r.

82   Paaw, *Hortus Publicus*, 152. URL=http://mdz-nbn-resolving.de/urn:nbn:de:bvb:12-bsb103 02693-3. I base the dating on a note added to a blank section, 152, indicating that the area immediately next to the Ambulacrum, constructed 1599–1601, did not allow much planting at the time. Tjon Sie Fat, "Clusius' Garden," 8. Otterspeer, *Groepsportret*, 1, 196. Compare to the 1594 official catalog: Molhuysen, *Bronnen*, 1, 317*–334*.

83   Paaw, *Primitiae Anatomicae*, *ijv.

84   Paaw, *Primitiae Anatomicae*, *ijv. Cooper, *Inventing the Indigenous*, ch. 2.

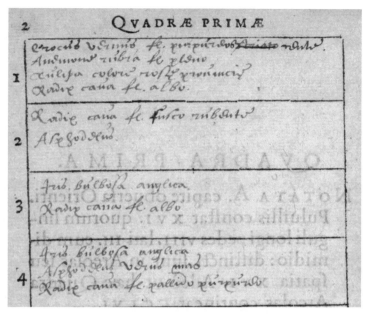

FIGURE 10   Entries for the first "pillow" of the first area of the garden, ca.
1601, listing plants such as crocus, anemone, radix cava (hollow
root), and asphodel. Paaw, *Hortus Publicus*, 2.
COURTESY, STAATS-UND STADTBIBLIOTHEK AUGSBURG, NAT
771-4# BEIBD. 2, P. 2, URN:NBN:DE:BVB:12-BSB11272075-1.

Dirck's son, Outgert Cluyt (1577–1636). Although he was only twenty-one at
the time, the students praised Outgert's expertise. Trained as an apothecary,
he also knew Greek and Latin well enough, and understood the seasons of the
plants. Further, Outgert knew foreign and local naturalists, and could teach
from the storehouses of specimens his father had used: over four thousand
simples, or dried plant samples, as well as many books of paintings of all sorts
of flowers. Lastly, the students claimed, Outgert was the only person who could
understand the full register of the garden.[85] As prefect of the garden, Outgert
would open the garden to students a full hour each day, and show dried plants
and minerals twice a week, as well as the six books of botanical watercolors,
which according to one contemporary estimate reached one thousand and
fifty figures or sheets.[86]

---

85   Molhuysen, *Bronnen*, 1, 380*–381*.
86   Letter of Anselm de Boodt to Clusius, 1602, quoted in Egmond, "Clusius, Cluyt, Saint
Omer," 28.

In their petition to the Curators, the students emphasized that the watercolors to be used in place of the garden in the winter were painted "from the life" (*near t leven*). As Claudia Swan has argued, this phrase and other terms, such as the Latin *ad vivum*, grew over from the natural historical tradition in the later 1500s into art practice then art theory around 1600.[87] We lack the set of paintings Cluyt used, but they may have followed similar practices found in a set of hundreds of botanical and zoological watercolors, the *Libri Picturati*. Florike Egmond has conclusively demonstrated that the core of hundreds of botanical paintings of this set come from the collection of Charles de Saint Omer (Karel van Sint Omaars), composed with the collaboration and annotations of Carolus Clusius in the 1560s. These watercolors, Egmond shows, emerged from the culture of "Bruges humanism," which united aristocratic patron-collectors like Saint Omer with artists and scholars such as Clusius.[88]

Across the sixteenth century, naturalists, collectors, and teaching physicians used a range of visualization techniques.[89] Watercolor paintings, such as those in the Saint Omer collection, and probably those used by Cluyt at Leiden, used color to show a range of seasonal appearances, with plants in bloom, or fruited and dried. Such colored images differed from Otto Brunfels' use of Hans Weiditz's "lifelike" images "imitated from nature" in their 1530s *Herbarum vivae icones*.[90] The Weiditz-Brunfels approach could obscure parts of the individual plant depicted with shading, and each could lack the range of growth stages or colors produced in nature—they were incomplete.

A decade after Brunfels, in 1542, Leonhart Fuchs published his own herbal, with illustrations exceeding the limitations of the singular specimen and artistic shading or arrangement. Instead, he took particular care to have illustrations done to match the text description exactly, and to include all important parts and stages of each plant: roots, stems, leaves, flowers, seeds, and fruits all together.[91] This resulted in a depiction as complete as possible (*absolutissima*), but yet not visible as such in the world, with flowers, fruits, and dried seed pods adorning the same plant. In contrast, the Saint Omer watercolors on which Clusius collaborated with scholarly annotations, showed the range

---

87   Swan, *Art, Science, and Witchcraft in Early Modern Holland*, 10–12, 36–51. Egmond's work joins with earlier scholarship to correct the claims of Claudia Swan that the *Libri Picturati* botanical watercolors came from Cluyt's collection, with his annotations. Swan, "*Lectura-Imago-Ostensio*."

88   Egmond, "Clusius, Cluyt, Saint Omer," 64. I thank two anonymous reviewers for help on this point.

89   Kusukawa, *Picturing the Book of Nature*, chapters 5–8.

90   Brunfels, quote and trans. in Swan, *Art*, 45.

91   Kusukawa, *Picturing the Book of Nature*, 114.

of the growth of vital plant parts—flowers, seeds, roots, leaves—with precise, naturalist colors and lines, but without depicting impossible specimens. Small spaces or cuts divided different branches with fruits and flowers, much like the compositions of plant parts on the dried herbal sheets.[92]

Students and professors wanted to see plants alive in their natural homes, too. At Leiden, students stressed that Outgert could lead herborizing trips to dunes, peat bogs, and forests, and teach them about the compositions of medicines. Although the Curators declined to appoint Outgert and turned the matter of the direction of the garden over to the medical professors Paaw and Bontius, the parallels in the activities between the students' earlier petition and Paaw's descriptions highlight the importance students placed on a range of first-person instruction. They could see plants in the garden and hear remarks about their names and medicinal properties, and then gather, touch, taste, and smell them on field trips.

What was in the garden and where did the plants and other *naturalia* come from? First of all, from naturalist collectors. The Leiden university garden became a place of collective expertise and experience, as did so many other gardens across Renaissance Europe.[93] They were also places of wonders which drew neighbors and notable visitors from afar. Such connections and displays were good for an ambitious university. In 1591, Curators offered the job of prefect of the garden, once it was built, to Bernardus Paludanus of Enkhuizen, but Paludanus protested he could not persuade his wife to make the trip to Leiden.[94] The Curators expressed strong interest in Paludanus's famed collection, with its "rarities, plants, fruits, sprouts, animals, shells, minerals, earths, poisons, stones, marbles, corals, etc."[95] When Paludanus and his collection could not make the trip, the Curators doggedly pursued the leading naturalist in Europe, Carolus Clusius (1526–1609), often sending messages through friends of Clusius such as the Leiden naturalist Johan van Hoghelande. Clusius first declined, citing his age (then 65) and ill health, but eventually agreed on the condition that he did not have to give lectures. He thought he might still enjoy herborizing trips to nearby sites, for then the chance for new knowledge and plants sufficed. The Curators appointed him in October of 1592.

Clusius, the erudite and epistolary leader of the naturalists focused on plants in the 1580s-1610s, had studied medicine but never practiced and preferred instead to follow his delight in collecting, growing, and describing

---

92   Swan, "*Lectura-Imago-Ostensio*," 196–7.

93   Egmond, *World*. Ogilvie, *Science of Describing*.

94   Molhuysen, *Bronnen*, 1, 62, 180*, 66.

95   Molhuysen, *Bronnen*, 1, 180*.

plants.[96] Like other naturalists of the growing community in roughly the last four decades of the 1500s, he prized novelty, rarity, beauty, and priority in discovering and describing new plants, as well as unknown properties of known plants—his major works of his time in Leiden were his *History of Rare Plants* (1601) and *Ten Books of Exotics* (1605). Decades before, in his earlier works, occasional comments on the medicinal properties of plants dropped away, crowded out by his descriptions of the appearance and varieties of plants, their locations, and his attempts to grow them.[97] Clusius trained his attention on the visual characteristics of plants, noting their shapes, growth over time, and especially color differences.[98]

Clusius also contributed two shipments of plants, and arranged for his contacts in Europe to send more. Two early shipments met the hazards of travel, confiscated by border soldiers and embezzled by an Amsterdam apothecary.[99] Dirck Cluyt helped to organize the garden, taught students from 1594–1598, and acted as prefect, though he technically assisted Clusius. And yet, he did not receive the recognition he deserved from the Curators; they paid less than a third of the value for his sizable contribution to the university garden (400 guilders for his estimate of 1,500).[100]

Leiden professor Petrus Paaw also practiced as a naturalist collector, even lending *naturalia* to Clusius and donating some of his own rarities, such as stuffed birds and animals, to the garden's Ambulacrum. Despite his busy schedule teaching anatomy and other medical courses, Paaw put his hand to the garden and his pen to the networks of naturalists. Before Clusius arrived in Leiden, Paaw corresponded with him and communicated through mutual contacts such as the Leiden apothecary Christiaan Porret. In a letter to Clusius from August 1593, Paaw sympathized with Clusius's suffering in ill health, and attempted to smooth over a perceived imposition from Heurnius and the Curators. He insists there must have been some miscommunication through Hoghelande, since the bits of conversation Hoghelande jotted down in his little daybook do not reliably reflect what conversants actually spoke (this may have been due to Hoghelande being hard of hearing).[101] Paaw also emphasized that he worked hard in the garden, eagerly awaiting Clusius's bulbs, so Clusius

---

96   Ogilvie, *Science of Describing*, 41–44, 160. Egmond, *World*, 1–8.

97   Ogilvie, *Science of Describing*, 44.

98   Ogilvie, *Science of Describing*, 149–150.

99   Kroon, *Bijdragen*, 74. Tjon Sie Fat, "Clusius' Garden," 4.

100   Egmond, *World*, 159.

101   Petrus Paaw to Carolus Clusius, August 1593, Leiden University Library, VUL 101:214. As Florike Egmond points out, Hoghelande was also quite deaf, which may have contributed to miscommunications. Egmond, *World*, 164–169.

himself would not have to labor to cultivate the plants. He also mentioned a monstrous garlic, much bigger than the one in Frankfurt, revealing a common interest in rarities.

Naturalists shared information relatively freely along their networks, even across social differences, and they had to earn their expertise in accurate identification of plants. One of Clusius's friends in town, the eminent naturalist and landowner Hoghelande, scoffed to Clusius earlier in 1593 that "I hardly know whether he [Paaw] is doing it [botany] seriously or as a joke."[102] According to Hoghelande, Paaw confused varieties of plants Hoghelande knew well, and seemed in dire need of practice: "[he] did not know any plant, however commonly known it is among herbarists...he was with Heurnius in my two gardens, so that I know with certainty how much he knows about it; nor did he deny that, because he and Heurnius together asked me if I was content to have them coming there often to practice."[103] We might not want to take Hoghelande's account of Paaw's initial knowledge as an accurate assessment, but his remark shows Paaw and Heurnius hard at work, practicing the sensory exercises necessary for the formation of reliable experience and knowledge of plant identification.

Professors joined larger networks through local experts as well as their correspondence. As Florike Egmond shows, Hoghelande's own social network of those interested and learned about plants extended to Antwerp merchants gathering exotics from the east and west Dutch commercial empires; naturalists in Leiden, Enkhuizen, Middelburg, and Amsterdam; princes; and noblewomen such as Marie de Brimeu and Marnix de St. Aldegonde, as well as the wife of Lipsius and wives of other professors.[104] His letters to Clusius reveal his passion for flowering plants, especially rare types in fashion such as anemones and tulips, as well as rare local types from the coastal dunes. Networks of naturalist learning connected professors, apothecaries, noblewomen, merchants, and households across the empire.

Second, local scholars such as Clusius, Paaw, and the Cluyts actively traded specimens, and students collected on their travels. The governors of the Dutch East India Company gave Paaw exotic nuts, a lizard, and the leg and claw of a dodo; a former student sent several rare birds from Scandinavia.[105] Clusius's 1602 instructions for non-academic collectors, sent to the lords of East India Company, repeatedly asked for branches, flowers, leaves, and fruit from plants,

---

102   Hoghelande to Clusius, 30 May 1593, in Egmond, *World*, 160.
103   Hoghelande to Clusius, 20 May 1592, in Egmond, *World*, 160.
104   Egmond, *World*, 166.
105   Egmond, *World*, 160.

especially "strange" or "foreign" (*vreemd*) ones, and to note their local names and uses as well.[106] Vital parts of the plants told more than drawings, which often misled when uneducated artists produced them. Only experienced naturalists produced reliable, credible knowledge, especially from personal experience.

Botanizing across early modern Europe and the sunny Mediterranean also threatened travelers with the perils of the period. Outgert Cluyt grew up around his father's apothecary shop in Delft and the local communities of naturalists, gardeners, physicians, and apothecaries. He matriculated in medicine at Leiden in 1601, and developed good Latin and Greek skills like other scholars. From 1602 to 1607, he traveled in Europe and around the Mediterranean, sending letters in Latin back to Paaw. He met anatomists of interest to Paaw, and collected hundreds of seeds, sending many back to Leiden, and noted some plants which promised "marvelous effects."[107] With his collecting, he hoped to fill out Clusius's catalog and also contribute to practical medicine— he mentioned visiting private patients with the professors at Leiden. He also asked Paaw to bear a greeting to his mother.[108] But between February and October of 1607, he had faced pirates and been jailed three times (and freed by the promise of a ransom). In North Africa "barbarians" seized and bound him, and he wore out his shoes on a forced march, only to be jailed again. Yet he still learned about medicinal herbs from Jewish doctors there, and managed to send many roots, bulbs, shoots, and seeds. Alas, other samples he had to commit to the sea; herborizing across the Mediterranean world offered rare treasures and frequent dangers.

These additions from travels and networks of correspondents augmented the first plantings, drawn mainly from the gardens of Dirck Cluyt, Clusius, and their network. The initial 1594 census of plants, drawn up by Dirck Cluyt and Clusius, listed 1,060 species of plants.[109] In the beds students could find hundreds of common and traditional medicinal plants such as dittany, chicory, digitalis, aconite, hellebore (in at least ten varieties), artemisia, salvia, and roses. From farther away, came Mediterranean cypress; Middle Eastern tulips, daffodils, and hyacinths; and American potato, tomato, and tobacco plants. Undoubtedly, Clusius and Cluyt included some of the plants for their rarity and beauty, independently of medicinal concerns.[110] This seems clear from the

---

106   Clusius, in Ogilvie, *Science of Describing*, 255.
107   Molhuysen, *Bronnen*, 1, 439*.
108   Molhuysen, *Bronnen*, 1, 440*.
109   Molhuysen, *Bronnen*, 1, 317*–334*. Tjon Sie Fat, 7–8.
110   Tjon Sie Fat, "Clusius' Garden," 7–8. Egmond, *World*, 158. Ogilvie, *Science of Describing*, 162.

twelve or more varieties of tulips. Yet even tulips, traded mainly for their rarity and beauty by naturalists and amateurs or *liefhebbers*, promised medicinal profits as well. In 1608, Joost van Ravelingen annotated Rembertus Dodonaeus's *Cruydt-Boeck*, affirming that tulip bulbs acted as a powerful aphrodisiac.[111]

Variety alone did not indicate a lack of medicinal powers, as shown by at least ten varieties of hellebore and ten varieties of aconite (one identified by Clusius) in the 1594 garden. These were both common drug ingredients, with hellebore a favorite purgative from the ancient pharmacopoieas. Yet the organization of the garden followed visual similarities in plant shapes and growth rather than medicinal powers. Unlike Dioscorides and earlier writers of other medicinal herbals, Clusius and other naturalists of his time tended to organize plants by morphology. Rare, exotic types stood out to the curious and acquisitive. By 1610, four beds with the rarest exotics—beautiful tulips, hyacinths, lilies, and more pedestrian but still rare types such as Hungarian wild garlic—sported stout fences against thieves.[112]

Thus even the university garden worked as a site for *two* overlapping communities defined by different communal practices: learned natural historians such as Carolus Clusius, who avidly studied and collected plants to learn about rare and new varieties and properties, and to develop and advertise his expertise as a naturalist; and physicians, medical students, apothecaries, and other healers who sought knowledge of plants primarily to learn and use their faculties or powers for preserving health and fighting disease. Of course, the Curators also wanted collections and experts for the prestige they lent to the young university.

4   Naturalists Knowing Plants by Experience and Experiment

Physician-naturalists learning about the medicinal powers of plants and naturalists interested more in description, novelty, and beauty differed in some practices, though they all grounded and tested their knowledge with experience and even some experiments. The two overlapping communities shared sites and members, and often individual actors shared allegiances and activities in both. Historians have highlighted the descriptive and aesthetic focus of later-sixteenth-century natural history, arguing that leading naturalists showed minimal interest in the plants for their medicinal properties.[113] Brian Ogilvie

---

111   Klerk, "Galen Reconsidered," 27 vs. Goldgar, *Tulipmania*, 39.
112   Ogilvie, *Science of Describing*, 161.
113   Ogilvie, *Science of Describing*, 29. Egmond, *World*, 4–5.

has traced the textual, collecting, communicative, descriptive, organizing, and social practices of the community of humanist, university-educated natural historians across the sixteenth century, stitching together printed texts, correspondence, and manuscript traces.[114] In explicit contrast, Florike Egmond deftly reconstructs the local communities of experts in *naturalia* which formed in different geographic centers and crossed some social lines, using for scaffolding the extensive correspondence of Carolus Clusius.[115]

In both approaches, naturalists and physicians alike trained in methods of precise and accurate identification of plants and other medicinal substances (though naturalists increasingly outstripped many physicians in the fineness of their descriptions and their zeal for such knowledge). Naturalists, more so than physicians, sought exact knowledge of plants, especially new and exotic types, for the pleasure and glory of knowing, describing, and growing them first of all. They tended to emphasize first-person, sensory "experience" of plants while on herborizing trips or working in gardens. But they also blended elements from encounters with multiple individual plants into single descriptions in their printed works.[116]

Physicians, especially teaching professors and students, emphasized the medicinal uses of plants, with accuracy in identification serving the end of the safe and effective use of the plants' powers or faculties to cure diseases and maintain health. While naturalists occasionally made trials, tests, or experiments by varying the conditions of plant growth or by anatomy of plants and animals, physicians relied on trials of drugs or "experience" in patients in order to know and fine-tune their capacities for effecting changes in bodies, especially drugs' higher-order faculties beyond heating, cooling, drying, or wetting.

Experimentation appears among the practices of both communities, though more commonly and explicitly in the testing of drugs among the medically-minded. Using the senses, especially taste, physicians could reason to the elemental qualities of simple substances, or medicinal "simples." Thus mint tasted cool, and so had an abundance of the basic quality of cold; pepper was sharp and hot. In this way, flavors, interpreted through a Galenic-Aristotelian philosophical matter theory of the qualities, provided an index of the basic qualities. But higher-order qualities or faculties, although generated from the basic elemental makeup, did not follow neatly from these elemental qualities. Many medicines contained multiple ingredients; the prized theriac (a medicine against venom or poison, often including viper flesh), consisted in forty to

---

114   Ogilvie, *Science of Describing*.
115   Egmond, *World*.
116   Ogilvie, *Science of Describing*, 12–21.

seventy or more ingredients. Thus, trying out medicines on patients remained essential as part of explicit methodology and daily practice.

Of course, many of the practitioners in these two analytical "communities" acted as respected members of both, even those without university degrees. Dirck Cluyt was a Delft apothecary with some Latin who worked closely with physicians and gardening naturalists to set up the university garden and teach students there for four years. Cluyt had established a flourishing apothecary shop in Delft, befriended the famed and royal physician Pieter van Foreest (and married into his family), and built a fine private garden and network of naturalist friends and correspondents.[117] His son Outgert gained more of the book-learning helpful for corresponding in Latin and training as a physician. And Paaw and Johannes Heurnius, though mainly professors of medicine rather than gardeners, helped to enhance, direct, and teach in the university garden, and even practiced plant identification in Hoghelande's expansive private garden just outside of Leiden.

These two overlapping communities shared more than common sites and objects of study; they shared a strong emphasis on first-person experience and expertise, which all understood as an epistemic virtue, a stance they drew in part from their engagement with ancient texts. The reform of scholarly natural history beginning in the 1490s grew out of medical professors' concerns about the apparent errors of the ancient Roman natural historian Pliny and Arabic authors in their descriptions of medicinal substances. Humanist scholars brought fresh energy and manuscripts to their engagement with the many obvious textual errors of Pliny's *Natural History*, especially as compared with the works on plants by Theophrastus and Dioscorides. Professors Ermolao Barbaro and Niccolò Leoniceno used keen philological erudition to cut away errors and corruptions in extant copies of Pliny's work.[118] While Barbaro always vindicated the correctness of the genuine Pliny, Leoniceno castigated the Roman historian for his mistakes against the senses. Should any authority receive credit against "our own eyes"? Aristotle, Galen, and Avicenna all agreed that compelling evidence from the senses rendered other sources of proof irrelevant, and "[w]hy did nature grant us eyes and the other senses, if not that we might see and investigate truth with our own resources?"[119] In order to train students to practice effective, safe medicine, they and their teachers had to

117   Egmond, *World*, 161. Molhuysen, *Bronnen*, 1, 435*–443*.

118   Ogilvie, *Science of Describing*, 122–133. Nutton, "The Rise of Medical Humanism." Nauert, "Humanists, Scientists, and Pliny."

119   Leoniceno, quote and trans. in Ogilvie, *Science of Describing*, 129.

combine textual precision and accuracy with first-hand sensory engagement: words and things together.

Scholars in other disciplines noticed the productivity and first-person authority of Renaissance natural history. As Sachiko Kusukawa has recently emphasized, physicians frequently practiced and published in both anatomy and medical natural history.[120] In his preface to the emperor Charles V, the anatomist Andreas Vesalius began his call for learned, humanist physicians to restore anatomy and its central place in medicine by praising the example of scholars studying medicinal simples. Through tireless labor and erudition, they had contributed to the restoration of the "pristine splendor" of botany; anatomists should do the same.[121] Leading anatomists such as Vesalius also studied, taught, and published on plants and other *materia medica*. Three years after his first edition of the *Fabrica*, Vesalius waded into the craze and controversy over using boiled "China root" for treating syphilis. He pointedly avoided categorizing the root according to Galenic theory, dismissed its popular use, and then spent even more time continuing his critique of Galen's anatomical errors.[122] Yet his dismissal and European commercial enthusiasm for the root provoked a wave of further investigations and publications.[123] In natural history as in anatomy, academic controversies over authoritative texts and personal experience drove auto-catalyzing cycles of the spread of first-person encounters with things, and even the making of trials to test claims and discover new phenomena.

For the most part, those who primarily practiced as naturalists, such as Clusius, "tried" or "experimented" with different soils, water, or lighting conditions when they attempted to grow and vary the plants in their gardens. Such practices and goals no doubt reach back far across human farming and gardening practices, but it is worth noting some of the explicit language and practices of making trials or experiments, as we build our panorama of medical trials at Leiden. Clusius continued language of "making a trial" widespread among physicians in the 1500s, mentioning in 1592 that he would be "making a trial" of some new anemones plants.[124] Two years later, he encouraged his fellow Leiden professor and gardener, the humanist Stoic philosopher Justus Lipsius, to try out an abundant variety of tulips by settling the seeds and

---

120   Kusukawa, *Picturing the Book of Nature*, 2012).

121   Vesalius, *Fabrica* (1543), *2v.

122   Vesalius, *Epistola*. Vesalius, *"The China Root Epistle."*

123   Winterbottom, "Of the China Root," 36.

124   Carolus Clusius to Joachim Camerarius II, Nov. 22, 1592. CLU C290. URL=https://clusius-correspondence.huygens.knaw.nl/edition/entry/588/transcription

immature tulips into wooden boxes, placed in sites warmed by the Sun. "To experience/try it [*experire*], perhaps you will take no less pleasure from those while they are springing up and from the growth of them each year than from the flowers themselves."[125] The busy Leiden apothecary Christiaan Porret (1554–1627), who also participated in the community of physicians, printers, and professors, used similar language, writing in French in 1611 that he "had experimented [*experimente*] for three or four years" with different bulbs and seeds, varying their locations, positions, pots, humidity, and light, and then checking especially for color stability in the flowers.[126]

Contemporary dictionaries synonymized the Latin *periculum facere*, the French *experimenter*, the Dutch *ondersoecken*, and similar terms, with all meaning "to Assay, Trie, Tempt, or to Enquire or Examine," in an "Experimen-tall" manner, "to find by trial," and similar expressions.[127] Of course, the French *expérience*, the Italian *esperienza*, or the Latin *experimentum* and *experientia* could all mean everyday experience *or* a deliberate trial or experiment. But investigators increasingly signaled deliberately carrying out tests with other words or phrases, too, especially those expressing the *making* of a trial or test.[128]

Such incidental or systematic variations in gardening conditions nicely characterize the "garden experimentation" identified by Florike Egmond as widespread in European Renaissance gardens of the 1570s–1590s, practices shared by professors, apothecaries, merchants, nobles, men, women, students, and artisans.[129] In general these activities were not tests of claims, let alone theories, but more "try and see" attempts to grow and vary plants. They tested some specific claims, such as when Clusius checked to see if carnation seeds placed in water with saffron produced red carnations (it did not). Instead, this sort of try-and-see variation usually followed closely the mundane demands of gardening.

In contrast, university-trained physicians inside or outside the university used trials to investigate more general questions about natural phenomena (which Egmond styles as "botanical experimentation").[130] Later in the century,

125 Carolus Clusius to Justus Lipsius, Oct. 8 1594, CLU C316. https://clusiuscorrespondence. huygens.knaw.nl/edition/entry/421

126 Christiaan Porret to M. Caccini, January 1611, in Egmond, *World*, 251, n. 34, 162–3.

127 Hexham, *Het groot woorden-boeck*, *345. "Experimenter" and "Espreuve" in Cotgrave, *A Dictionarie of the French and English Tongues*. "Experiment. To finde by trial," in Cockeram, *English Dictionarie*.

128 Ragland, "'Making Trials.'" Eamon, *Science*, 55–58, 150, 221. Schmitt, "Experience and Experiment." Garber, "Descartes and Experiment." Findlen, *Possessing Nature*, ch. 5.

129 Egmond, "Experimenting with Living Nature."

130 Ragland, "'Making Trials.'" Egmond, "Experimenting with Living Nature," 29–33.

eminent naturalist Ulisse Aldrovandi (1522–1605) used a trial to adjudicate a running debate between philosophers over the preservative powers of honey. He tried walnuts, figs, peaches, and pears. Only the walnuts did not putrefy, though once a sour peach showed preservation all winter in Mantua, and the dregs of wine helped to keep another preserved (though inedible).[131] In the 1590s, Onorio Belli grew young baobab trees from fruit imported from Cairo. His careful attention revealed steady variation of the leaves, as well as daily turning toward the Sun (heliotropism), a matter "wonderful and worthy of observation."[132]

Physicians likely made many more trials, but they were hardly the only ones. Around the same time in the Low Countries, Tobias Roels, a physician in Middelburg and friend of Clusius, moved from comments on coconut sprouts to philosophical speculations about why oil floats, engaging the long debate over heaviness and lightness reinvigorated by professors such as Borro and Galileo. Curiosity drove these investigators, as well as the desire for credit for priority in discoveries from their colleagues. As Egmond details, the Dutch fish merchant and auctioneer Adriaan Coenens (1514–1587) filled notebooks with his dissections and investigations, dissecting hundreds of fish and marine mammals, and carefully observing the change of caterpillars into butterflies and tadpoles into frogs.[133] His deep curiosity about the origins of life extended to making a test of the origins of maggots on meat. Even when the flies seemed to remain separate from the meat for three hot days, maggots still emerged. With only village school training and some encounters with Dutch translations of works of natural history, Coenen fed his curiosity with tests similar to those of the eminent Mattioli on galls a few decades earlier, or even Francesco Redi on galls and maggots a century later.[134]

For naturalists, it seems, experimentation was not yet a self-conscious practice which they set out intentionally to cultivate or discussed in their reflections on practice. Experimentation appears incidentally, on the way to a communal goal. Only very rarely did experiments or trials reach beyond trying out different ways to grow plants to touch on theory. Usually, other, non-theoretical motives inspired these tests or attempts. Describing new plants and natural phenomena, controversies among claims ancient and contemporary, the desire for credit and glory, the practicalities of growing and varying plants,

131   Ragland, "Making Trials,'" 514.
132   Belli, quote and trans. in Egmond, "Experimenting with Living Nature," 31.
133   Egmond, "Experimenting with Living Nature," 36–8. Egmond, *Het Visboek*.
134   Ragland, "Making Trials,'" 513. Parke, "Flies from Meat and Wasps from Trees."

and the passion of curiosity all inspired people to engage in experimentation in and around gardens. At the university, the demands of medical practice drove students and professors to develop the skill of precise plant identification with exacting knowledge of their medicinal powers.

5   God's Medicines and Models of Making Trials

Making medicines from plants in the garden or imperial commerce demanded far more widespread and frequent trials.[135] As noted above, healers could discover or check most of the healing powers of plants only through making trials. The higher-order faculties of plants followed from their primary qualities, or from their "total substance," but only in ways apparently opaque to reason. Early modern commerce and empire brought a deluge of new substances, which provoked wider, more frequent, and novel testing. A vibrant Christian providentialism imbued physicians with the firm belief that God had given remedies for all diseases throughout the world of plants. But the basic models and language of making trials, and the matter theory that embraced the search for qualitative indexes for guessing about plant faculties all continued from ancient sources. Renaissance expansions and corrections of the ancient Greek herbal of Dioscorides and the books on medicines by Galen formed the core of teaching and learning about drugs in universities. Despite our present-day skepticism about the efficacy of pre-modern remedies, all of this combined to make most physicians confident that they could find effective, safe, and agreeable remedies for their patients.

Naturalists, apothecaries, merchants, physicians, and naturalist-physicians all hoped for new remedies from global empires. These dreams became more vivid after the widespread investigation and debate around drugs such as the high-priced Peruvian bark (guaiacum, cinchona), new balsam, sarsaparilla, sassafras, and other promising substances adopted from indigenous peoples in the "New World," and then collected, tested, and brought back by Spanish officials and physicians.[136] After all, God made plants for just this purpose, and now a whole New World of them promised new remedies.

---

135   Cook, *Matters of Exchange*, chs. 5, 8, 9. Rankin, *Panacea's Daughters*. Leong and Rankin, eds., "Testing Drugs and Trying Cures." Ragland, "'Making Trials,'" 509–519.
136   Cook, *Matters of Exchange*, 98, 128, 203, 305, 365. Egmond, *World*, 155. Estes, "The European Reception of the First Drugs from the New World," 3–23. Huguet-Termes, "New World Materia Medica in Spanish Renaissance Medicine." Barrera, "Local Herbs, Global Medicines." Wear, *Knowledge & Practice*, ch. 2.

That so many plants and other natural substances promised treasures of healing powers was not in doubt. Like other healers across Europe, Leiden physicians endorsed a monotheistic version of the maxim of the ancient Alexandrian anatomist, Herophilus, that drugs were nothing in themselves, but used rightly acted as "the hands of the gods."[137] Scripture concurred with this providential vision of natural remedies, per Ecclesiastes 38:4. "The Lord hath created medicines out of the earth; and he that is wise will not abhor them."[138] At Leiden, teaching physician Johannes Heurnius added an epigram to many of his works: "If God had not been present, and poured powers into plants, / What, I ask, would dittany, would panaceas help?"[139] While the face of Nature constantly changed, God had instituted an "unbroken and fated law," of opposing elemental qualities, that "the cold things fight with the hot, the humid things with the dry."[140] The "kindly parent Nature" was nothing other than a "living power of GOD," and produced at God's command the effective powers of remedies to fight diseases.

God had created many plants for use as ingredients which produced targeted effects in bodies. For example, the liver played an important role as one of the principal or chief organs of the body, turning nutriment into venous blood and acting as the seat of the natural faculties. So, God had provided a "great supply" of remedies for correcting its diseases.[141] Chicory, for example, cooled an overheated liver but did not cool the nearby stomach, acting as an effective, targeted simple. Yet these medicinal "simples" could have contrary effects: roses loosen and constrict; rhubarb purges out stagnant bellies, yet also holds back excessive flows. Depending on the strength of a disease located or "seated" in a given part, one might have to mitigate the power of an ingredient, or strengthen its qualities and faculties, by mixing it precisely with other ingredients. For instance, scammony itself acts as a powerful purgative and de-worming drug, but grows mild when mixed with roses; similarly, anise tempers the violence of the explosive purgative hellebore, and crocus weakens the soporific effect of opium.[142]

A strong sense of Providence undergirded early moderns' optimism about natural remedies and combined with traditions of ancient excellence and long use to create what Andrew Wear describes as an "ethos of certainty" about the

137   Johannes Heurnius, *Aphorismi*, 8. Von Staden, *Herophilus*, 400.

138   KJV.

139   Johannes Heurnius, *Institutiones*, 554. Heurnius, *De morbis qui in singulis partibus humani capitis insidere*, 351.

140   Johannes Heurnius, *Nova Ratio*, Preface.

141   Johannes Heurnius, *Nova Ratio*, 193.

142   Johannes Heurnius, *Nova Ratio*, Preface.

efficacy of traditional remedies and even new medicinals for new diseases.[143] Dutch physicians joined the optimistic, faithful chorus. Johannes Heurnius quoted Galen about the foolishness of putting aside already-approved remedies, calling them "sacred" on account of their greater agreeableness for the patients.[144] He stuffed the majority of his course and textbook on medical practice with discussions of specific "medicines proven by use," targeted at different diseased parts of the body.[145] Vernacular medical books agreed. In his widely-read Dutch *Treasure of Unhealthiness*, Dordrecht city physician and cultural "institution" Johan van Beverwijck (1594–1647), who had studied medicine at Leiden and Padua, expressed common confidence in the long experience of physicians from the ancient period on: "All the powers of medicines, which have been described by the Ancients, and are still passed on, have by them first been proven, and found, on the whole."[146]

How, then, could Renaissance physicians and naturalists come to know these medicinal powers or faculties? The answers usually depended on experience, reason, and the senses. Here, "experience" referred to both one's own uses and observations of medicines, and the centuries of long, collective use of remedies and attention to their effects. Quite often, "experience" referred to singular or repeated instances of the use of drugs, or even deliberate trials of drugs in sick patients, and frequently appeared as *experientia* or *experimentum* in Latin, or *empeiria* (and sometimes *peira*, or trial) in the Greek.[147] Reason usually meant the use of natural philosophy, especially inferences to the principal qualities of medicinal substances, and the expected effects of those qualities on the qualitative states of body parts. The senses, especially taste and, to a lesser degree, smell, acted as indexes of the qualities of medicines in rational accounts.[148]

Another option found a vocal proponent in Paracelsus, who declared that God revealed the uses of plants to worthy healers through "signatures." In Paracelsus's anti-Galenic Christian philosophy, the active agents in Creation are more spiritual, and share correspondences with each other. God has made potential medicinal substances resemble parts of the body as signs of their mutual sympathy, made for our use since similars cure similars. Thus Eyebright (Eufragia) bears the image or signature of the eye, so it cures eyes

---

143   Wear, *Knowledge & Practice*, 67, 91.

144   Johannes Heurnius, *Institutiones*, 548.

145   Johannes Heurnius, *Nova Ratio*, 147–456.

146   Johannes an Beverwijck, *Schat der Ongesontheyt*, 73. Van Gemert, "Johan van Beverwijck als 'instituut.'"

147   Ragland, "'Making Trials,'" 509–515.

148   The most extensive treatment is Klerk, "Galen Reconsidered."

sympathetically.[149] Sharing this signature, Eyebright and eyes also corresponded with the Sun, which ruled vision. Since the natural world is a network of correspondences and similars indicated by signatures, some Paracelsians and other investigators depended on the science of signatures to reveal "all hidden things."[150] Although the conception of "the" early modern worldview as one of such signatures and correspondences has found influential proponents such as Michel Foucault, it did not achieve anything approaching universal acceptance in the early modern period, even among those drawing on the Paracelsian tradition.[151] Important Renaissance naturalists such as Conrad Gessner and Rembertus Dodonaeus stridently rejected this view.[152]

Dodonaeus (or Dodoens, 1517–1585) gives us a good introduction to the more common thinking of physicians and the textbooks they used. He wrote popular Dutch and Latin herbals, or detailed descriptions of plants and their medicinal faculties, in the second half of the 1500s. At the end of his life, he taught for just over two years in the new medical faculty at Leiden, from the end of 1582 until his death in early 1585. Like Galen, Dodonaeus wrote that physicians needed to know the faculties or powers of plants and other medicinal simples such as minerals. One came to know these by the effects evident in bodies after administration of the drugs, or, in the language of his tradition, after "experience" or "trials" (*experimenta*).[153] The recent idea that humans can discover and recognize the medicinal faculties of plants from their appearance or other signs, he wrote, is a "fabrication." Such powers and faculties, especially the hidden or occult ones, cannot be known in the way that human character can be read off from a person's appearance, or physiognomy. Yet physiognomy finds approval from Aristotle and other ancient philosophers, while "the doctrine of signatures of plants receives testimony from no one of any value among the ancients, and also is so unstable and uncertain that it seems that it cannot at all be held as a science or doctrine."[154] Similarly, for the Leiden professor Johannes Heurnius the doctrine of signatures or resemblances did not offer help to the physician, although it did not reach to the

149   Pagel, *Paracelsus*, 149.

150   Findlen, "Empty Signs?" 513.

151   Ashworth, "Natural History and the Emblematic Worldview." Ashworth endorses Foucault's interpretation, e.g., 306, 317–318.

152   Ogilvie, *Science of Describing*, 277, n. 64; 128, 130, 236. Maclean, "Foucault's Renaissance Episteme Reassessed," 157.

153   Lindeboom, *Dutch Medical Biography*, 453–454. Dodonaeus, *Stirpium Historiae Pemptades Sex*, 7.

154   Dodonaeus, *Stirpium Historiae Pemptades Sex*, 16.

level of "superstition" as incantations and other "abracadabra," which really only worked by naturally stirring the imagination and the bodily spirits.[155]

Instead, like the authors of their ancient textual sources Galen and Dioscorides, physicians and naturalists had to make trials of medicinal substances in patients. From the 1490s into the later 1500s, Renaissance naturalists and physicians increasingly took Dioscorides as a model. By far the most common textbook for medicinal substances—used at Leiden and just about everywhere else in tens of thousands of copies—came from the pen and press of Pietro Andrea Mattioli (1501–1577), who wrote an extensive commentary and expansion of the herbal of Dioscorides, and even styled himself the successor to Dioscorides. He claimed that his commentary appeared in over thirty thousand editions, and gained enough fame for him to serve as the physician to the Holy Roman Emperor, Maximilian II.[156]

As in other areas of Leiden academic medicine, ancient texts, supplemented with recent additions and critiques, formed the foundation of instruction. The work on *materia medica* of the first-century physician Dioscorides, translated into Italian then Latin, and greatly expanded by Mattioli in the middle of the 1500s, became a widespread teaching text at Leiden and across Europe. For professors and working physicians, Dioscorides offered an ancient pedigree, attestations in subsequent sources, and a catalog of over a thousand medicinal ingredients, buttressed by his personal expertise.

Renaissance physicians adopted Dioscorides and Galen as exemplars for their work in medicinal botany. The ancient authors' self-presentations provided models for emulation in pedagogical communities. Dioscorides rejected top-down systematizing and strongly emphasized seeing for oneself (*autopsia*) and trials in order to identify plants and investigate the powers and faculties of drugs. In contrast, he wrote, some of his sources and rivals relied only on words, and gathered accounts of the effects of medicines "without any trial [*experimentum*]" and with empty zeal for reaching causes, they poured out only words.[157] Some reported things plainly false, which indicated they accepted too much from the reports of others, not by "ocular confidence," or their own eyes. They then often arranged the histories of the plants in

---

155   Johannes Heurnius, *Institutiones*, 660.

156   Ogilvie, *Science of Describing*, 25, 34–35, 45. Findlen, "The Formation of a Scientific Community," 373–374.

157   Dioscorides, "Preface," in Mattioli, *Commentarii* (1565), 1. I have used the most common Latin translation and commentary of the time, and the one professors and students had on hand in Leiden. Cf. Scarborough and Nutton, "The *Preface*," 196.

alphabetical order, for ease of memorization, but this scheme split up substances with similar properties and uses.

In contrast, Dioscorides traveled throughout many regions, partly through his "soldier's life," and "came to know the greatest number of plants very exactly by sight itself." He asked his prefatory friend and future readers to judge not his verbal facility, but rather look to his careful, skillful application to things. His work described the kinds of individual medicinals and their powers (*vires*). Such knowledge is necessary, since it is joined to the whole of the art of medicine, and gives efficacious help to all its parts. Moreover, knowledge of compositions and mixtures of medicines extends to trials (*pericula*) done in diseased patients. In order to know the powers of drugs and their ingredients, one needed all this, as well as first-hand knowledge of plants, and to attend closely to variations in their growth, weather, seasons, sites, sunlight, collection, and storage. As ancient and early modern authors often cautioned, different varieties of plants could produce dangerously different effects in patients, and the soil, moisture, season, collecting vessels and other circumstances also contributed to this perilous variation.[158]

Dioscorides' close attention to the powers or faculties of drugs carried over into his organization of the medicinal substances. Beginning with individual or "simple" substances, he grouped the folk and elite medicines he encountered, in texts and in person, not by systems or theoretical features but by their preparation methods and observable effects or "faculties" (*dunameis* or *facultates*). This organization by faculties overlapped with grouping by natural characteristics, since in general faculties followed on natures.[159] Dioscorides wrote of "testing" drugs on sick patients, and used a word (*dokimasia*) that usually meant a legal examination of a person for status or rights, but more generally a test, including a test of substances by the senses.[160]

Scholars' recovery and use of Dioscorides' descriptions and method sparked serious worries and controversy in the later 1400s and early 1500s. Lack of a shared system of names, troubles of translation, and a flood of additions through the long fourteen centuries complicated the work of botanists and physicians by the 1500s. Medieval Arabic physicians and scholars had drawn from their wide regional resources around the Mediterranean and pieces of medical culture from India and China. They *added* more plants to the Greek pharmacopoeias than they found in them. By the late 1400s, translation posed a stubbornly tough problem, especially given the wide variety of

---

158   Dioscorides, "Preface," 2.
159   Touwaide, "Therapeutic Strategies," 266.
160   "*dokimasia*" in LSJ. Scarborough and Nutton, "The *Preface*," 201.

names for the same plants, or the same name for different plants, as well as Dioscorides' terse descriptions and what Renaissance humanists saw as Arabic corruptions of the original Greek sources.[161] Matching up physical plants and ancient names, descriptions, and powers met three main problems: naming, recovering ancient ingredients, and understanding new ones from new places. There were promiscuous and unreliable ingredient-name associations. Many of Dioscorides' identifications of medicinal plants remained mysterious or contentious. Worse, a host of vital ancient drugs listed in his book remained missing from early modern European apothecaries' stores, while the plants of northern Europe and Arabic sources often escaped the ancient Mediterranean catalogs.

Solving these puzzles demanded philological erudition, encounters with plants, and making trials of substances. Scholars debated identifications and drew on their learning to make glossaries. They pointed to substitutions for missing or mysterious ingredients in recipes. Around 1500, violent controversies proved that piecemeal scholarship no longer sufficed. Travelers and foreign healers and correspondents gradually filled in the gaps, topping up the many dozens of ingredients needed to reproduce the prized antidote theriac from the 1540s through the 1560s.

When Mattioli presented himself as a second, modern Dioscorides, he could collect information and samples from a vast European and Mediterranean network, and occasionally made his own investigations and trials.[162] He tested the efficacy of poison antidotes and remedies for intestinal worms, checked oak galls for spiders and insects, and made trials to identify the faculties of substances such as viper fat, chickpeas, and white beetroot.[163] In Leiden, an edition of Mattioli's translation and expanded commentary on Dioscordes' book appeared in the covered gallery of the garden, chained alongside Theophrastus's work on plants, with commentary by J. C. Scaliger, and the works of Galen and Hippocrates.[164] The official Leiden curriculum stipulated that Paaw used Mattioli's commentary version of Dioscorides' herbal in his lectures, at least from 1598, and likely as early as 1592.[165] Like Dioscorides, Mattioli almost always described what the various medicinal substances did when administered to human bodies, without giving explanations of why or how

---

161 Siraisi, *Medieval*, 143. Palmer, "Medical Botany." Ogilvie, *Science of Describing*, 131. Kusukawa, *Picturing the Book of Nature*, 101–3.

162 Palmer, "Medical Botany." Findlen, "The Formation."

163 Ragland, "'Making Trials.'" Rankin, *The Poison Trials*.

164 Molhuysen, *Bronnen*, 1, 154.

165 Molhuysen, *Bronnen*, 1, 113, 192*.

they did it. And, as Sachiko Kusukawa points out, other Renaissance naturalists' insistence on seeing for oneself (*autopsia*) and thorough examination to
gain the necessary precise knowledge of plants likely echoed Dioscorides' own
preface.[166]

As the new reports and collective experience grew, medical natural historians' confidence and self-regard swelled along with a selective embrace of
ancient claims. For instance, Mattioli's skepticism about early modern "theriac" turned to enthusiasm. As Richard Palmer details in an exemplary case,
a decades-long controversy over the identification of the poison Aconitum
moved from humanist invectives to testing one candidate, Doronicum, a medicine borrowed from Arabic practices as a heart remedy.[167] Paduan scholar Giacamo Antonio Cortusio tested precise doses of Doronicum on wolves, dogs,
and pigs, killing them all. His readers, including Mattioli, carried out their
own tests on a host of unfortunate animals. The humanist naturalist Conrad
Gessner tried on himself *twice* the dose deadly to dogs and survived with only
illness and stomach pains. Ignorance and mistaken identifications could be
deadly. Physicians and scholars increasingly used philological expertise, first-
hand experience, and some trials to sort the medicinal helps from the harms.

In his long commentaries added after his translations of Dioscorides' text,
or simply appended for accounts of new substances unknown to the ancients,
Mattioli often referred to his own practice of "making trials" (*periculum facere*).
He tested a variety of chickpea and found no medicinal properties, but his trials identified "wonderful effects" for a colleague's poison antidote.[168] He also
used trials to test claims from Dioscorides, Pliny, and Galen, for example confirming Pliny's recommendation of white beetroot for killing bowel worms.
Students, trained in this practice, continued making trials later, while working
as physicians. Michael Stolberg describes how the Bohemian physician Georg
Handsch first studied under Mattioli and Gabriele Falloppio, and then made
frequent trials of simples and compound medicines. Occasionally he used parallel trials, such as testing powdered "unicorn horn" as an antidote to a poison
(mercury sublimate) by giving the poison to two pigeons but the antidote to
one, and recording differential effects of medicines on patients.[169]

Of course, making trials of drugs and other remedies also extended well
beyond academic physicians. Women provided most of the medical care in
early modern Europe yet were routinely excluded from university medical

---

166   Kusukawa, *Picturing the Book of Nature*, 108.
167   Palmer, "Medical Botany," 155.
168   Mattioli, quoted in Ragland, "'Making Trials,'" 514.
169   Stolberg, "Empiricism," 502.

schools.[170] As Alisha Rankin shows, sixteenth-century noblewomen acted as courtly practitioners, making, assaying, testing, repeating, and witnessing medicinal cures. In the sixteenth century, non-academic medical writings flooded private homes and marketplaces, and the great majority of medical manuscripts consist of collections of recipes. As Elaine Leong, Sara Pennell, and other scholars show, seventeenth-century women and men elaborated on these practices, making, using, tweaking, recording, and sharing recipes for medicines and all sorts of household products.[171]

6 Galen's Models for Knowing Drugs and Making Trials

Elaborations and critiques of ancient texts became the main conceptual framework for the academic trials. After all, professors and students read, discussed, critiqued, commented on, memorized, and skimmed such texts daily. Galen's writings, which formed the foundations and framing of Renaissance academic medicine, provided professors, students, and physicians with sophisticated philosophical and methodological models for making trials and knowing the powers or faculties of drugs. Galen's *On the Faculties and Mixtures of Simple Drugs* (*De simplicium medicamentorum facultatibus ac temperamentis*), in particular emerged as a favorite of Renaissance physicians, appearing in sixteen European editions from 1530 to 1592.[172] Medieval Arabic and Latinate writers usually depended on adaptations and extracts from *Simple Drugs*, despite a complete translation by Niccolò da Reggio in the early 1300s.[173] But university curricula increasingly embraced the book from the early 1400s through the 1500s, at places ranging from Ferrara and Montpellier to Bologna and Leiden.[174] At Leiden, it appeared in course lists and lectures alongside Mattioli's edition and commentary on Dioscorides' work.[175] Professors such as Johannes Heurnius also relied on Galen's *Simple Drugs* and other medicinal works for their own textbooks and lectures.[176]

170   Rankin, *Panaceia's Daughters*.
171   Leong, *Recipes and Everyday Knowledge*. DiMeo and Pennell, eds. *Reading and Writing Recipe Books, 1550–1800*.
172   Siraisi, *Medieval*, 142. Durling, "Chronological Census." Karen Reeds, *Botany in Medieval and Renaissance Universities* (New York: Garland, 1991), 22, 42–43, 56, 61–62. Findlen, *Possessing Nature*, 159, 60, 254.
173   Ventura, "Galenic Pharmacology in the Middle Ages."
174   Grendler, *Universities*, 343, 346, 350. Findlen, *Possessing Nature*, 159, 250, 254.
175   Molhuysen, *Bronnen*, 1, 384*.
176   E.g. Heurnius, *Institutiones*, 69, 134

The importance of Galenic pharmacological texts for the development of early modern experimental practices and methodological reflections is very often overlooked by present-day historians, but they flourished as a widespread and ineliminable call to make trials among early modern universities and practicing physicians.[177] Since Galen's works on drugs informed nearly all academic Renaissance discussions of drug action and testing, and we still lack translations of *Simple Drugs* and other key texts, or even much scholarly engagement with them from historians of medicine, it is worth spending a few minutes reviewing its key models and concepts. Importantly, Galen's *Simple Drugs* explicitly articulated his epistemology and method of combining reason and experience, and provided models in the form of reports of his own first-person trials.

Like Dioscorides, Galen advocated and described making personal trials. He advertised his own experience working as a physician to gladiators, noting that those under his care and using his wound plaster suffered a low number of deaths. He sent recipes out for other doctors to try, "so that their efficacy could be confirmed by use."[178] Other remedies he attested from his own experience traveling, gathering herbs, testing medicines on patients, and circulating remedies among patrons, friends, and family.[179] Galen of course borrowed many of his remedies from elder doctors, and gleaned them from Hippocratic works, as Dioscorides did, but he frequently emphasized his methodology of making trials and instances of his actual trial-making.[180]

Unlike Dioscorides' book, Galen's *Simple Drugs* gave few tips for identifying the plants or other medicinal substances by their visual characteristics. Instead, he listed them by the hundreds, giving their common names and describing their temperaments, flavors, qualities, and medicinal faculties. He began with his broadly Aristotelian matter theory, and then spent several sections detailing his qualitative temperament theory in relation to the intensities and qualities of drugs. Then he catalogued hundreds of individual "simples," especially about four hundred and forty different plants, but also some two hundred and fifty

177   See, e.g., the lack of attention to Galen's *Simple Drugs* and pharmacology in Maclean, *Logic, Signs, and Nature*, and the reliance on Fernel's *De abditis* as the inspirational text in Klerk, "The Trouble with Opium." Compare Rankin, "On Anecdote and Antidotes" and Ragland, "'Making Trials'" for brief nods.

178   Galen, *Comp. Med. Gen.* 3.2, 13.599–603K, quote and trans. in Mattern, *The Prince of Medicine*, 262.

179   Scarborough and Nutton, "The *Preface*," 190.

180   Vogt, "Drugs and pharmacology," 311–313.

other substances such as earths, stones, minerals and metals, and animal products or parts used in medicines.[181]

Trials played indispensable roles in Galen's epistemology and practice. Along with his anatomical tests, they also appeared as exemplars of experimentation and even experimentalism.[182] Trial-making (*peira*) tested and confirmed the teachings of reason (*logos*), judged disputes in medicine, and often was the only means for reliably discovering the powers or faculties of drugs.[183] Alongside or as part of experience (*empeiria*) more generally, trials acted as a necessary part of Galen's method of joining reason and experience to produce a rational, effective practice.

One parallel trial stands out for its method. Galen narrated his own experience to describe his "method" by which one could settle the question of whether vinegar is hot. Since human bodies were at the midpoint of hot-cold temperaments, and skin possessed a moderate temperament in the human body, one should use a human's skin. First try a healthy, temperate body and then a body made unnaturally hot. Galen suggested using "unlearned" healthy subjects since "their judgment in things of this sort will be uncorrupted, namely since they not bound servilely to any dogma."[184] Immediately they would sense a manifest coldness, but after a few hours, gradually, they will feel something like a phantom or rumor of the beginning of heat.

In the next stage, he smeared the plant *thapsia* on himself and tried out different antidotes in different spots. He self-consciously followed a careful "method" to learn by "experience [*experientia*]...we made on ourselves, by which we could try more accurately the powers of the medicine."[185] Galen described how he made this experience or trial in specific, historical terms: "We spread [*thapsia*] on our thighs in different points, and after four or five hours, when they began to burn and become inflamed, we bathed one point with vinegar, another with water, another with oil; on a fourth, we spread rose-oil, and other specimens...[v]inegar proved to be more active."[186] Vinegar did

---

181   Vogt, "Drugs and pharmacology," 310.

182   Van der Eijk, *Medicine and Philosophy*, ch. 10. Ragland, "'Making Trials,'" 509–511.

183   R. J. Hankinson, "Epistemology," in *Cambridge Companion to Galen*, 176–177.

184   Galen, *De simplicium medicamentorum facultatibus libri XI*, 33. The Latin (*quia nulli videlicet dogmati serviliter sunt addicti*) puts me in mind of the Royal Society's Horatian source (*Nullius addictus iurare in verba magistri*).

185   Galen, *De simplicium medicamentorum facultatibus libri XI*, 34.

186   Galen, *De simpl. med. fac.* 1.21, quote and trans. in Gourevitch, "The Paths of Knowledge," in *Western Medical Thought*, ed. Grmek, 132. Galen, *De simplicium medicamentorum facultatibus libri XI*, 34–35.

this, according to all the sensory evidence, by cooling the heat of the *thapsia*, not merely blunting its bite, as an oil might.

This sophisticated parallel trial, and others made according to specified conditions or "qualifications" (*diorismoi*), appeared in *Simple Drugs*, which also articulated his general method combining reason and the right sort of experience, one informed by reason. Again and again in this work, Philip van der Eijk shows, Galen presented qualified or properly-conditioned experience as the best way to discover and test the faculties of drugs. He presented his system of the powers of drugs based not on plausible theory but on "qualified experience."[187] As he put it in *Simple Drugs*, "[T]he best addition to theory, as has been said many times, is to discover them on the basis of qualified experience. For you won't go wrong in this, even though before detecting the power by experience, taste provides most indications, with smell...providing some additional evidence."[188]

The goal of such properly-conditioned or qualified experience was to discover and refine *knowledge* of the capacities or faculties of medicinal substances. Aristotle's philosophy and the work on poisons by Diocles of Carystos in the fourth century B.C. pushed Greek attention to such capacities or faculties (*dunameis*), beginning a vocabulary and set of concepts carried on by Dioscorides, Galen, and many others into the early modern period.[189] For example, even a small amount of venom bears a hidden power to bring about great effects, including qualitative changes of a patient's entire body. So, too, medicinally-active substances have capacities or faculties for causing effects in living bodies.

The effects and abilities of drugs relative to specific body parts exemplified what Galen meant by "faculty" (*dunamis, facultas*). We have already examined this concept in detail in chapter three; a short summary review will suffice here. In his work on the mixtures and faculties of simple drugs, he defined a faculty as "an efficient cause" characterized by its effects: purging drugs have purgative faculties, sneeze-inducing drugs sneezing-inducing faculties, etc.[190] A spirited introduction to his work arguing that the passions of the soul follow (or just are) the changing mixtures of the body also took drug action as a model for faculties, and clarified his thinking. Faculties were not extra entities which "inhabit" substances as people inhabit houses, but relative concepts used to

---

187   Galen, *De simpl. med. fac.* 3.13 (11.573K), trans. in Van der Eijk, *Medicine and Philosophy*, 284.

188   Galen, *De simpl. med. fac.* 3.13 (11.573K), trans. in Van der Eijk, *Medicine and Philosophy*, 284, n. 15.

189   Touwaide, "Therapeutic Strategies: Drugs," 262–263, 270. See also chapter three above for more discussion of faculties in general.

190   Galen, *De simplicium medicamentorum facultatibus libri XI*, trans. Theodoricus Gaudanus (Leiden, Gulielmus Rouillius, 1561), 2. Kühn XI, 381.

track the bundles of effects substances have when applied to different objects.[191]
There are just as many faculties as there are relative effects. Thus, "aloe is *able* to
cleanse and strengthen the stomach, and bind wounds, to scar over grazes, to
dry moist eyes, there is no difference between the statement that it is *able
to cleanse* and the statement that it *has a cleansing faculty*; similarly, *being able
to dry wet eyes* means the same thing as *having a drying faculty for the eyes*."[192]
As Galen asserted in another work, "so long as we are ignorant of the true
essence of the cause operation, we call it a faculty."[193] Given the explanatory
power and everyday confirmation of their theory of the qualities, Galen and
most of his followers remained firmly convinced that a substance's faculties
derived from its basic mixture of hot, cold, wet, and dry qualities. Thus, talk of
faculties allowed physicians to correlate effects and ingredients, through what
they understood as the best matter theory of the time.

Understanding the properties of drugs required the marriage of reason and
experience. Experience can show us, through our senses, what happens, but
it cannot supply the rational causes *why* something happens, Galen repeats
in his work on medicinal simples.[194] Reason directed the physician toward
the proper method for using these rational qualifications or conditions. Using
reason, one could set up the trials in order to avoid confounding causes or accidental variations. According to reason and the best natural philosophy, these
faculties and effects had to result from the mixture or temperament of the drug
interacting with the mixture or temperament of parts of the patient's body.

Across his works, Galen defined the basic qualitative mixture, or temperament, as the essence of a drug's faculty. His approach here relied on the matter
theory he found in the "best" or "most distinguished" doctors and philosophers,
especially Hippocrates and Aristotle.[195] He noted that some deny the possibility of such knowledge altogether, namely the "Skeptic philosophers, and those
who among physicians are called Empirics."[196] Others think such knowledge
is possible, yet ascribe it to the "sizes, figures, and positions of particles and
pores," as did Galen's rival and frequent target Asclepiades.[197] The best philosophers, though, used careful reasoning and the everyday phenomena of the
senses to conclude that all things consisted of the principal qualities of hot,

191   Galen, *The Soul's Dependence on the Body* (QAM), in P. N. Singer, *Galen: Selected Works*
       (Oxford: Oxford University Press, 1997), 151. Renaissance Latin editions used similar
       language: Galen, *Galeni Omnia, quae extant*, (1562), 9v.
192   Galen, *Soul's Dependence*, trans. Singer, *Galen: Selected Works*, 151.
193   Galen, *On the Natural Faculties*, 1.4; Brock trans., 17.
194   Galen, *De simplicium medicamentorum facultatibus libri XI*, 11.5, 81–83.
195   Galen, *Mixtures*, trans. Singer, in *Galen: Selected Works*, 202.
196   Galen, *De simplicium medicamentorum facultatibus libri XI*, 2.
197   E.g., Galen, *On the Natural Faculties*, trans. Brock, 1.14.

cold, wet, and dry. These constituted the material stuff of the four elements fire, air, water, and earth, a theory Galen elsewhere attributed to Hippocrates.[198]

Galen's qualifications for experience, or rules for making trials, appear across his works on dietetics and drugs, as Van der Eijk demonstrates.[199] His book on simples used at Leiden and across Europe for centuries listed several qualifications for judging the effectiveness of a drug or assessing faculties from the phenomena following its administration to a patient. The physician had to consider whether the drug's particles were thick or thin; whether the patient's body is healthy and naturally has a good temperament, or naturally has a bad temperament but is not otherwise ill, or the body is ill and accidentally poorly tempered (by an external source of heat or cold, for example); to test the drug's power one must apply it to a sick body suffering only from a simple disease with a simple bad temperament or mixture of a part or parts; different kinds of a medicinal simple may have different powers; the cause of the diseased state may vary; the season, location, sex, age, custom of life, and other Hippocratic characteristics may influence the outcome of the test; some drugs act immediately on contact with the human body, others must be cut into pieces; one should consider whether the substance acts as a food preserving the state of the body, a poison harming the body, or a drug altering the body; some drugs act by their "total substance" in a way hidden from the senses rather than by one or more of the principal qualities; most fundamentally, a drug might have an effect by virtue of a quality it has acquired accidentally, or a quality it has primarily and by itself (e.g., opium, which induces sleep by its own cooling power might be accidentally very hot if heated).[200]

Each of these qualifications is a thoughtful attempt to connect the administration of a given medicinal substance with later observed phenomena, ideally linking causes and effects by avoiding confounding variables. Some of these qualifications clearly depend on theory, such as the requirement about testing a drug's essential versus accidental qualities, or another one stipulating that the physician take into account the natural temperament of the patient. Temperaments of parts varied, so the physician had to establish the natural,

---

198   Galen defended this case in his *On the Elements According to Hippocrates*, which deployed rhetorical sleights to credit Hippocrates, rather than Empedocles or Aristotle, with the discovery and articulation of the four-element theory. Hankinson, "Philosophy of nature," 211–217.

199   Van der Eijk, *Medicine and Philosophy*, ch. 10.

200   I am collecting and paraphrasing the qualifications attributed to *Simple Drugs* (*De. simp. med. fac.*) in Van der Eijk, *Medicine and Philosophy*, 287–289. Since the faculties followed from the mixtures of the substances involved, Galen discussed many of his qualifications or conditions in his work *On Mixtures*.

healthy baseline for each patient. In every person, the heart was the hottest part, but people had relatively colder or hotter hearts, brains, livers, and other parts, according to each person's natural variation of the qualitative mixtures of the parts. Other qualifications or conditions for assessing drugs attend more strictly to the phenomena, such the observation that some drugs act on immediate contact while others need to be diced. The goal, though, in each trial is to show that a certain kind of medicine has a certain kind of effect when administered to certain sorts of patients and diseases.

Quite strikingly, Galen explicitly stressed that these qualifications enabled the physician to reach the necessary goal of conducting *reproducible* trials.[201] Setting up the rational conditions or qualifications moved physicians from the realm of chance experience to deliberate, contrived experimentation. Throughout his works on drugs, Galen wrote of the necessity of deliberately setting out to "make a trial" (*facere periculum* in the Latin) in order to confirm, disconfirm, or even discover a drug's faculties.[202] This inspired similar language from physicians in the Renaissance, especially those making drug trials and anatomical tests.[203]

Deliberate, careful trials not only distinguished the faculties of drugs, they also marked Galen's method as superior to other approaches. A rival sect, the ancient Empirics, laudably used experience but failed to make well-qualified, reproducible trials.[204] The Empirics took up ancient Skeptic arguments against believing in entities or causes demanded by theory but hidden from the senses. Different competing schools of medicine all claimed to know the fundamental, hidden stuff or causes of bodies—atoms; humors; *pneuma*; the elements earth, water, air, and fire; the principal qualities—yet they all disagreed. Empirics rejected this doomed search for hidden causes and instead claimed to rely on "the phenomena" alone, as collated through experience and memory. Effective healers needed only experience (*empeiria*), supplemented by reports of other healers' experiences collected and passed on (*historia*). Experience, in turn, they divided into three sorts of trials: involuntary trials, made by chance or nature (such as using whatever happens to be at hand when sick); voluntary trials made in order to try out a remedy; and imitative trials in which healers over time learned from experience how to apply similar cures to

---

201   Van der Eijk, *Medicine and Philosophy*, 292–3.

202   Galen, *De simplicium medicamentorum facultatibus libri XI*, 423, 175, 139, 562–563.

203   Ragland, "'Making Trials.'"

204   Van der Eijk, *Medicine and Philosophy*, 291–293. Galen's early *On Medical Experience* attacked a caricature of Empiricists, while his later *Outline of Empiricism* presented a more balanced account. Hankinson, "Epistemology," 171–173. Hankinson, "Causes and Empiricism."

similar diseases in similar patients.[205] Empiric medicine produced collective guides to practice, in terms of correlations of phenomena, with theory and theory testing proscribed, and no unnatural conditions set up for their own trials.

Galen agreed with the Empirics on the necessity of grounding medicine in the phenomena as witnessed by the senses. Importantly, he united this with the use of reason in ways the Empirics rejected. Galen's core texts on drugs also presented his epistemology of reason and experience, in which all knowledge and demonstrations take their foundations in the senses. *Simple Drugs*, for instance, rebutted Skeptics by arguing that if they "overturn what is plainly apparent through the senses, they will have no place from which to begin their demonstrations."[206] Others, Sophists, spurned the senses and tangled themselves up in "philosophical disputes," conjecturing about uncertainties and quarrelling over words.[207] Following reason (and poor logic), they could reach insane conclusions, viz., that substances took their brightness and light color from elemental fire—all the while leaving out the obvious counterexample of cold, white snow. In contrast, "unreasoned perception" (in the Latin, "irrational senses") is the means by which we learn that the sun is bright, flames orange, and other qualitative phenomena.[208]

Of course everyone making knowledge-claims about the phenomena had to depend on their (generally reliable) senses; only fools and hick Skeptics ("Pyrrhonnian boors") would be idiotic enough to suggest otherwise.[209] We need the senses and their general reliability for *any* sort of natural philosophical demonstration. The best philosophy, too, taught that our senses acted in such a way that we directly perceive objects in the world. After all, there are continuous causal chains of like-to-like interacting substances, from objects out in the world to sense organs and the brain, the seat and ruling organ of the rational and sensitive soul.[210]

Reason and Galen's philosophical matter theory adopted from the best philosophers allowed him to attempt to build philosophical explanations for drug actions. Like every other substance, plants and other medicinal ingredients

---

205   Hankinson, "Causes and Empiricism." Von Staden, "Experiment and Experience in Hellenistic Medicine."

206   Galen, *De simpl. med. fac.*, quoted in Hankinson, "Epistemology," 163. Galen, *De simplicium medicamentorum facultatibus libri XI*, 71.

207   Galen, *De simpl. med. fac.* quoted in Hankinson, "Epistemology," 170, cf. 161. Galen, *De simplicium medicamentorum facultatibus libri XI*, 69.

208   Galen, *De simplicium medicamentorum facultatibus libri XI*, 70.

209   Galen, *De simplicium medicamentorum facultatibus libri XI*, 48. Galen, *Prognosis*, 98.5, in Lehoux, "Observers, Objects, and the Embedded Eye," 466.

210   Lehoux, "Observers, Objects, and the Embedded Eye," 459–464.

essentially were mixtures of the principal qualities hot, cold, wet, and dry, with hot and cold more active and wet and dry more passive. Faculties or derivative qualities resulted as the effects of the predominant principal qualities on specific bodies: heating, cooling, moistening, and drying, of course, but also softening, purging, burning, hardening, loosening, constricting, etc. He divided medicines into four orders depending on the intensity of their effects. As he put it in *Simple Drugs*, firstly there were those whose effects were hidden from the senses so one needed reason to discover them, next those clear to the senses (e.g., warming), thirdly those with strong effects (e.g., making hot), finally those with massive effects (e.g., burning).[211]

Yet reason remained in a supporting role to experience. The sure principles of rational demonstrations—the universal qualities of hot, cold, dry, and wet—always were "more certain than those things which are demonstrated by them."[212] Throughout this widely-used textbook on simple drugs, Galen warned that physicians who wandered away from these sense-based principles of demonstration always failed, with disastrous consequences for their patients.

Usually, the two "methods" complemented each other. Using reason, one could move from the nature of a medicinal substance (its temperament or mixture) to its effects in this or that part of a living body. Following the way of experience (*experientia* or *experimentum*), one would apply a substance to a body and note its perceptible effects.[213] Ideally, nothing would escape the senses, but some things, such as faculties of the total substance or form of a drug, inevitably did. There reason went only as far as the senses and experience allowed.[214]

The senses of taste, smell, and touch could act as indexes of the faculties. They allowed the physician to connect the sensory qualities and effects to the substance's principal temperament, running through the four principal qualities. Thus, tasting went through "reason" to reach faculties, rather than through "experience." Galen remarked on the flavors of specific ingredients here and there in his books. But in book four of *Simple Drugs* he provided a systematic treatment, giving a rational account of how different combinations of the principal qualities produced characteristic flavors across over sixty-nine pages in the common Latin edition of the later 1500s. Galen had tied his philosophical

---

211   Galen, *De simplicium medicamentorum facultatibus libri XI*, 344–345, 428–429. Cf. Vogt, "Drugs and pharmacology," 313.

212   Galen, *De simplicium medicamentorum facultatibus libri XI*, 71.

213   Galen, *De simplicium medicamentorum facultatibus libri XI*, 491–2.

214   Galen, *De simplicium medicamentorum facultatibus libri XI*, 72.

use of flavors to Plato's authority, refining the categories of flavors Plato had laid out in his *Timaeus*.[215] Plato had given six or seven flavors (astringent, harsh, bitter, salty, pungent, sour, and sweet), which he explained by the interaction of particles of different properties and shapes with the tongue and mouth. Galen, ever fussy about proper distinctions, at times numbered the astringent and harsh together, and added a "fatty" flavor to the list.[216]

Galen may have been concerned to defuse the close association of flavors and powers found in a dissident Hippocratic text. While Galen read the specifics of his own theory of qualities, matter, and humors back into the Hippocratic *The Nature of Man*, it provided a relatively easy text for doing so. There, the author defended understanding the solid parts of the body as anatomical containers for four fundamental humors, blood, phlegm, yellow bile, and black bile, which interacted with each other, food, medicines, and the environment by a principle of like affects like. So, phlegm is clearly abundant in winter, as it and the weather are cold and wet. The author of *On Ancient Medicine* took a strong contrary stance, objecting to the entire project of making speculative "hypotheses," and specifically rejected taking hot, cold, dry, and wet as the fundamental causes.[217] Instead, this author argued for the origins of medicine in basic cookery, each person learning what substances acted to help or harm her own body in health and disease. Bread and barley cakes good for healthy humans would harm a sick patient who needed barley gruel. Flavors matched powers, and diseases, in bodies: "there is in the human being salty and bitter and sweet and acid and astringent and insipid and myriad other things having powers of all kinds in quantity and strength."[218] Blunted by cooking and blended together, these flavor-powers did not harm; when one stood out its strength caused disease and even death.

For Galen, flavors gave some indications of the primary qualities more reliably than touch or smell: pepper is cold to the touch but hot to the taste, and clearly heats the body.[219] Through tasting, the physician can learn to "discern the natures" of ingredients, though he has to train his tongue and reason to work together. In tasting, all the particles of tastable bodies fall on the tongue, and move the sense according to their own individual nature.[220] Other parts of

---

215   Galen, *De simplicium medicamentorum facultatibus libri XI*, 62. Plato, *Timaeus*, trans. Bury, 167–169.
216   Galen, *De simplicium medicamentorum facultatibus libri XI*, 62–63, 205.
217   Schiefsky, *Hippocrates*, 57.
218   Hippocrates, *On Ancient Medicine*, 14, trans. Schiefsky, *Hippocrates*, 93.
219   Galen, *De simplicium medicamentorum facultatibus libri XI*, 4, 48. 255.
220   Galen, *De simplicium medicamentorum facultatibus libri XI*, 205, 273.

the body can respond to the faculties or powers of medicines in similar ways, as when they become ulcerated from a sharp, powerful faculty or constricted from a cold one.

The tongue makes better distinctions, and some flavors are sensed clearly, such as the harsh or acerbic flavors acting more slowly and less deeply on the tongue than the sour or acidic. In other cases, one needed to triangulate or perform "induction" from other phenomena.[221] The "biting" effect of a substance might be from accidental coldness, hotness, or from intrinsic harshness or acridity. When soft bodies containing watery stuff grow colder, for example sponges, they are compressed and condensed, pushing out the thinner watery stuff and leaving many small empty spaces. Biting hotness, though, dissolves and fuses things, and acts more quickly and more deeply.

Galen's association of flavors with faculties was far more sophisticated, and traveled through his philosophical matter theory. To learn an ingredient's faculty from its flavor, use a studious program of tasting. For example, take garlic or onions and by long use and "assiduous tasting" infix the sense of present passions to memory—then you will know what "acrimony" is. Similar acrimonies caused diseases when they attacked, eroded, or altered parts of patients' bodies. Classifying by flavors and indexing with the hot, cold, dry, and wet primary qualities gives some good indications of temperaments. All bitter things are hot, such as bile, nitre, very old wine, and many seeds.[222] Every sweet thing is not immoderately hot, and can be watery and somewhat cold.[223] Salty flavors are from hot and earthy temperaments, sour from a predominance of coldness (as indicated by their constrictive and biting sensations).[224] Acerbic or sharp flavors, found in many fruits, show themselves by manifestly drying, contracting, and roughening the tongue to the touch. This indicates constriction by a predominance of coldness. It dries the tongue unequally, rather than penetrating deeply as with substances made up of watery parts or particles (*particulae*), and so is wholly earthy.[225]

Yet making careful, qualified trials gave much better knowledge than flavors. If the flavor is unclear, or there are mixed and contrary flavors, or the flavor seems contrary to an ingredient's other sensory properties, then one must make a trial. The real judgment of the faculty of any given medicine is "discovered by experience alone abundantly beyond recognition of flavors." Galen claimed

---

221   Galen, *De simplicium medicamentorum facultatibus libri XI*, 221, 207–209.

222   Galen, *De simplicium medicamentorum facultatibus libri XI*, 227.

223   Galen, *De simplicium medicamentorum facultatibus libri XI*, 227–230.

224   Galen, *De simplicium medicamentorum facultatibus libri XI*, 267.

225   Galen, *De simplicium medicamentorum facultatibus libri XI*, 220.

he discovered faculties by experience for six hundred ingredients.[226] For difficult cases, the physician ought to use Galen's conditions or qualifications for
experience, giving the medicine to someone of the best, moderate constitution, and then in patients with simple diseases (only a hot intemperance, only
a cold one, etc.).[227] Galen reiterated the necessity and reliability of making
such trials according to experience, and closed his long discussion of flavors as
indications or indexes of the temperaments by again elevating testing through
qualified experience. Even colors might allow some conjectures about medicinal powers (all white plants are hotter), and taste may indicate more, and smell
a little. But "clearly it is best (as I have very often both said and shown) to find
the faculties by qualified experience."[228]

When he transitioned from plant, earth, stone, and mineral ingredients to
animal products, Galen gave a summary of his treatise:

> It has been shown that medicines act by their named efficient qualities,
> namely hotness, coldness, wetness, and dryness, and those produced by
> their mixture, the sharp, the harsh, the salty, the saltish, the bitter, the
> acrid, the sweet, and, beyond these, wiping, striking, attracting, softening,
> burning, putrefying, encrusting [faculties]: after these follow other, more
> special actions, the flesh-growing, scar-forming, agglutinating, fistulating
> or ulcerating, or drawing excretions from flesh. It has been shown also
> how a faculty of the whole may be found demonstrably by experience
> alone, and not common experience of any sort, but with the specified dis-
> tinctions applied. Of the rest, the faculty of the whole having been found,
> there is no experience needed beyond that which is aimed at particular
> actions, except for the confirmation of those which reason discovers.[229]

This careful, intentional trial-making allowed the physician to isolate causal
linkages. Reason could move along the path from primary qualities to flavors,
and to secondary and tertiary qualities, but it always remained subordinate
to the refutation or confirmation of the outcomes of trials. For faculties of
the total substance, reasoning from perceptible qualities to the ingredients'
temperament was impossible, making trials unavoidable.

---

226   Galen, *De simplicium medicamentorum facultatibus libri XI*, 225
227   Galen, *De simplicium medicamentorum facultatibus libri XI*, 223.
228   Galen, *De simplicium medicamentorum facultatibus libri XI*, 224, 273.
229   Galen, *De simplicium medicamentorum facultatibus libri XI*, 620–621.

7   **Medieval and Early Modern Debates over Sensing and Knowing**
       Medicinal Faculties

Early modern physicians embraced and vigorously debated Dioscorides'
and Galen's foundational texts on drugs. They eagerly followed their recommendations to see for oneself and try out new remedies. Yet, despite Galen's
sense-based realism, the capaciousness and fineness of his explanations in
terms of the basic qualities, and his cultivation of long experience with simple
medicines—through his own direct tasting and sensing, the reports of other
healers, and carefully qualified trials—there remained serious tensions or gaps
in his pharmacology. Did flavors really allow one to reason back to primary
qualities? How could one *measure* the intensities of qualities reliably? Further,
how could one explain the faculties of *compound* drugs, made up of even several dozen simple ingredients?

To sketch early modern answers to these questions, I will give three brief
histories showing the continuities and elaborations of Galenic methods on
three different themes: using flavors for knowing and administering drugs,
making trials of compound drugs, and making trials of poisons and antidotes.
Although Galen had advocated the use of the sense of taste as a primary index
of the faculties of medicinal ingredients, the connections between flavors
and faculties were never certain. Early modern physicians engaged in never-
ending debates over the reliability of flavors, especially for crucial drugs such
as opium, whose bitter flavor seemed to indicate a hot temperament in opposition to its assumed cooling faculty. Second, the complexity of compound drugs
demanded that physicians make trials, since their philosophical principles and
actions escaped understanding. Rational programs to quantify ingredients'
qualitative intensities, notable in medieval university medicine, demonstrate
physicians' attempts to bolster the philosophical status of the medical art,
but were far too cumbersome to use in practice. Third, poisons and antidotes
seemed to work with violent powers that defied rationalization in terms of
temperament theory, so physicians had to resort to trials. In the sixteenth century, they allied with increasingly powerful states to test poisons and possible
antidotes on condemned criminals.

In these three themes, Galen's works and methods inspired debate and
increasingly sophisticated developments in matter theory, quantification, and
the performance of deliberate trials, including parallel trials with what look to
us like "control" subjects. Lines of making trials ran from Galen's texts, through
medieval elaborations and refinements by Arabic and Latinate physicians, and
into the early modern universities. These short histories will then help us to

put the Leiden practices with drugs in their historical place, as well as work toward a richer history of experimental activities in academic work with and about medicines.

First, there was quite a bit of disputing about tastes. Over the sixteenth century, reasoning by flavors came in for serious criticism. Earlier on, some physicians gloried in the reliability of taste for identifying plants. Euricius Cordus of Marburg, who had learned the value of correct identification from Leoniceno, took his own students on herborizing trips. For Cordus, the colors of plant species often changed by regions, but "flavor, however...cannot be mistaken."[230] For Leonhart Fuchs, where the three ancient authorities Galen, Dioscorides, and Pliny the Elder agreed on the medicinal faculties of plants, one could trust their claims. In disagreements, Fuchs followed Galen over Dioscorides, and Pliny last. Galen "knew the faculties of plants by a certain sure reason and method, which he entrusted repeatedly to writings, and partly learned them even further by experience."[231] Thus, Fuchs included descriptions of the taste, smell, and medicinal faculties of plants, as well as rational accounts of their temperaments, following Galen.

As usual, other scholars mounted a counter-attack. The brilliantly caustic Aristotelian physician Julius Caesar Scaliger argued across his works in the 1550s and 1560s that temperaments formed from the "fight" of the four qualities or elements could not explain flavors (or other faculties such as sensation, growth, or intellection).[232] Many hot mixed bodies remained insipid, and it would be absurd to say that the elements themselves had flavors. Instead, it seemed that plants and other mixed bodies consisted of a hierarchy of forms, in which smaller parts or particles retained distinct forms subordinate to a higher form, and so retained and expressed their powers, all orchestrated by the higher form.

Other eminent scholars extolled anti-materialistic philosophies, in which the active qualities and powers remained always hidden from direct sensation. The physician and Platonizing philosopher Jean Fernel resisted much of the rational system of drugs and their actions, which relied on an Aristotelian-Galenic matter theory of the principal qualities and "thick" or "thin" material parts. Instead, he insisted on experience, or making trials, for knowing the medicinal qualities and faculties of drugs, which were otherwise hidden or "occult" from the senses, much like the insensible power of a

---

230   Cordus, *Botanologicon*, 92. Ogilvie, *Science of Describing*, 135.
231   Fuchs, *De Historia Stirpium Commentarii Insignes*, a6v.
232   Ragland, "Chymistry and Taste," 7. Lüthy, "An Aristotelian Watchdog as Avant-Garde Physicist."

magnet to draw iron.[233] Many diseases did not arise from qualities available to the senses, but rather from the "total substance"—scabies, plague, phthisis, venereal disease, rabies, etc. all took their powers from less material, more formal causes. Fernel greatly expanded the ambit of Galen's notion of the "total substance" beyond the actions of poisons, purgatives, amulets, and attractive drugs to include a wide range of poisonous, pestilential, and contagious diseases.[234] Similarly, Fernel resisted crass materialistic explanations and held that the actions of parts of the living body followed not from their elemental temperament, but from the activity of the unitary soul or form, through the semi-material *spiritus*, which was the vehicle for a divine, celestial, vital heat.[235] After all, the anatomical structures and temperaments of dead and living bodies were the same, but only the living body displayed its proper functions.[236] These must proceed from some source beyond the material temperaments.

Like Scaliger, another scholar, the physician Laurentius Gryllus (Lorenz Gryll, 1484–1560), drew on corpuscularian thinking to attack the idea that flavors derived from substantial forms. Gryllus may well have written the first treatise dedicated to the sense of taste and flavors. He was a Bavarian physician and botanist, educated at Vienna in 1540, who toured Italy, France, the Low Countries and Germany on the Fuggers' dime, and later taught *materia medica* at Ingolstadt, where he corresponded with Clusius on botanical matters.[237] In 1566, Gryllus published what seems to be the first treatise focused on taste.[238] He borrowed the idea of relating the faculties of medicines to the little material seedlets of contagion of things from Fracastoro, arguing that the four qualities explain medicinal faculties only somewhat.[239] The actions and faculties do not flow from a single substantial form, but from different qualities and seeds.[240] Gryllus dismissed the solution of the eminent physician Jean Fernel for rushing away from the senses to insensible occult qualities.[241]

According to Gryllus, Galen and the other ancients often made mistakes or even "hallucinated" about the flavors of plants, and the connections they alleged between flavors, primary qualities, and faculties do not withstand

233   Deer Richardson, "The Generation of Disease."
234   Deer Richardson, "The Generation of Disease," 182–3.
235   Hirai, *Medical Humanism*, 70.
236   Deer Richardson, "The Generation of Disease," 179.
237   Cunningham, "The Bartholins, the Platters and Laurentius Gryllus."
238   Gryllus, *De sapore dulci et amaro*.
239   Gryllus, *De sapore dulci et amaro*, 24a, 50a, 79a, 88b.
240   Gryllus, *De sapore dulci et amaro*, 28b.
241   Gryllus, *De sapore dulci et amaro*, 50a.

scrutiny.[242] Opium is clearly bitter, but Galen and Dioscorides claimed that it induced sleep due to extreme coldness.[243] Yet Galen insisted that all bitter things are predominantly hot. Nor was the bitterness artificially produced by roasting the poppy head or seeds on sheets, since its parts are naturally bitter, prior to processing. Gryllus then expanded his attack: bitter plants cut, thin, heat, and burn. One scholar who ate a whole head of bitter absinth in honey for his stomach got instead excruciating pains and despaired of life. Unlike the sweet things, which nourish, they taste horrible and their nature opposes the nature of the human body—"Nature herself" abhors bitter things, as demonstrated in the careful separation and excretion of bile in living bodies, out through the intestines and urine.[244] This broadside against bitter medicinal plants, as opposed to nourishing sweet ones or cleansing salty, sharp, or sour ones, aimed not only at common purgatives such as dittany or hellebore, but the substantial majority of plant ingredients in sixteenth-century medicinal herbals.[245] About two-thirds to three-quarters were bitter.

Despite such attacks on sensory and philosophical grounds, many physicians and most at Leiden continued to follow Galen's basic approach to making rational inferences to the qualities of medicinal ingredients based on their flavors. Yet they also criticized Galen's specific claims while following his method. As Saskia Klerk has argued, a number of physicians who taught and studied at Leiden rejected Galen's claim that opium was a strongly cold soporific, in large part because it tasted so bitter. Following Galen's general approach, early modern professors such as Dodonaeus, Johannes Heurnius, and others attributed greater certainty to the conclusions about temperaments and qualities drawn from the flavors of plants versus those based on their smell or colors.[246] But like Mattioli before them, they noted the strongly sharp and bitter flavors of opium, sure signs of a strong hot quality in stark contrast with its assumed cooling power. In response, they could take the hint from Galen and Fernel and offer explanations for opium's sleep-inducing faculty in terms of its the "total substance," or substantial form, or some occult quality.

Dodonaeus, from 1582–1585 the first Leiden professor of medical ingredients, carried the Galenic baton into the lecture room. He gave students and colleagues a brief summary of Galen's pharmacology, citing *Simple Drugs*

---

242   Gryllus, *De sapore dulci et amaro*, 3a.
243   Gryllus, *De sapore dulci et amaro*, 88b–90a. Dioscorides, *De materia medica*, trans. Beck, 273. Klerk, "The Trouble with Opium," 309.
244   Gryllus, *De sapore dulci et amaro*, 94b–95a.
245   Teigen, "Taste and Quality in 15th- and 16th- Century Galenic Pharmacology," 60–68.
246   Klerk, "The Trouble with Opium," 304.

liberally.[247] Medicines display a hierarchy of faculties: primary, secondary, tertiary, and quaternary. Primary faculties derive from the elements, and so do the primary qualities: heating, cooling, humidifying, drying, and the non-contradictory combinations of these. Secondary faculties follow intelligibly from the primary qualities or temperament, too: softening from heating and humidifying, hardening from drying and cooling or heating, and attracting from medicines with thin, penetrating, and heating parts. Tertiary faculties follow from the secondary. Quaternary faculties, though, do not depend on the material temperament, but only the total substance or form—these can be known by trials alone. Knowing by flavors is similarly mixed. Narcotics such as opium work, according to Galen and other ancient witnesses, by stupefying through coldness in the highest, fourth degree. Yet Dodonaeus did not sense this cooling directly, and even when opium is mixed with hot ingredients of thin parts, it still has a "violent power of stupefying," and a sharp, hot taste. So it must have its stupefying power from its total substance. Though he mostly followed Galen on the sharp, bitter, salty, harsh, sour, sweet, and fatty flavors and their indications of the primary qualities, Dodonaeus made a point of privileging trials. Experience "alone, beyond recognition of flavors, can discover the faculty of a given medicine." One could seem to know the faculty of some medicine by "taste or reason," but "that which reason has proven, experience refutes."[248] Trials trumped reason.

Second, compound drugs were a trial, at least in theory. Experience or trials came to be accepted as the only way to know the faculties of compound drugs. Trials discovered the faculties of compound drugs, and refuted or confirmed claims about them.[249] Galen himself, for all his love of logical systems, could not provide a quantified or clear account of how compound medicines worked. Although compound medicines stocked most of the Galenic pharmacy, Galen himself offered only lists of ingredients.[250] Instead, the best physician took on the remedies already affirmed by trials, and any indicated by reason (based on elemental theory or flavors) ought to be confirmed by experience and trial. As Michael McVaugh has shown, around 1300 at Montpellier, university physicians crafted careful elaborations of Galen's rules for qualified experience, drawing on Avicenna's medieval synthesis.[251]

---

247   Dodonaeus, *Stirpium Historiae Pemptades Sex*, 6–16.
248   Dodonaeus, *Stirpium Historiae Pemptades Sex*, 16.
249   Van der Eijk, *Medicine and Philosophy*, 280.
250   Vogt, "Drugs and pharmacology," 315.
251   McVaugh, "Determining a Drug's Properties."

Following Galen's "qualifications" for experience, Avicenna articulated seven conditions for generating knowledge of a drug's medical properties from the "footpath" of experience: 1) the medicine must be free of any acquired or accidental quality, such as heat or cold; 2) the test must be done with a singular, not a composite disease; 3) the medicine tested must be tried on two contrary diseases, since some medicines, such as scammony, can cure by their own faculties (by heating a cold sickness) and accidentally (by evacuating yellow bile in a hot tertian fever); 4) one must test a medicine first on the weakest diseases of a contrary quality, and then proceed to the stronger gradually; 5) the time of operation of the medicine should be noted, since it could have an initial effect accidentally and then a later effect by its own operation; 6) the effect of a medicine must be observed either always or for the most part, since this would show it was not accidental, but proceeded from the medicine's principles; 7) the medicine must be tested in a human body, since a medicine might be hot compared to a human body but cold compared to a horse (as is rhubarb), and because it might have a distinct property in relation to one body but not another.[252] Galen stated clearly the first and second rules, and major parts of the fourth and fifth, and his other qualifications and approach included or implied the rest. As repeated in Avicenna's *Logic*, these rules became the major point of departure for later medieval philosophers' debates over how to reason back from manifest effects to hidden causes.[253]

At Montpellier, teaching masters such as Arnau de Vilanova and Bernard de Gordon thought carefully about these rules, and offered elaborations and refinements. Bernard followed up Galen's important conceptual innovation of the neutral mid-point, which came to influence medieval thinking on dynamic balancing in systems from medicine to politics and economics.[254] In his new rule, one had to test the sample on a truly temperate body. He also broke Avicenna's final rule, suggesting a cautious test of an unknown substance on birds, then beasts, then on patients in hospitals, and then on the "lesser brethren" (or Franciscans)![255] After all, it might kill.

As Michael McVaugh shows, Arnau re-thought the rules and theory from Galen, Avicenna, Al-Kindi, and Bernard, producing the most sophisticated

---

252   Avicenna, *Liber Canonis Avicenne revisus*, f. 82r, Bk. 2, tract. 1, cap. 2. For a translation of the medieval Arabic text, see Nasser, Tibi, and Savage-Smith, "Ibn Sina's *Canon of Medicine*: 11th century rules for assessing the effects of drugs," The James Lind Library (www.jameslindlibrary.org). Accessed Monday 23 February 2009.

253   The list includes Robert Grosseteste, Albert the Great, Duns Scotus, and William of Ockham. Ragland, "'Making Trials,'" 510.

254   McVaugh, "Determining a Drug's Properties." Kaye, *A History of Balance*.

255   McVaugh, "Quantified Medical Theory," 403.

protocols for testing drugs. Arnau needed a neutral qualitative midpoint, so he specified the body for testing in greater detail: Galen's perfectly temperate human, healthy, of moderate body type and diet. He insisted that the medicine had to be tested on this sort of healthy body in the same way one administered it to a sick patient. Nor should the medicine show any signs of decay or improper processing. Most important, Arnau stipulated that the *dose* of the medicine must be precisely specified. In this he described an application of his elaborate quantitative schemes for specifying numerically the intensities of medicines, and calculating the intensities of even the compound medicines Galen had found so vexing. Arnau adapted Al-Kindi's quantification of a simple drug's intensity, arguing that they act in an increasing geometric ratio to a unit of the opposite quality. Thus, temperate ingredients have an intensity of one unit equal to that of one unit of the opposite quality (1:1). Those of the first degree, 2:1; the second degree, 4:1; the third degree, 8:1; the fourth degree, 16:1.[256] Moreover, there should be a basic unit—related to the Aristotelian *natural minimal parts* (*minima naturalia*), the smallest part at which a substance produced perceptible effects. Simples hot in the fourth degree, such as pepper, had this "prime quantity" of one drachm.[257] First degree medicines, three drachms. Compounding a medicine of one drachm of pepper with something cold in the first degree (4:1 hot to cold "parts"), such as three drachms of rose (1:2), then, by addition would produce a medicine with a hot to cold ratio of 5:3.[258] With this method, a physician could predict the degree of new compound medicine, or make a medicine to order for the precise degrees needed for a patient's disease.

It seems no one used this quantified, careful theory in practice. Bernard's later use of Arnau's quantification of intensities is a purely descriptive illustration of an existing recipe, and Arnau himself seems to have used recipes at hand from traditional collections without the quantified gloss.[259] On their own, the rules for testing a drug would have been labor-intensive and time-consuming—perhaps reaching even Haly Abbas's prediction of a thousand men taking a thousand years to determine drug properties by trial.[260] Before 1600, physicians lacked instruments for measuring these qualities other than their own bodies, and Galen mounted a strong case for taking the human body as

256   McVaugh, "Quantified Medical Theory."
257   McVaugh, "Determining a Drug's Properties," 200–201.
258   McVaugh, "Quantified Medical Theory," 401–404.
259   McVaugh, "Quantified Medical Theory," 404. McVaugh, "The *Experimenta* of Arnau of Vilanova."
260   McVaugh, "Quantified Medical Theory," 402.

the best reference, since its temperament occupied the midpoint on the scale of living bodies.[261]

In the early modern period, innovative programs of quantification in university medicine aimed to shore up the venerable edifice of Galenic medicinal temperament and faculty theory. Santorio Santorio, moving in Galileo's circles in Venice and teaching medicine at Padua from 1611 to 1624, raced ahead in the vanguard of medical quantification of qualities.[262] Santorio spent years and many publications describing and defending his use of instruments to quantify heat, humidity, daily changes in weight, and even otherwise insensible perspiration.[263] He announced that his teaching relied on "statics experiments [*statica experimenta*]" as well as "instruments and the art of statics" to make medical philosophy "clear and manifest."[264]

Quantification allowed for the establishment of precise ranges of hotness, wetness, pulse rates, and other variations for healthy and diseased bodies and bodily parts, which could rid medicine of errors and establish demonstrative certainty.[265] His thermoscope, a glass tube equipped with a quantified scale to measure the changes in volume of the air bubble trapped inside, could determine the range of temperaments of body parts. He also used his instruments to attack astrologers.[266] He and his students tested the effects of the heat of rays of the full Moon and the rays of the Sun on his thermoscopes, rays concentrated by a concave mirror. The Moon's rays changed the measurement two degrees over ten beats of the pulsilogium (a pendulum device for measuring pulses). The Sun's rays, on the same thermoscope, brought a change of a hundred and ten degrees in two pulses. Strikingly, Santorio used this cutting-edge instrumentation to *confirm* rather than dispute the major lines of temperament theory central to the union of medical theory and practice.[267]

Third, poisons and antidotes especially demanded physicians make trials, as attested by evidence from ancient, medieval, and early modern sources. No methods of quantifying perceptible intensities seemed to work with poisons; physicians had to make trials. Texts on poisons frequently discussed parallel trials of antidotes. For Galen, poisons seemed to act without material penetration, and although many likely acted by extreme cooling, quickly chilling

---

261   Galen, *Mixtures*, trans. Singer, in *Galen*, 217, K I 541.
262   Siraisi, *Avicenna in the Renaissance*, 237, 304, 314.
263   Siraisi, *Avicenna in the Renaissance passim*.
264   Santorio, quoted in Siraisi, *Avicenna in the Renaissance*, 210, n. 104, my trans.
265   Siraisi, *Avicenna in the Renaissance*, 237, 304, 314.
266   Siraisi, *Avicenna in the Renaissance*, 289.
267   Siraisi, *Avicenna in the Renaissance*, 304.

a body to death, they caused death seemingly regardless of the dose.[268] One influential Galenic treatise on theriac, the royal antidote made from honey, water, viper's flesh and dozens of other ingredients, described how "we take roosters...wild ones, and with a rather dry constitution, and we put poisonous beasts among them, and those who have not drunk theriac die immediately, but those who have drunk it are strong and stay alive after being bitten."[269]

Later commentators, beginning with Avicenna and Averroes and on into Latin texts in the fourteenth and fifteenth centuries, argued poisons acted by the "total substance" or "specific form" in ways that resisted sensory perception and rational understanding.[270] Other violent diseases, such as plague, seemed to be produced by the communication of poisons, raising the stakes for testing antidotes. Just after 1300, Bernard de Gordon drew on Avicenna to suggest using pheasants instead, and in a more controlled setting: "take two pheasants, cut off their crests, apply a poison to the wounds (or administer it orally) and wait until they begin to stagger. Then put theriac on the crest wound and in the drink of one of them: if this lives and the other dies, the theriac is good."[271] Since the powers of poisons and antidotes remained hidden from direct sensation, one had to try them both in living subjects, with the parallel structure allowing for an inference about causation.

In the early modern period, as Alisha Rankin very recently shows, poison trials and historical anecdotes describing them became much more widespread.[272] They also became increasingly expansive in their choice of subjects, putting even live humans to the test in parallel trials. Richard Palmer already pointed us to the parallel trials of doronicum, testing whether it was a medicine or poison; there were far more trials of supposed antidotes.[273] Mattioli recounted a story from 1524 in his influential book on medicinal ingredients. Pope Clement VII placed two criminals condemned to decapitation in the hands of his physicians, in order to test a purported antidote. Both took poisonous wolfsbane, one received the antidote; he lived, while the other, not so treated, died in agony. In the 1560s through the 1580s, emperors, counts, and kings tested antidotes on condemned prisoners from Prague to Paris and German lands. Many trials sacrificed only individual criminals, others used two birds or dogs. In the 1580s, Wilhelm IV of Hesse-Kassel directed his physicians to test a controversial new

---

268 Hankinson, "Philosophy of Nature," 235. Vogt, "Drugs and pharmacology," 307.

269 Ps.-Galen, *On Theriac to Piso*, trans. Leigh, 71. Leigh argues against Galen's authorship of this text. Nutton argues for it: Nutton, "Galen on Theriac."

270 Gibbs, *Poison, Medicine, and Disease in Late Medieval and Early Modern Europe*, chs. 2–4.

271 Bernard de Gordon, trans. McVaugh, quoted in Ragland, "'Making Trials,'" 510–511.

272 Rankin, "Of Antidote and Anecdote." Rankin, *The Poison Trials*.

273 Palmer, "Medical Botany."

antidote on eight dogs of different breeds, arranged in parallel pairs, with each pair ingesting a different poison but only one given the antidote, terra sigilita.[274] The hiddenness and violence of powers of poisons raised the epistemic and existential stakes: physicians, especially when directed by vulnerable rulers, had to make trials.

Even at Leiden, deeply personal stakes and pressing crises urged physicians and students to understand antidotes and poisons, and make the needed trials. In the mid-1590s, the professor of anatomy and medicinal botany Petrus Paaw faced a horrible series of deaths by suspected poisoning. His post-mortem anatomies confirmed the diagnosis of poison in some of the horrible cases, but also cleared his accused colleague Johannes Heurnius.[275] Two decades earlier, during his own medical education in Italy, Heurnius had fallen into mortal danger three times, twice from venomous animals.[276] Taking a summer break in the garden of his hosts, Heurnius lounged in the tall grass, petting a captive tortoise. A snake slipped from the river into the grass, seeking, Heurnius thought later, the bovine shape of the reclining medical student. Running up and yelling, the host scared off the murderous snake. Later, staying in a room in Crete, Heurnius noticed a small crack in the wall nearby, and shined in his candlelight to examine its secrets. A furious "phalangium," either a wandering spider or solifugid, jumped out onto his hand. Without a thought, he retracted his hand and threw his candle at the creature. In response to his cries, the servants rushed up and killed the "insect," warning him about its fatal venom. His life was likely in greater danger when he later stayed with a murderous, thieving host in the countryside around Padua, but the threat of deadly poison made an impression. Back in Utrecht, he diagnosed a fatal poisoning of a local lord, and paid careful attention to the powers of poisons in his own works. In his work on the plague, for example, he followed medieval tradition in ascribing the action of theriac to its total power rather than temperament, and he recommended a "proven" four-ingredient theriac against the exhaled or perspired poison of the plague.[277] Even with much simpler compound medicines, early modern physicians followed Galen's lead in theory and practice.

---

274   Rankin, "Of Antidote and Anecdote," 296–297.
275   See chapter six.
276   [Otto Heurnius], "Vita Auctoris."
277   Johannes Heurnius, *Opera Omnia*, Book 2 (1658), 82–83.

8   Making and Knowing Medicines with Johannes Heurnius'
         New Method

Johannes Heurnius' *New Method* and practical medicine courses presented
students with a vast storehouse of medicines, and methods for their making,
as well as a broad range of therapeutic operations and a Galenic theory of their
qualities and uses against diseases. We have already seen his close attention
to chymistry in his *practica* lectures and textbook. Now we will look beyond
the lengthy discussion of chymistry to take in an overview of his teachings
on the production and use of medicines. Even in his courses and textbooks
on the theory of medicine, Heurnius' rational method of healing (*methodos
medendi*) put a summary of Galenic pharmacology at the center of the therapeutic art. Drugs also headlined the long section dedicated to the method in his
Institutes textbook and course. Echoing Galen, he foregrounded the "mutual
connection" between the method of healing and the different faculties of medicines.[278] Although he cited Galen's pharmacological works liberally, Heurnius
smoothed over the gaps and tensions in Galen's system, providing a simplified,
optimistic introduction for aspiring physicians.

Faculties came first, illustrated by medicinal simples, such as chicory, which
work an effect by themselves. Just as in Dodonaeus's summary, there are primary, secondary, tertiary, and quaternary faculties. The four elements and
qualities produce the primary faculties (heating, cooling, humidifying, drying),
which singly or in combination produce the secondary and tertiary faculties
such as rarefying, opening, thinning, attracting (which all act by heat), or repelling, condensing, closing, thickening (which act by cold), or softening or drying
(by humidity and dryness).[279]

Heurnius delved into Galen's *Simple Drugs* and borrowed his four degrees
of qualitative intensity across fourteen centuries.[280] He also expressed casual
optimism about measuring their intensities. Taste and touch could distinguish
these degrees: drugs of the second degree of heat rarefy, concoct, and restore
innate heat; third-degree hot drugs increase thirst, dry, thin, drain, and bite;
fourth-degree hot drugs enflame, erode, and burn membranes. Secondary faculties, as Galen noted, depend on the primary qualities and the matter of the

---

278   Johannes Heurnius, *Institutiones*, 462–464. See also his *Nova Ratio*, discussed more in
      chapter five.
279   Johannes Heurnius, *Institutiones*, 463–471, 479.
280   Johannes Heurnius, *Nova Ratio*, 379, and elsewhere, cites Galen's *Simple Drugs*. Heurnius,
      Institutiones, 471–476.

medicine, whether it has thick or thin parts, which affects how deeply it penetrates into patients' bodies. Heurnius listed pages of medicinal ingredients by their degrees of heating, cooling, drying, and moistening, all supposedly attested by long experience through reliable sources.[281]

Flavors show the primary and secondary faculties only, since flavors emerge from the temperament and matter of the ingredient. Like his predecessor Dodonaeus, Heurnius gave nine flavors: three hot (sharp, bitter, and salty), three cold (harsh, austere, and sour), and three temperate (sweet, fatty, and insipid).[282] He also neatly connected flavors and faculties. Bitter-tasting substances have a more moderate heat than acrid ones such as pepper, and their hot, dry, earthy qualities and dense matter clean, thin, and open up internal blocked passages in the body. Sour or acidic medicines cool, penetrate, repress inflowing fluids, and restrain hemorrhages by drying. The other flavors correspond with sets of secondary faculties, so that "the powers of remedies are easily apprehended, when they emit one sole tastable quality."[283] Here, as elsewhere, Heurnius generally passed over theoretical debates. He knew and recommended to students J. C. Scaliger's works, but gave only a simplistic, and optimistic, evaluation of flavors as indexes of faculties. Odors, as Galen noted in *Simple Drugs* with the example of the rose, are unreliable due to the matter of the ingredient; colors indicate nothing certain.[284]

Discoursing about the tertiary faculties and the multiple faculties of ingredients distinguished the learned physician from the empiric, who knew only to supply a given remedy for a given disease. Primary and secondary faculties together produce tertiary faculties, such as flesh-producing, maturing, or stone-breaking faculties, the latter of which cut and liquefy through heating and drying, just as milk is coagulated.[285] Multiple faculties must be referred to the primary and secondary qualities, not any peculiar powers. As Galen taught, aloe is bitter, and opens obstructions of the liver and promotes expectoration of the chest; it can open and close vessels in different parts of the body due to its temperament. In contrast, only the unlearned "empiric" skips over the knowledge of temperaments, ascribing each effect to a separate power.[286]

Only an abbreviated set of rules for testing drugs appeared in Heurnius' medical theory courses. He followed precedent to insist that only trials produced

---

281   Johannes Heurnius, *Nova Ratio*, 649–655, 183, 379, etc.

282   Johannes Heurnius, *Institutes*, 472.

283   Johannes Heurnius, *Institutiones*, 476.

284   Johannes Heurnius, *Institutiones*, 476.

285   Johannes Heurnius, *Institutiones*, 479.

286   Johannes Heurnius, *Institutiones*, 482.

knowledge of the effects of quaternary faculties, since they flowed from the substance or essence, as the magnet draws iron or the venom of the asp poisons a human. "For by experience the faculty of a simple remedy is known. With these cautions for this work: Let the remedy examined not be mixed, and be given to a healthy human, or one occupied by a simple disease. Let it be a pure remedy, not imbued with any other quality than its own: and discern what is exerted by its own power, and what by another. If you bring judgment to this matter, experience will be more steadfast. However, many things escape judgment, such as those which follow from substance or essence, and are to be explored by use alone."[287] The rest of the method of healing involved careful reasoning from indications to the disease "seated" in the "sick part," as discussed further in chapter five.

Heurnius' *New Method* began with very practical guides for making medicines in "Book 1" of the work, reaching nearly one hundred and fifty pages. He covered weights and measures from ancient and modern sources in detail, with a handy symbol guide and unit conversion lists. Then, he described in detail the operations and instruments physicians and apothecaries used to make medicines and administer other treatments, as well as proper cautions for known dangers and errors. We have already seen his detailed descriptions and illustrations of chymical apparatus and procedures. Following this, in "Book 2," Heurnius worked exhaustively through the diseased body, noting the qualitative variations of impaired organ temperaments from head to toe, and describing the medicinal simples and compounds "proven by long use" which could restore the proper temperaments of the organs, and so return them to healthy functions.

With Heurnius' book and lectures, physicians could hunt through ancient or more recent texts, or visit gardens or apothecary shops, and precisely make their own medicines. Careful attention to the qualities and faculties of medicinal simples, compounded together to make each remedy, allowed Heurnius to set out rules for precisely weighing quantities of ingredients and estimating their effects based on the dose. Precise weights and measures were essential. For instance, he adopted a "more certain rule [*ratio*]" from the humanist scholar Georgius Agricola (1494–1555), whose work on weights and measures had demonstrated that the ancient *denarius* weighed seventy-two moments of the early-modern goldsmiths.[288] In this way, Heurnius used his linguistic skill to set up a humanist compendium of conversions for weights and measures,

---

287   Johannes Heurnius, *Institutiones*, 482.

288   Johannes Heurnius, *Nova Ratio*, 2. Agricola, *Libri quinque de Mensuris & Ponderibus*.

mining ancient, medieval, and recent sources for the exact measures of the best recipes.

Next, Heurnius detailed the different procedures for compounding various recipes (pessaries, suppositories, decoctions, potions, infusions, pills, baths, oils, distillations, ointments, etc.). Decoctions, for example, steeped roots, leaves, seeds, flowers, and other parts of plants in pure water, alcohol, or some other distilled liquor. He always gave students rules and tips for better practice, passing on the hard-won knowledge from long experience preparing and mixing drug ingredients. One should begin with a pound of material, but increase the amount with harder substances, such as roots. One should use lighter or stronger fires depending on the resistance of the substance, and cook in order: first roots, then leaves and seeds, then fruits, and finally flowers. Otherwise, the thinner parts vanish into the air from excessive cooking. As usual, he added a practical caution: one should not use decoctions from purgatives in fevers, since they produce violent bodily reactions and enervate the patient's strength. Recipes concluded the section. He took a similar approach, with more attention to apparatus and variations in theory, in his long section on chymistry.

In Book 2, reaching over three hundred pages, Heurnius provided a synthesis of his precise quantitative pharmacy with the medical *practica* approach to catalogue "Medicines Proven by Use."[289] He handed on medicines from the Galenic-Hippocratic tradition as well as those he found personally effective. As he noted, these medicines, proven by long use by centuries of physicians, or by his own practice and those of recent named physicians, are "dedicated to the individual parts."[290] He divided his directions for practice by organs: heart, liver, brain, stomach, spleen, intestines, kidneys, bladder, uterus, etc.; some locations such as the chest; and, as a postscript, the four humors. For each organ, Heurnius gave careful descriptions of disease states and precise remedies, with cautions for dosages and mitigating factors. He divided the practical instructions by theory even further, according to the primary causal qualities of hot, cold, dry, and wet. The theory often focused on the alteration, movement, and local collection of qualities and humors which changed organ temperaments, e.g., with excess yellow bile making organs too hot, phlegm, too cold, and black bile, too dry. External causes, such as the qualities of the air, also affected and impaired organ temperaments.

Here, qualitative anatomical theory constructed the divisions of practice. For each organ or bodily location, Heurnius described the remedies to be

---

289   Johannes Heurnius, *Nova Ratio*, 147.
290   Johannes Heurnius, *Nova Ratio*, 147.

used to alter and strengthen the qualitative state of each part: e.g., a hot liver, a cold liver, a humid liver, a dry liver. The next step was to select a precisely-targeted remedy, and in the right qualitative degree. For a hot liver, God has happily supplied a set of plant simples which cool the liver without affecting the nearby stomach. Chicory, endives, sow thistles, and other plants all cool the morbidly hot liver, and can be mixed with other ingredients for enhanced effects. The physician also had to follow Galen to consider how to get the right medicinal ingredient, in the right amount, to the impaired organ. In the case of an intempered liver, some honey added to half an ounce of plant juice helps to carry the medicine to the liver. Adding acid mineral waters increases the coldness (the sharp sour taste of the acids is a clear index of their basic coldness). If the increased heat of the liver is due to bile rather than a simple intemperance of the organ, the physician will have to cool the openings from which the bile flows, using plants such as Venus's hair, but avoiding sweet, bitter, or salty plants. If there is pain, Heurnius noted, the physician should also add a drachm of opium, in a syrup of absinth.[291] Heurnius taught his students to target precisely each major intemperance of an organ, or even strong symptoms such as pain, with calibrated drug ingredients and helping vehicles such as honey.

Compared to the importance of precisely-targeted drugs, other means for preserving health and fighting disease played minor roles in his method of medical practice. For instance, the six non-naturals appeared as a standard classification of the causes of bodily change that patients cannot avoid: contact with the air, motion and rest of the body, sleeping and wakefulness, food and drink, substances excreted and retained, and the passions of the soul. The list appears in Galen's *The Art of Medicine*, and the category of "non-natural," as opposed to "natural" and "preternatural" causes, also appears in Galen's works, though he did not use the term "non-naturals" for these six categories.[292] Even from Galen's time, and before, these causes or conditions of bodily activity and change were important means for preserving health and for understanding the origins of disease states.

While Heurnius certainly acknowledged the traditional importance of the non-naturals, he concentrated much more on restoring patients to health by the use of drugs and other therapeutic interventions, as we will see. The non-naturals appeared in his teaching as causes that sap the natural powers of patients, and make some interventions such as bloodletting potentially dangerous. Excessively hot or cold air, too much exercise or not enough food all

---

291   Johannes Heurnius, *Nova Ratio*, 193–195.
292   Galen, *Art of Medicine*, trans. Singer, 374. K I 367. Niebyl, "The Non-Naturals." Siraisi, *Medieval and Early Renaissance Medicine*, 120–123.

exhaust the body, just as too much wakefulness, excesses of sexual activity, grief, or even happiness can exhaust the body's *spiritus*.[293]

Heurnius followed Galenic precedent in dividing the interventions physicians made into three genera: turning away or removing, alteration, and evacuation. Since many of the changes in the temperaments of organs developed from excess or altered local humors, purgation through medicinal purgatives or bloodletting were especially helpful. As Michael Stolberg and Andrew Wear have shown, early modern healers and patients thought about curing primarily in terms of the purgation and evacuation of some local morbid matter.[294] Heurnius taught this principle in his courses and textbooks over several decades.

Even bloodletting and other forms of turning away or removing a flux from a sick part depended on local anatomical structures. Cutting a vein, cupping, rubbing, or other procedures drew humors from where they flowed and built up in morbid amounts and states. Heurnius taught his students to draw or remove humors from sick parts in "straight lines...according to the fibers and filaments of the veins."[295] These were not the straight lines of mathematicians, he noted, but direct vascular paths. If the bulge of the liver had a morbid swelling, the physician could draw the morbid buildup out through the straight portal vein directly connected to that part of the liver, into the vena cava and then the kidneys, into the urine. The physician should draw out localized morbid collections in the lower part of the liver through the mesentery veins into the intestines. Similarly, physicians could draw blood from veins opposite to a sick part, but always through the straight courses of the veins and fibers. For example, pleurisy, or inflammation of the pleural membrane around the lungs, on the right side of a patient should *not* be treated with cutting veins on the right side, since there are no such straight courses for the humor to flow. Of course, in all this physicians had to avoid drawing a contaminated humor from the sick part through a vital "noble member" such as the heart, liver, brain, etc.[296]

At times, Heurnius recommended to students and readers remedies for specific diseases he attested from his own use or those of acquaintances. He used ointments made from almond oil, herbs, and spirit of wine to good effect against pestilent fevers, and other ointments "always with happy success" for treating baldness.[297] At other times, changes to regimen sufficed, such as stopping a pathological flow of phlegm from the head (catarrh) by abstaining from

---

293   Johannes Heurnius, *Nova Ratio*, 567.
294   Stolberg, *Experiencing Illness*, 95. Wear, *Knowledge & Practice*, 90, 117–118, 124.
295   Johannes Heurnius, *Nova Ratio*, 518.
296   Johannes Heurnius, *Nova Ratio*, 519–520.
297   Johannes Heurnius, *Nova Ratio*, 104, 12.

drink for three days, or cutting a very turgid vein to treat head pains caused by too much blood (plethora).[298] Usually, though, he agreed with the therapies of what he understood as a unified school of medicine, the "Asclepian" school, which enfolded Hippocrates and Galen.

The deeply Galenic drug theory and practice taught by Dodonaeus, Heurnius, and their colleagues formed the core of Leiden pharmaceutical instruction for some sixty years or more. Only by the 1650s do we see very slight modifications, for example in the courses of Albert Kyper (1614–1655), a former Leiden medical student and then philosophy lecturer appointed to teach medicine in 1650.[299] By 1654, he taught in the public hospital, and lectured on his own medical *Institutes* for a year before dying of plague. Kyper's textbook for the course contains no mention of the hierarchies of drug faculties, so confidently prescribed by earlier professors.[300] Although he remained an Aristotelian in his physical theories of elements and qualities, he arranged drugs by their observable effects: diuretics, sudorifics, purgatives, etc.

In contrast, Henricus Regius (1598–1679), teaching at the rival school of Utrecht, embraced a variant, empiricist form of Cartesian mechanism.[301] Perhaps drawing on his teacher Santorio, Regius built an original epistemology in which all knowledge comes from the senses, and experiences are prior to theory, yet he kept a commitment to matter-as-extension and other teachings of Descartes. His 1647 textbook, *Medical Foundations (Fundamenta medica)*, rejected the senses as reliable indicators of drug faculties or effects, noting contradictory cases such as opium. Instead, invisible particles of variable shapes made up medicines, bodies, and all other stuff, and one had to learn drugs' effects from experience.[302] Yet his practice remained famously traditional, with Galenic and Hippocratic remedies for traditional diseases at times described in corpuscular terms.

9 Conclusions

Making medicines built upon sophisticated philosophical and rational understandings of faculties, qualities, and matter, yet always demanded that students and professors integrate rational schemes with direct sensation and testing of

---

298 Johannes Heurnius, *Nova Ratio*, 344, 73.
299 Molhuysen, *Bronnen*, III, 40, 26*, 31*.
300 Kyper, *Institutiones Medicae*, 305–346.
301 Bellis, "Empiricism without Metaphysics."
302 Klerk, "Galen Reconsidered," 151–154.

ingredients and remedies. After all, the senses acted as the grounds of knowledge. These specific practices reflected the general commitments to reason and experience, and the procedures of ancient sources, but also embraced some surprising developments.

At Leiden, there was a great deal more enthusiasm for chymistry, and actual chymical teaching, much earlier than suspected by historians. Yet it was less hands-on than at other universities at the time, especially German medical faculties at Marburg and Wittenberg. But Heurnius brought chymical teaching into the lecture hall at least by 1587, and likely earlier, and seems to have performed some of his own distillations, which suggests that students could learn more in private courses with their professors.

The two overlapping communities engaged with knowing and growing plants both displayed the making of tests and emphasized first-person experience with plants as an essential source of expertise. Making trials or experimenting, though common among naturalists practicing the more descriptive, aesthetic botany, appeared mostly as incidental results of practical goals such as finding ways to grow plants and maintain or diversify the colors of their blooms. Increasingly, as Brian Ogilvie and others have detailed, natural history consisted in experience-based, descriptive practices.[303] There were only hints of systematic experimentation or experimentalism among the natural historians more distinct from the medical community, in contrast to the explicitly experimentalist methodologies for studying drugs medical professors borrowed from ancient Greek and Roman sources.

Through their courses, students could see the plants in person in the garden, and match them to textual descriptions of their forms and lists of their medicinal faculties. On herborizing field trips to the coastal dunes or local fields and forests, students could see plants much more closely, and touch, smell, taste, and try them for their effects. In the barren winter, Dirck Cluyt's thousands of exquisite watercolors were treasured as lifelike representations of plants, most of which were vital for knowing and making medicines.

Learning about medicinal substances and their faculties had much higher stakes. Human senses and reason could not reliably pick out a drug's effects without making trials. Following Galen, students learned to index flavors and faculties, a doctrine expressed with confident brevity but explicit limits; trials of drugs, made in patients or in the physician's own body, were more certain. Professors and students used the best available texts on medicines, such as Galen's *On the Faculties and Mixtures of Simple Drugs*, which demanded that physicians

---

303   Ogilvie, *Science of Describing*.

make trials or experiments of drugs to know their faculties for acting on bodies, poisons, or morbid matter, and presented descriptions of Galen's historical trials and rules for making new ones.

At times, Galen narrated accounts of his own trials, which acted as warrants for his general claims about the powers or faculties of medicinal substances. His systematic parallel trial of the purported cooling power of vinegar by spreading burning *thapsia* on his own thighs presented a single, well-qualified trial by which he established the power and principal quality of vinegar. *Simple Drugs* demanded physicians make trials under the right conditions or qualifications, which alone could isolate causal relations between a drug's temperament and its faculties. Galen's rules, carried into Arabic and Latin medieval sources and, in simplified form, Leiden lectures and textbooks, also demanded reproducible trials. In contrast, the Empirics had neither reproducible trials nor knowledge of causes. Following Galen, Heurnius and other professors set the knowledge of drug properties in the center of their rational method of healing.

This experimental, even experimentalist, methodological tradition should not be overstated. These trials did not reach to tests of fundamental natural philosophy or theory; they were not tests of core Galenic or Aristotelian natural philosophy, but usually instances of its application. In general, physicians had four main avenues for explaining drug action: an Aristotelian-Galenic matter theory of hot, cold, wet, and dry principal qualities (with the emphasis on the more active first pair, hot and cold); recourse to "occult" qualities or action of the "total substance" when the first approach did not seem to work; attention to chymical, especially Paracelsian, matter theory; very occasionally, reasoning along corpuscularian lines. Usually, physicians at Leiden teaching the basic *theoria* or *practica* courses presented the Galenic matter theory as historically proven, still resilient in the face of new substances and theories, and indispensably useful in daily practice.

Yet Galen's very sophistication and erudition, advertised in the textbooks used at Leiden and across Europe, pre-empted the need to carry Galen's experimentalist methodology into practice and make *systematic* tests of most or all the drugs at hand. After all, Galen, Dioscorides, Mattioli, and a host of named and unnamed sources for recipes had already done so much work to provide the medicines "proven by use" and long experience. Unless they acted as natural historians or tested poison antidotes, apothecaries generally avoided making intentional trials, relying instead on public displays of authentic ingredients and learned fidelity to ancient recipes.[304] In general, physicians expressed

---

304   Pugliano, "Pharmacy, Testing, and the Language of Truth in Renaissance Italy."

similar confidence in their shared stores of remedies from Hippocrates, Galen, or other expert physicians. At Leiden and other universities, physicians made trials of drugs when the situation raised the stakes against assuming the substances worked as advertised, when they encountered new substances or diseases, or when they wanted to see the effects for themselves. Suspected poisons and purported antidotes, especially, demanded trials, from ancient stories to contemporary cases of murder and suspected murder. Leiden professors made occasional references to their own trials and recommended remedies, but there is no strong evidence for systematic trials of known drugs or attempts to test the foundations of Galenic-Aristotelian matter theory, as done in the medical school at Wittenberg around Daniel Sennert in the 1610s and 1620s.[305]

Renowned historian of medicine Owsei Temkin influentially described Galenic pharmacology as the least "empirical" part of Galen's medicine, especially compared with his observations in anatomy.[306] Temkin was probably right that it is unlikely that most of Galen's remedies, so confidently attested in his writings, actually did much good for his patients.[307] Yet this is to take a very narrow meaning of "empirical," and one which applies standards from modern testing protocols to premodern medicinal knowledge. In contrast, Galenists' steadfast reliance on temperaments reveals their commitment to grounding knowledge in the principles accessible to the senses. In this sense, the Galenic methodology of testing drugs was likely far *too* empirical. It often put direct sensation of primary qualities and flavors, and conceptions of temperaments accessible to the senses, before the results of tests on carefully-distinguished classes of diseased patients. Similarly, the causal connections he claimed to identify between remedies and diseases through his trials or "qualified experience," no doubt were often due rather to the natural recovery of his patients. On the other hand, the careful qualified trials, designed to connect hidden causes with particular effects, broke starkly with the chance trials and phenomenal histories of the Empirics, who rejected knowledge of causes in favor of descriptions of the phenomena alone.

If students wanted the tools for discovering new knowledge and testing claims about plants, medicinal ingredients, and compound drugs, they certainly had a wealth of models and methodological reflections available. What is more, personal sensory engagement with ingredients and medicines, as well

---

305   Klein, "Alchemical Histories." Klein, "Daniel Sennert." Newman, *Atoms and Alchemy*.
306   Temkin, *Galenism*, 114.
307   See, e.g., Brennessel, Drout, and Gravel, "A Reassessment of the Efficacy of Anglo-Saxon Medicine."

as incidental trials of drugs with various patients, and one's self, remained an unavoidable practice in an early modern marketplace teeming with new plants, drugs, claims to cures, and constant threats to health and life. That neither the students nor their professors yet set up systematic *programs* for such testing is telling evidence of their confidence in God's remedies, proven and preserved by long traditions of use.

Knowing and Treating the Diseased Body

> Therefore one must always begin from the organ of the injured action, and then seek what is the manner of the injury.
>
> —GALEN, *De Affectorum Locorum Notitia* [*De locis affectis*] (1520), 6r

• • •

> Diseases, as we said, dwell in the parts. However many ways therefore those become faulty, there are just so many diseases.
>
> —JOHANNES HEURNIUS, *Institutiones Medicinae* (1638), 516

• •
•

Bodies, sick and healthy, whole and dissected, drew scholars' investigating eyes, hands, ideas, and, in unfortunate cases, scalpels. After all, bodies were the meeting point of all this learning and practicing, and the point of studying medicine. Restoring bodies to health when injured and diseased, and preserving healthy bodies, were the ends for which physicians and other healers practiced their art. Taken together, this chapter and the next two chapters describe a vigorous tradition of routine post-mortem anatomical practice in a university up close, situated prominently and quite naturally *within* Galenic medicine. Even in its early stages, students often attended bedside teaching and care of living patients, and viewed the states of diseases displayed in the post-mortem dissections of the bodies of those who died. The argument and evidence here directly challenges widespread and longstanding narratives about the nature of Galenic medicine and the history of pathological anatomy.

University-trained physicians claimed to know the true causes of health and disease, and to follow a rational method for diagnosing any given disease and matching it with just the right therapy, or predicting an inevitable death. But how could one find universal, rational causes for an overabundant diversity of individuals' diseases? If patients varied in their own temperament, and the temperaments of all their parts, and diseases just were injurious variations of one or more body parts, how could physicians reach the universality of reason?

© EVAN R. RAGLAND, 2022 | DOI:10.1163/9789004515727_007

Knowledge of diseases, like all natural knowledge, began with the senses. Students trained their minds to look for the actions of faculties grounded in material temperaments, and disciplined their senses to track the signs of different organs' changing and morbid temperaments. As Aristotelian and Galenic philosophy had it, repeated direct sensations of a thing built up experience, putting flesh to concepts and systems learned through lectures, books, and disputation practice. Following Galen and early modern Galenic physicians, Heurnius and his colleagues taught students to identify the sick parts (*partes aegrae*) of their patients' bodies. As elsewhere, pulse-taking and uroscopy allowed students to identify and classify changes to the major vital and nutritive faculties, per Galen and later Galenic elaborations. But the sensory search for signs and symptoms embraced a wide field of color changes, smells, tangible variations, and even some quantification.

Leiden medicine, and the widespread Galenic-Hippocratic medicine of the period, was far more focused on specific anatomical changes, especially those revealed in post-mortem dissections, than is nearly always assumed. The view in Leiden gives us insights into the academic medicine of the late 1500s and early 1600s, since professors and students across Europe often traveled and communicated with each other widely, and shared similar practices, interests, networks, and sources.[1] Leiden professors and students studied ancient sources used widely in university classes on pharmacy and medical theory, as we saw in chapters three and four. Leiden diagnostic and anatomical instruction and practice, discussed in this chapter and the next two chapters, also give us a broader view of major issues and trends in academic medicine. Moreover, they provide strong reasons to revise some long-established assumptions. The final chapter examines the practices of hospital teaching and regular post-mortem dissections there, and the innovations in pathology and therapy developed from these pedagogical practices. Together, these next three chapters provide a new, explicitly revisionist account of early modern Galenic ideas and practices of knowing and treating patients' diseases.

Repeated throughout scholarship on the history of early modern medicine we find confident, even dismissive repetition of the claim that early modern physicians were not really concerned with anatomy for medical practice, since the primacy of some sort of humoral theory and ideals of individual temperament rendered detailed knowledge of the solid parts of bodies less important

---

1 Wear, *Knowledge & Practice*. Grell, Cunningham, Arrizabalaga, eds., *Centres of Medical Excellence?*

or even useless.[2] We hear that Hippocratic writers and Galen "often ignored the solid parts of the body," and that it was only in the mid-to-late eighteenth century that doctors included the analysis of the "seats" of diseases by attending to localized lesions in cadavers.[3] Supposedly, attention to the anatomical "seats" of diseases "directly opposed" thinking in terms of humors.[4] A recent expert summary maintains the standard line, in which Giovanni Battista Morgagni is the pioneer in the mid-1700s who sought to anchor "disease in specific organs of the body [which] provided for anatomically localized approaches to diseases such as cancer, as opposed to the global, humoralistic approaches to diagnosis and treatment still dominating the thinking of most physicians."[5]

Very recent scholarship has begun to call this master narrative into question, pointing to the interplay of thinking about organs and humors in early modern medicine, as well as the correlation of patients' symptoms and anatomical lesions in Padua in the mid-1500s, other Italian cities in the early 1600s, and especially Rome in the first decade of the 1700s.[6] Yet the older narrative persists in influential scholarship, in large part because we lack a comprehensive view of how thinking in terms of impaired parts fit with Galenic theory and practice. How did diseased and healthy organs and parts make sense *within* the Galenic medicine flourishing among university medical faculties, and cultivated by students during their education and later medical practice?

Organ-based pathology was not new in the 1700s; it was the core of Galenic pathology for centuries before. Here and in the two following chapters I argue that we have seriously misconstrued both the broader history of pathology *and* Galenic medical theory and practice, ancient and early modern. Galenic bodies were not mere containers for humoral changes, and while morbid humors and their qualitative changes often *caused* diseases (by causing changes in simple parts and organs), they did not usually *constitute* diseases. Organ-based, anatomical-clinical approaches to pathology were not opposed to Galenic medicine. They were essential and *primary* parts of Galen's own medicine and that of his students in the 1500s and 1600s. Galen and his early modern followers at Padua, Leiden, and across Europe frequently focused their diagnostic, pathological, and therapeutic attention on the "seats" of diseases in organs and

2   *Pace*, e.g., French, *Dissection and Vivisection*, 1–2; Cook, *Matters of Exchange*, 37, 393–4; Cunningham, *Anatomist Anatomis'd*, 196–198; Lindemann, *Medicine and Society*, 18; Bynum, *History of Medicine*, 15, 55.

3   Maulitz, "The Pathological Tradition," 169–170. Cf. Maulitz, "Pathology."

4   Reiser, "The Science of Diagnosis," 827.

5   Maulitz, "Pathology," 370.

6   Bylebyl, "The Manifest and the Hidden." Stolberg, *Experiencing Illness*. Stolberg, "Postmortems." De Renzi, "Seats and Series." Donato, *Sudden Death*.

other solid parts. After all, they defined diseases in terms of impaired or damaged bodily functions, and organs acted to produce most of these functions.

Previous scholarship has occasionally flashed glimpses of this view of Galenic medicine, against the prevailing narrative. Owsei Temkin followed Walther Riese in very briefly pointing out the "anatomical bent" and "localistic interpretation of disease" of Galen's pathology.[7] In Riese's summary, Galen's pathology depended on identifying the impairment of the specific function of the part, examination of the part, and examination of the type of lesion (inflammation, swelling, stones, etc.).[8] He suggested that the rise of Renaissance anatomy made anatomical localization the most significant part of pathology, but that organ-based lesions became primary only in the 1700s. Galen's approach to disease informed and inspired these early developments. For Riese, Vesalius was "even more Galenic than Galen" in insisting on the total primacy of the parts and their functions, and *"anticipated the anatomical conception of disease."*[9] But Riese's history leaps from Vesalius to Morgagni, leaving behind without a backward glance two centuries of pathological anatomy.

Building on the discussions of the temperaments and faculties of organs and drugs built up over the previous chapters, this chapter and the two following show how Leiden physicians, students, and surgeons put this localist Galenism into practice in their teaching and engagement with patients. Evidence of Leiden's sustained, regular practice of post-mortem dissections challenges the canonical view of the uses of post-mortem dissections for pathology in early seventeenth-century Europe. In this view, which stretches from Esmond Long's *A History of Pathology* (1965) to recent overviews of early modern anatomy, post-mortem dissections before the eighteenth century are supposedly *rare*, about rarities or marvels, and of little use for understanding diseases.[10]

As the story goes, only slowly, and in the later-seventeenth century or early eighteenth century, did physicians take up mechanical philosophies and surgical ways of thinking and so focus on solid parts and perceptible lesions. This shift depended on the beginnings of regular, first-hand, systematic dissections of patients' cadavers in order to reveal and catalog morbid lesions. This established narrative often turns on influential but deeply problematic histories of the discrete "birth" of modern anatomo-clinical medicine based on hundreds of post-mortem dissections in the Paris hospitals around 1800. This rough

---

7   Temkin, *Galenism*, 138, n. 10. Cf. pp. 17–18.

8   Riese, *The Conception of Disease*, 41–45.

9   Riese, *The Conception of Disease*, 57, italics in original.

10   Long, *A History of Pathology*. Cunningham, *Anatomist Anatomis'd*, 196–198.

chronology, popularized in works by Foucault and Ackerknecht, still shapes
many historians' periodization of early modern European medicine.[11]

The main pedagogical sources of evidence from Leiden, and other major
teaching universities, contradict this story. Even commonly-used textbooks
of medicine plainly argue the contrary. So do student disputations and
records of anatomical practices from the public dissecting theater to private
post-mortems and hospital post-mortems. Students and professors prized
post-mortem dissections, especially clinical anatomies done in the hospital, as
the touchstone of clinical teaching, from at least 1636 on. Reading some of the
ancient texts used most extensively by our Leiden scholars, combined with a
close study of their own publications and notes of dissections, tells a story that
cuts deeply against the reigning narrative of diagnosis, pathology, and anatomy
in early modern Europe. It shows that even late-Renaissance academic *teaching* was not the merely bookish, rational exercise of ancient Greek categories
and methods, which supposedly depended predominantly on the narrative of
the patient rather than the physician's observations.[12]

Rather than looking at Galenists searching for the anatomical seats of diseases as exceptions, I argue that a comprehensive picture of academic medical
thinking shows that they likely were the rule, and certainly were at Leiden.
This strongly corroborates and expands beyond Michael Stolberg's very recent
argument for Renaissance anatomists' occasional interest in localized pathological changes revealed in post-mortem dissections.[13] After all, as I argue,
Galen's own definition of disease emphasized localization in an organ or simple part, since diseases just were injured actions or functions of the body, and
organs and simple parts performed most actions or functions. Galen certainly
claimed great prestige for anatomy, and his pathological works often organized
diseases by parts and localized their seats. Widely-used works by Galen, read
and cited at Leiden and elsewhere in Latin translations, explicitly demanded
physicians locate the diseased part of the body, the "seat" (*sedes*) of the disease,
and organized diagnosis, prognosis, and therapy by bodily parts.

I go beyond Stolberg's excellent short survey to show in detail the variety
of anatomical practices which constituted the core of the Leiden pedagogical *tradition* of anatomically-localized pathology. I also build on the previous
chapters to situate these practices *within* the rich medical theory and practical medicine courses which helped to motivate and make intelligible those
practices. My work here from traditional and influential pedagogical sources

11   De Renzi, Bresadola, and Conforti, "Pathological Dissections in Early Modern Europe."
12   *Pace* Nicolson, "The Art of Diagnosis," 805–6.
13   Stolberg, "Post-mortems."

provides a comprehensive intellectual complement to Stolberg's findings from patients' records across the early modern period. As he has already shown, patients themselves did not explain diseases by whole-body excesses of one of the four humors, but by "more or less specific, harmful, and corrupt matter" flowing into or building up in a specific part or parts.[14] Such localization and organ-based approaches, including regular post-mortem dissections, were not foreign imports into Galenic medicine, but valued practices growing naturally from its key texts, pedagogical traditions, and theories (with added motivation for legal determinations of the causes of death).

This Galenic focus on the impaired organ or part appears consistently across the sources from professors and students. Reading Leiden's main textbook from the course on practical medicine in context, and pairing it with student disputations and records of dissections from Paaw and Otto Heurnius in the next chapters, reveals a programmatic insistence on tracking diseases as localized disturbances of one or more organs or parts. Dozens of post-mortem dissections of patients, around three each year, gave eager professors, and sometimes students, the chance to see the hidden causes of diseases they learned to imagine and trace from a distance based on external signs. Even student disputations, a formal practice carried on from medieval academic life, aimed at proving students' knowledge of knowing and curing localized diseases.

With the evidence from the detailed autopsy records of Paaw and Otto in hand, I have distinguished the interrelated practices of dissection into three types, by locations and audiences: public anatomies in the anatomy theater, private anatomies in homes and other sites, and clinical anatomies performed as part of the regular diagnosis, treatment, and post-mortem dissection of poor patients in the local hospital. In all three, professors and surgeons collaborated to cut and observe the phenomena of healthy and diseased bodies. Students regularly attended the public anatomies and clinical anatomies (after 1636), and appear occasionally in the records of the private anatomies.

Public anatomies, performed in official sites of the university such as the theater constructed in 1593, were decorous spectacles and learned investigations. The university cancelled classes and professors gathered with students, visitors, and curious Leideners. The professor described the structures as the surgeon busily cut and probed the dead. They followed the lines of God's craftwork displayed in anatomical structures and functions, and traced the tracks of disease in patients' cadavers. Even public anatomies primarily served to

---

14   Stolberg, *Experiencing Illness*, 95.

educate students about the nature and actions of healthy and diseased body parts. Moral or pious readings of human mortality, rightly noted by historians, played a distinct secondary role.[15]

Private anatomies occurred at the request of a recently deceased person's family or the local civic authorities, with the goal of establishing the hidden causes of death by visual and tactile sensation. These often occurred in patients' homes, though sometimes in the public hospital or even, it seems, a building in the marketplace. Records of these anatomies usually lacked even the smallest mentions of patient narratives or histories of their lives and diseases, against the expectations of influential historiography.[16] In the standard view, before around 1800, physicians often had less social power to control the narrative of disease and patients' own interpretations of their bodies dominated bedside diagnosis. Yet these canonical studies, which emphasized a story of bedside medicine changing to clinical medicine around 1800, lacked serious engagement with sources from the long seventeenth century and earlier.[17] Nor were the frequent post-mortem dissections of the later 1500s and 1600s merely passive canvases on which these Galenic-Hippocratic physicians painted stories of their preconceived diagnoses. Post-mortem dissections could confirm or disconfirm diagnoses, as in several cases of suspected poisoning.

Clinical anatomies, discussed in chapter seven, happened as part of the instruction of students, as well as the pursuit of the causes of disease and death in patients' opened bodies. At least by 1636, and perhaps earlier, professors gave weekly instruction at patients' bedsides in the municipal hospital. While the patients lived, professors and students discussed diagnosis, prognosis, and therapy for each one. If patients died and their family consented, professors and surgeons dissected the bodies to check diagnoses and inspect diseased parts. Across these sites and audiences, professors connected evidence for diseases and morbid matter, demonstrating again their ultimate, coordinating goal of understanding and curing localized diseases.

Although the physicians and anatomists worked deeply within the tradition of Galenic-Hippocratic medicine, they still tried to make new discoveries. They prized recent, new anatomical findings, and tried to enhance their own expertise with their own claims to novel structures. Most of all, they greatly expanded the store of first-hand, sensory descriptions of disease lesions found in cadavers. This led slowly toward innovations in pathology, such as their

---

15   Pace, e.g., Cook, *Matters of Exchange*, 164–167; Lunsingh Scheurleer, "Un Amphithéâtre"; Huisman, *Finger of God*, 37–42.

16   Pace e.g., Jewson, "Disappearance"; Fissell, "Disappearance."

17   Foucault, *Birth of the Clinic*. Jewson, "Disappearance." Fissell, "Disappearance." Nicolson, "Art of Diagnosis." Maulitz, "Pathological Tradition."

encounters with the variety of tubercles and ulcers causing the constant and deadly disease of phthisis or consumption, as described in chapter seven.

Dissections in the theater, in private homes, and the anatomy room of the hospital represented the culmination of students' learning, and were treasured experiences for students and professors. Patients' families often demanded private anatomies to find the causes of death. The act of dissection *itself* was not always morally or socially abhorrent, especially given the stakes of understanding the loss of a loved one (or suspected murder). This evidence is strongly contrary to ongoing stories about the social and cultural violations supposedly inherent in the act of cutting human bodies, but is corroborated by similar findings from studies of Italian anatomical theaters and teaching.[18] In private anatomies, dissectors anatomized all sorts of bodies, from members of noble families to unnamed vagabonds, and even professor Johannes Heurnius himself! Surgeons socialized and collaborated frequently with the academic professors and students, and acted as expert witnesses for the recorded historical facts of the autopsies. Even though licensed surgeons had their own exams and guilds, surgical books and learning formed part of the curriculum for physicians, and physicians showed productive interest in surgical techniques, especially in relation to anatomical learning. Scholars presented the public anatomies, in particular, as places of republican leveling, in which all who behaved soberly could see and learn the secrets of God's artistry in the human fabric.

1   **The Malfunctioning Seats of Diseases**

The theory of practical medicine at Leiden, and its model Padua, demanded the development of anatomically-based understandings of disease and treat-, ment. The Galenic-Hippocratic medicine taught at Leiden did not depend on vague assertions about diseases as total-body imbalances of the four basic humors, blood, phlegm, yellow bile, and black bile. In the core courses on practical and theoretical medicine, students learned to think about diseases as local changes in specific parts, concentrating on the specific qualitative and structural characteristics of each organ or part of the body. Johannes Heurnius (1543–1601), who taught at Leiden from 1581 to 1601, led this pedagogical program through his textbooks and matching lecture courses on the theory and practice of medicine. His colleagues used his books as the core of medical instruction into the 1640s.

---

18   E.g., *Pace* Sawday, *Body Emblazoned*. Cf. Klestinec, *Theaters of Anatomy*.

In his *New Method of the Practice of Medicine* (1587–1650) and his popular textbook, *Institutes of Medicine* (1592–1666), Heurnius advanced his "new method" (*nova ratio*) for curing diseases based on the precise location and quality of the affected part and the nature of the affect.[19] As Heurnius put it in his course and textbook on medical theory, the *Institutes of Medicine*, "a disease is a constitution beyond nature of the living body, primarily and in itself wounding an action."[20] Diseases, for Heurnius, "dwell in the parts," while the causes of diseases frequently "dwell in the humors."[21] His new method connected specific parts and precise remedies proven by use. As he rhetorically framed the project in the preface, "Does not the varied nature of the parts, their sense, nobility, and location, require a varied idea of the remedies?" Heurnius' rational, methodical attention to all the causes of a disease, its local changes of parts revealed through impaired functions, and his precise compounding of small amounts of medicinal ingredients all show innovative gradual changes. But his approach was solidly Galenic.

In his "new" method, Heurnius followed the example of Galen, who brought his therapeutic theory to bear on localized diseases, diseases understood through organ temperament theory and anatomy. Heurnius framed his own contribution in both of his major books by invoking Galen's admonition from the sixth book of his *Simple Drugs*: "medicine is not able to be performed without medicines and their perceived powers, and, as Galen writes, the method of healing and the contemplation of the faculties of medicines are so associated by mutual connection. Neither, really, can be understood without the other."[22]

Galenic medicine depended on local anatomy: one must know the hidden parts to know their diseases, so a true physician must be versed in anatomy.[23] Galen even agreed with his frequent punching bag, the earlier anatomist Erasistratus, to insist that a physician must know "not only the quality of that affect, but know rightly the affect and also its location."[24] A physician had to know first of all the wounded action or function of the part (*actio laesa* or *functio laesa*,

---

19   Johannes Heurnius, *Institutiones Medicinae* (1592). Johannes Heurnius, *Institutiones Medicinae* (1609). This second edition was re-issued in 1627, 1638, and 1666. With some corrections, the main text is the same for editions 1609–1666, and substantially the same as the 1592 edition. The 1638 edition contains additional front matter, including an oration by Heurnius on the historical origin of medicine. I have compared the editions, but primarily use the 1638 edition: Johannes Heurnius, *Institutiones Medicinae* (1638).

20   Johannes Heurnius, *Institutiones*, 188.

21   Johannes Heurnius, *Institutiones*, 516, 492.

22   Johannes Heurnius, *Institutiones*, 464. Cf. Johannes Heurnius, *Nova Ratio*, 1. Compare Galen, *De simplicium medicamentorum facultatibus libri XI*, 163, 347–348.

23   Galen, *De Affectorum Locorum Notitia, libri sex*, 3r.

24   Galen, *De Affectorum Locorum Notitia*, 5r.

with both *actio* or action and *functio* or function common Latin translations for Galen's term *energeia*).[25] Indeed, rather than beginning from a person's general temperament, as some approaches to medical theory demanded, Galen argued here, and elsewhere, for a method of anatomical localization of diseases:

> Therefore one must always begin from the organ of the injured action, and then seek what is the manner [*modus*] of the injury, namely whether the disposition is constant, or is still coming about, so that it is not yet made to persist. And if it is now coming about, whether the cause which brings about the affect is contained in the part itself, or passes through it, must be investigated.[26]

The strong emphasis here on diseased parts of the body should not come as a surprise for readers of Galen's works. After all, he most often conceived of diseases as dispositions of the body that harm or impede its proper, healthy actions.[27] Since different organs acting individually and in concert produce the body's actions and functions, most diseases find their locations or seats in specific organs or parts of the body. His comprehensive definitions across several works did *not* define diseases as general imbalances of the humors, but in terms such as these:

> A disease is an affect of the body, primarily impeding some action. Affects which precede this [impeding affect] are not called diseases. If other things supervene on these affects, following as shadows, we will not call these diseases, but symptoms. Thus whatever occurs in the body beyond nature should not straightaway be named a disease. But only that which primarily wounds an action, while that which precedes it will be called a cause of disease, but not a disease.[28]

---

25   Galen, *De Affectorum Locorum Notitia*, 22v. Latin texts generally translated the Greek *"energeia,"* which Galen used to refer to the action or activity of a part, as *"actio"* or *"functio."* Galen himself blurred distinctions between the two terms *ergon* (action) and *energeia* (function), though at other times he made sharper distinctions between action (*ergon*), function/activity (*energeia*), and use (*chreia*). Distelzweig, "The Use of *Usus* and the Function of *Functio*," 380. Johnston, "Introduction," in *Galen: On Diseases and Symptoms*, 28–30.

26   Galen, *De Affectorum Locorum Notitia*, 6r.

27   Hankinson, "Philosophy of Nature," 230, citing *Symp.Diff.* VII 50. Bylebyl, "The Manifest and the Hidden," 45. Maclean, *Logic, Signs, and Nature*, 261.

28   Galen, *De Symptomatum Differentiis* in Galen, *De Morborum et Symptomatum Differentiis et Causis libri sex*, 39. Cf. Galen, *De Differentiis Morborum*, in the same work, 3: "a disease is a fault either of an action or a constitution." Cf. Galen, *On the Differentiae of the Symptoms*, in *Galen: On Diseases and Symptoms*, trans. Johnston, 182.

Similarly, in his comprehensive, *On the Differentiae of Diseases*, Galen defined "disease" as "a constitution beyond nature, or the cause of a damaged function."[29] Thus, if we could find out all the ways in which bodies are impaired so that they cannot perform their natural actions or functions, we would find out the number of all the simple diseases. Since health is the proper "balance" (*symmetria*) of the hot, cold, wet, and dry *qualities*, then "disease is a departure from this."[30]

Although distinguishing causes, diseases, impaired functions, and symptoms was not always clear or easy for Galen or early modern Galenic physicians, his basic scheme remained consistent.[31] Galen's comprehensive and influential *Method of Medicine* (or *Method of Healing, Methodo medendi*) is nicely explicit, and included the relations of cause, disease, and symptom: "The disease damages function, the cause precedes the disease, and the symptom follows it, its nature being twofold—the one being damage of function [*energeia*], and the other being some condition which follows the disease."[32] Thus, the goal of medicine is "to restore the functions of the parts to nature wherever they should happen to have been damaged."[33]

In his work on diseases according to the parts of the body, Galen emphasized especially the impaired action of an organ or part: "In the first place one must examine whether some action is injured, since of course the proper instrument of the action must necessarily be affected."[34] A damaged action or function gave the surest indicator of a disease and its "seat" in the body, but as usual Galen had a long list of things to notice: "Therefore affected seats [*sedes*] are discerned from the symptoms, from the wounded action, from the quality of the excrements, from swelling beyond nature, from pains, from a fault in the color of something that follows, either in the whole body or in one part, or in two, and especially in the eyes and the tongue."[35] Renaissance physicians debated the ambiguities in Galen's formal definitions (Did an affect—*affectus, diathesis*—have be persistent and unchanging? Were all alterations, including changes of color, affects?) but agreed on the main lines of diseases as

---

29   Galen, *De Differentiis Morborum*, in Galen, *De Morborum...Differentiis* (1546), 3. Cf. Galen, *On the Differentiae of Diseases*, 134.

30   Galen, *De Differentiis Morborum*, 4.

31   On the difficulties, see Siraisi, "Disease and Symptom." For Galen, see Johnston, *Galen: On Diseases and Symptoms*, 21–125.

32   Galen, *Method of Medicine*, bk. 1, ch. 9, ed. and trans. Johnston and Horsley, vol. 1, 116–117.

33   Galen, *Method of Medicine*, 67. I have amended the translation, substituting "nature" for "normal" to better render the Greek "*phusin*."

34   Galen, *De Affectorum Locorum Notitia*, 22v.

35   Galen, *De Affectorum Locorum Notitia*, 22r–22v.

impairments of functions, usually of a localized part or parts.[36] Early modern medical pedagogy at Leiden and elsewhere followed the major Galenic models, as we will see.

Galen's method used all sorts of evidence to identify the injured part, including pains. As we can still attest, where it hurts, there is something wrong. Pain indicated clearly injury to a specific part, especially when analyzed according to Galen's exhaustive list of distinct sorts of pain. Pain indicates inflammation of a part when the part is moved.[37] Different types can be pulsating, heavy, biting, inherent, pointlike, fierce, harsh, fixed, lacerating, constricting, ulcerating, acute, turgid, and on and on. Pulsating pains often indicate trouble with the arteries and heart, and those suffering from migraines feel the fullness of turgid pain, which begins as if in roots and quickly moves to nearby parts.[38] Different pains indicate both the part affected and the morbid affect: inflammation, ulcer, abscess, etc.[39]

Other, even more influential works, carried forward this localizing program. Galen's summary teaching work, *The Art of Medicine* (*Techne iatrike* or *Ars medica* or *Ars parva* or *Tegni*), was a major teaching text from the Late Antique period, through Arabic medieval medicine from the ninth century on, and appears as a mainstay of Latin learned medicine from the later twelfth century versions of the *Articella* through the seventeenth century.[40] In that work, Galen discussed the signs of the mixtures or constitutions of the chief parts which departed from the "best" or midpoint constitutions, but were still "natural" given their idiosyncratic temperaments generated through fetal development. Humors play very minor roles throughout the text. First of all, he defined a healthy body "in the general sense" as one that "has from birth a good mixture of the simple, primary parts, and good proportion in the organs composed of these."[41] These simple, primary parts are the homoiomerous ones (those of a single qualitative mixture, alike in every part) such as arteries, veins, nerves, bones, ligaments, flesh, and membranes.[42]

---

36   Siraisi, "Disease and Symptom."

37   Galen, *De Affectorum Locorum Notitia*, 14v.

38   Galen, *De Affectorum Locorum Notitia*, 17v.

39   Galen, *De Affectorum Locorum Notitia*, 47v.

40   Kaye, *History of Balance*, 137–8. Ottoson, *Scholastic Medicine*, ch. 1. Even after extended debate, most scholars accept this work as genuine, and medieval and early modern scholars certainly accepted it as Galen's own work. See Hankinson, "Philosophy of Nature," 237 n. 28.

41   Galen, *The Art of Medicine*, in *Galen: Selected Works*, trans. Singer, 347.

42   Galen, *On the Differentiae of Diseases*, in *Galen: On Diseases and Symptoms*, 137.

Throughout *The Art of Medicine*, Galen worked systematically through the *qualitative* variations of simple and composite parts, and especially the chief *organs*, describing the signs and symptoms found when patients' brains, hearts, livers, and testes were hotter, colder, drier, and wetter than the "best" mixtures. He considered a range of other parts such as muscles, lungs, stomachs, etc. As elsewhere, he diagnosed the morbid states from the changes in action or function: "the distinguishing mark [of morbid bodies] is the perceptible impairment of function."[43] Lumps, swellings, inflammation, and pain indicate diseased parts, and healing comes about through the destruction of the state impairing natural function, especially by applying opposing qualities.[44] Since "organs have acquired their particular nature by virtue of their mixture," mixtures were responsible for every faculty, and thus for healthy or impaired functions.[45] Symptoms followed these changes in mixture (or structure): e.g., a diseased heart revealed its morbid state through difficulties in breathing, palpitations, pulses, excitement or depression of the spirits, fevers, chills, changes in color, and pains.[46]

Even Galen's frequent invocation of the proper "mixture" (*krasis*) or balance in patients' bodies did not aim primarily at a proportional balance of the humors. In *The Art of Medicine*, Galen discussed in detail the proper "balance" of the four qualities of the homogenous parts, and the proper composition of the organic parts.[47] Imbalances are not generally in terms of the four humors, either, but of the proper qualitative mixture of each part.[48] "Each of the other parts, similarly [to the stomach], might be too moist, too dry, too hot, or too cold; and each of these will require its own regimen for this imbalance."[49] Similarly, the qualitative mixtures or balances of drugs or other therapeutic materials are the means by which they possess faculties and affect the qualities of bodies, as we have seen in the previous chapter.[50] Humoral balances and imbalances play more important roles for wound care, and for abnormal fluxes of humors into morbid *parts*.[51] Thus, the morbid movements and states of the humors, for Galen

---

43   Galen, *The Art of Medicine*, in *Galen: Selected Works*, trans. Singer, 350.

44   Galen, *The Art of Medicine*, in *Galen: Selected Works*, trans. Singer, 369, 381.

45   Galen, *The Art of Medicine*, in *Galen: Selected Works*, trans. Singer, 366-7.

46   Galen, *The Art of Medicine*, in *Galen: Selected Works*, trans. Singer, 368-9.

47   Galen, *Art of Medicine*, 349, 353, 354, 356, 357, 362. Pages 374-5 also mentioned the "balance" of what later physicians called the six non-naturals: air, motion and rest, sleep and waking, ingesta, excretion and retention, and passions of the soul.

48   Galen, *The Art of Medicine*, in *Galen: Selected Works*, 357, 359, 363, 365.

49   Galen, *The Art of Medicine*, in *Galen: Selected Works*, 378.

50   Galen, *The Art of Medicine*, in *Galen: Selected Works*, 375, 376, 382.

51   Galen, *The Art of Medicine*, in *Galen: Selected Works*, 385, 390.

and Galenic physicians, were often the *causes* of imbalances and diseases of parts, with treatments aimed differently at humors or solid parts: "the treatment of the effective causes of imbalance of mixtures is through evacuation, while the treatment of imbalance itself is merely alteration."[52]

As Joel Kaye has shown in a recent, detailed exposition of Galen's notion of "balance," the Galenic model emphasized the proper "balanced" temperament or complexion of the four *qualities* of all the body's parts, their dynamic, multipart systems of relations, and their complex relations with the ingesta and the environment. As Kaye summarizes, "[Galen] never drew a simple equation between health and the balance (or the proper blending) of the four humors themselves, and in his most direct and technical discussions of complexion, he refers solely to proportional mixtures and their possible permutations, involving the four primary qualities."[53] Early modern physicians from Padua to Leiden closely followed Galen's emphasis on the multiple sites of balanced qualitative temperaments for patients' bodies.

In sum, Galen's matter theory linked diagnosis, anatomy, drug theory, and therapy by ascribing the same natural philosophical understanding to all the different substances—organs, humors, plants, the physician's sensory organs—and so establishing an interacting network of qualities. Galen, like his Renaissance students, adopted the best "science" of his time, taking on the opinion of the "best philosophers and doctors" that the qualities hot, cold, wet, and dry mixed to compose all things.[54]

In his *On the Affected Places* (*De locis affectis*), and other works, Galen hewed to the definition and diagnosis of diseases by their diseased parts. This book traversed the major organs and activities of the body from the head (including memory, melancholy, mania, headaches, and disorders of smell, sight, hearing, and the voice), through the chest and abdomen to the groin. Other medical texts, from ancient Egyptian sources through a few Hippocratic works, compiled standard reports of diseases from the head to the chest, but Galen's approach thoroughly systematized diseases as seated in the simple parts and organs and defined by impaired actions or functions.[55] Galen began with the wounded function of the patient's body (pain and swelling of the liver, impaired breathing, poor nutrition, impaired reasoning, etc.), then moved from the function to the part performing the function, then on to the nature of the impairment

---

52   Galen, *The Art of Medicine*, in *Galen: Selected Works*, Singer trans., 382.

53   Kaye, *A History of Balance*, 168. His analysis agrees with that of Ottoson, *Scholastic Medicine*, 130–132.

54   Galen, *Mixtures*, in *Galen: Selected Works*, trans. Singer, 202.

55   Jouanna, *Hippocrates*, trans. DeBevoise, 145.

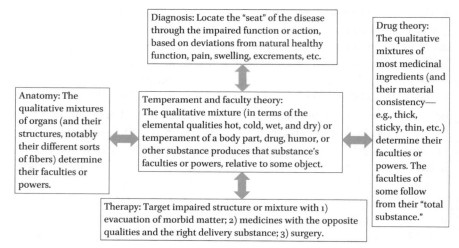

Diagnosis: Locate the "seat" of the disease through the impaired function or action, based on deviations from natural healthy function, pain, swelling, excrements, etc.

Drug theory: The qualitative mixtures of most medicinal ingredients (and their material consistency— e.g., thick, sticky, thin, etc.) determine their faculties or powers. The faculties of some follow from their "total substance."

Anatomy: The qualitative mixtures of organs (and their structures, notably their different sorts of fibers) determine their faculties or powers.

Temperament and faculty theory: The qualitative mixture (in terms of the elemental qualities hot, cold, wet, and dry) or temperament of a body part, drug, humor, or other substance produces that substance's faculties or powers, relative to some object.

Therapy: Target impaired structure or mixture with 1) evacuation of morbid matter; 2) medicines with the opposite qualities and the right delivery substance; 3) surgery.

FIGURE 11   Diagram showing the centrality of Galenic qualitative mixture or temperament and faculty theory to the causal relations and powers of body parts and plants, and the perceptions and actions of diagnosis and therapy.

(usually described in terms of Galenic qualitative matter theory), and finally to the causes of this impairment. As in his other works, he emphasized the qualitative temperament of the simple parts and organs, reiterating that "the essence of each of the primary bodies consists in the temperament of the four qualities."[56] He drew on Hippocratic texts and his own experience—including observing and treating gladiators—to list the signs and descriptions of various ailments according to their seats in faulty or wounded parts.[57] For instance, an inflamed and enlarged bulging part of the liver can and should be known by manually palpating the patient's abdomen, but inflammations of the enclosed hidden side should be diagnosed by the patient's disgust, nausea, bilious vomiting, and great thirst.[58] *On the Affected Places* enjoyed wide reception and influence in the early modern period, appearing in at least eight editions in the sixteenth century, and serving as a regular part of university teaching from Spain to German lands, Italy, and the Low Countries.[59] In Leiden, in 1634, Otto Heurnius described his teaching commentary on Galen's *On the Affected Places* as embracing "the whole of practice."[60]

---

56   Galen, *De Affectorum Locorum Notitia*, 60v.
57   Galen, *De Affectorum Locorum Notitia*, 51v.
58   Galen, *De Affectorum Locorum Notitia*, 58r–58v.
59   Durling, "Chronological Census," 245, 264, 264, 267, 271, 272, 275, 279.
60   Molhuysen, *Bronnen*, 2, 191.

Galen's vastly influential *Method of Medicine* expressed a similar approach, arguing that the rational approach, one common to all the Greeks, was to define health as the absence of impediments to functions or actions (*energeias*) "of all the parts of the body," and to identify a person as diseased when any natural action is impaired, "at least in that particular part of the body whose function they see to be damaged."[61] The goal of therapy, then, is "to restore the functions of the parts according to nature, wherever they should happen to have been damaged."[62] Leiden professors such as Johannes Heurnius cited this work often, too, especially on how to recognize the "sick part" (*pars aegra*) by impaired functions and symptoms.[63] Galen's pharmacology matched this vision of diseases as localized impairments, and Galen's *On the Composition of Drugs according to the Parts* also arranged reports of drugs and personally-tried medicines by their uses from head to toe.[64]

Some of Galen's other works, notably *On the Causes of Diseases* and *On the Differentia of Diseases*, display an even more elaborate accounting of diseases as localized impairments of organs and simple parts, caused by qualitative or structural changes. These texts appeared in multiple editions from the 1520s to 1560, and professors at Leiden and elsewhere cited them frequently.[65] In *On the Causes of Diseases*, Galen set up two competing hypothesis, the doctrine of Asclepiades, in which diseases are caused by the passage or blockage of tiny corpuscles through channels (*poroi*), and the doctrine of diseases as qualitative bad temperaments (*dyscrasias*) of the parts.[66] Both hypotheses also described some diseases in terms of changes in structure, or the dissolution of continuity.

As in his other works, the morbid temperaments appear most often in terms of harmful qualitative changes to simple parts, organs, and humors, not imbalances of humors in general. Thus, bodies can become too hot from movement, putrefaction, closeness to a hotter body, constriction, and the ingestion of

---

61   Galen, *Method of Medicine*, trans. Johnston and Horsley, 65, cf. 97, 107. For the influence of this work in the early modern period, see, e.g., Johannes Heurnius, *Institutiones Medicinae*, 489, 495, 503, 519, 527, 533. 539, 542, 543, 544. See also Boss, "The 'Methodus Medendi' as an Index of Change." Jerome J. Bylebyl, "Teaching *Methodus Medendi* in the Renaissance."

62   Galen, *Method of Medicine*, trans. Johnston and Horsley, 67. I have emended the translation to give "according to nature" for "*kata phusin*," rather than "to normal."

63   Johannes Heurnius, *Institutiones* (1638), 539–544. Johannes Heurnius, *Nova Ratio*, 328, 622–624, 628, 637, 640, 681.

64   Vogt, "Drugs," 311.

65   Durling, "Chronological Census," 254, 254, 265, 266, 269, 274. Johannes Heurnius, *Institutiones* (1609), 96, 222, 223, 279. Fuchs, *Institutiones* (1555), 506, 507, 527.

66   Galen, *On the Causes of Diseases*, trans. Johnston, 159. Cf. Johnston, *Galen*, 70, 99, 113–114.

certain foods with heating faculties, such as garlic and onions.[67] Galen's preferred matter theory comes into play throughout his discussions, especially
when he uses examples of the qualitative change of non-living things as exemplars for change in living things. Stones rubbed together become warm just
as excessive bodily movement can heat the heart and cause a fever, or heat
another body part or parts. Putrefying feces and seeds clearly generate heat
(Galen claimed to have seen the feces of pigeons catch fire), just as putrefying matter generates erysipelas, pustules, and inflammations in living bodies.
Similarly, "constriction" or closing up the doors or air vents of bathhouses and
furnaces causes excess heat just as extreme ambient cold or astringent water
can cause the skin to close its "air vents," producing morbid heating.[68] Galen
went on to consider diseases caused by excess cold, dryness, and hotness, with
inaminate examples grounding and illustrating his arguments. They also displayed the complex causation of disease. Just as the same external cause, such
as excess ambient heat, did not always cause a fever in every person, due to the
natural variations of their bodies, so fire was slower to burn very cold hands, or
wet wood, as compared to dry reeds.

Galen spent much more time considering the various changes of structure
in relation to diseases than he did to the movement or changes of the humors.
External injuries, changes in cavities or channels, abnormal roughening or
smoothing of surfaces, decrease or increase of parts of organs, dislocations,
and changes of simple parts in terms of dissolution of continuities—either
surface or interior dissolutions, or both—all feature prominently in his
accounting. The humors appear in bit parts, since they "sometimes" cause
qualitative changes of simple parts or organs as they flow into and around
them, bearing the qualities hot, cold, wet, and dry which act on the parts.[69]
Morbid conditions are likely to arise when there is a flux of too much of a
humor, or one too hot or cold, and especially if a humor becomes blocked,
builds up, and putrefies.[70] Humors clearly sometimes caused diseases,
but these diseases almost always appear as causes of impairments of the
actions or functions of the simple parts, organs, and organ systems, or as the
impairments themselves.

---

67   Galen, *On the Causes of Diseases*, trans. Johnston, 160–162. Cf. Johnston, *Galen*, 114. Galen,
      De Morborum et Symptomatum Differentiis et Causis, 20–22.
68   Galen, *On the Causes of Diseases*, trans. Johnston, 160–162.
69   Galen, *On the Differentiae of Diseases*, trans. Johnston, 141. Galen, *De Morborum
      Differentiis*, 8.
70   Galen, *On the Causes of Diseases*, trans. Johnston, 171. Galen, *De Morborum Causis*, 30.

2   Seats of Diseases after Galen

Galen's approach to localized diseases, defined primarily as qualitative imbalances and structural faults of organs and simple parts, flourished after him. Many ancient, medieval, and early modern writers followed a head-to-toe format for diseases and the recommended (or not) remedies, organized by the impaired organs and parts: Paul of Aegina, Rhazes, Avicenna, Constantine the African, the Salernitan writers Gariopontus and Petrocellus, as well as later medieval writers such as Arnau of Vilanova. This focus and organization continued through the sixteenth and seventeenth centuries with books by influential writers such as Leonhart Fuchs (1501–1566) and Theophile Bonet (1620–1689).[71] The major Galenic textbook compendium of at least the first half of the sixteenth century, Avicenna's *Canon*, also included an extensive Book Three on particular diseases, from head to toe (though mostly on the head and chest), according to whether the disease resulted from an intemperance or structural disorder of one or more parts.[72] Specifically, Avicenna organized diseases by the signs taken from the dispositions and hot, dry, cold, wet and other mixed intemperances of the matter of the parts, as well as pains and signs of more specific diseases of one or more parts. Before Avicenna, the head-to-foot mapping in Rhazes' influential text, *Ad Almansorem*, also limited the discussion of diseases largely to diagnostic signs and the appropriate remedies, bypassing the wide-ranging rational method for inferring causes advocated by Galen.[73]

Medieval Latin physicians and professors followed the lead of the Arabic writers. They even classified the ever-present fevers in terms of the bodily substances or parts affected (ephemeral fevers by the spirits, putrid or humoral fevers by the humors, hectic or chronic fevers by the solid parts).[74] Treatises on "practical medicine," read far more widely by later medieval and Renaissance physicians than university textbook-style works on theory, also used head-to-toe organization schemes, with diseases arranged according to specific impairments of specific body parts.[75] Most courses and texts in "practical medicine" (*practicae*) presented systems of diseases and treatment (diagnosis, prognosis, and therapy), rather than directly recording the actual practice of encountering and treating patients.

---

71   Wear, "Explorations in Renaissance Writings," 127.
72   Siraisi, *Avicenna in the Renaissance*, 77–106. Avicenna, *Liber Canonis, de medicinis cordialibus, et cantica* (1544), 176r–416r.
73   Bylebyl, "Teaching *Methodus Medendi* in the Renaissance" 167.
74   Jacquart, "Anatomy, Physiology, and Medical Theory," 605.
75   Demaitre, *Medieval Medicine*.

Thus, strong Galenic precedents provided ample justification for bringing together anatomy, pathology, therapeutics, and philosophical understandings of qualitative change to know localized affects and make remedies for them. Yet for some physicians earlier in the sixteenth century a new *ratio* of *practical* medicine might well have appeared as a contradiction in terms. This was a contested and difficult topic at the time. The goals of pedagogical clarity and long philosophical training motivated professors to develop systems for thinking about diseases and treatments, rather than grab-bags of Empirical histories. But the variations of patients, diseases, medicines, climates, food, drink, and all the rest threatened to bury clarity and reason under an avalanche of confounding factors. Still, leading early modern physicians and professors, notably the famous Paduan professor and Galenist Giambattista da Monte (d. 1551) in the first half of the sixteenth century, had strongly insisted on the rational basis of medical practice. This rational basis sought to measure up to Galenic ideals by insisting that the physician understand every individual's idiosyncratic temperament, or proper balance of the bodily qualities, especially hot, cold, wet, and dry. Leiden professors such as Johannes Heurnius, who had studied in Padua, carried on this quest for a rational, philosophical, practical medicine, yet strongly de-emphasized idiosyncratic temperament.

Bridging the universals of philosophical matter theory and natural causes and the specifics of *this* particular patient remained a thorny problem, then as now.[76] Da Monte attempted a solution by constantly running from a patient's "appearances which offer themselves to the senses" through universal functions of bodies and parts established by Galenic explanatory principles. A vast, iterative system of divisions did much of the work, beginning with the chief functions, then the parts, then the temperaments and structures, then causes, and so on. In this way, "as under a cloud," one could understand how universals apply to particulars.[77] Galenic principles of causation, which fit with the Aristotelian natural philosophical emphasis on the hot, cold, wet, and dry qualities, supplied the universal causes through which students learned to interpret particular cases.[78] Anatomical expertise across individual bodies and species grounded further universals. The organs performed functions based on the action of their faculties, which in turn derived from their temperaments. Knowledge gained across bodies showed, for example, that the liver generated nutritious venous blood (after all, the hepatic veins connecting the large, red liver with the vena cava must indicate the origin of the flow of

---

76   Temkin, "The Scientific Approach to Disease."
77   Da Monte, quote and trans. in Bylebyl, "Teaching *Methodus Medendi* in the Renaissance," 180.
78   Bylebyl, "Teaching *Methodus Medendi* in the Renaissance," 180.

venous blood, and the liver nestled above the organs of digestion, linked to them by the huge portal vein). Like so many other organs, and many natural and artificial processes from the formation of stones to baking, the liver needed the right amount of heat to properly concoct this blood. Changes in its temperament altered its blood-making faculty, potentially causing a serious disease state. Yet most of these changes remained hidden from direct sensory perception, and patients varied in the natural temperaments of their organs and parts.

Given this complexity, and the ongoing problem of explaining how, exactly, universals related to particulars, it should come as no surprise that the medical *practica* courses from the medieval period on had almost exclusively treated the method of curing in terms of handy, head-to-toe reference works which pointed the user to the right remedy based on the disease and the bodily location.[79] Gestures to a rational method through philosophical, qualitative matter theory and calibration to each individual's temperament often remained just that—prefatory nods before a more Empirical approach connecting common signs and remedies, organized by specific parts rather than disease states in general (e.g., "inflammation").[80]

Ideally, Galenic medicine ought to unite rational, philosophical medicine and local causation. Da Monte, Gabriele Falloppio, and other medical professors of the mid-sixteenth century in northern Italy sought to provide this integration by joining bedside and hospital instruction with anatomical localization. Leading anatomists contributed to this endeavor. Teaching in Bologna in 1540, Vesalius advised students on proper palpation technique for abdominal organs during his anatomical demonstrations.[81] At Padua, Falloppio performed post-mortem dissections to make the retrospective diagnoses more certain, through students' direct sensation of the internal appearances of patients' organs and humors.[82]

Medical instruction at northern Italian universities such as those in Padua, Ferrara, and Bologna already prized bedside teaching by the middle of the sixteenth century. From around 1540 up to his death in 1551, Da Monte practiced bedside teaching for students at Padua. His published *Consultationes*, many of them transcribed by students, pair well with student notes to reveal his Galenic practice, as Jerome Bylebyl and Michael Stolberg have demonstrated.[83]

---

79   Bylebyl, "Teaching *Methodus Medendi* in the Renaissance." Wear, "Explorations in Renaissance Writings."

80   Bylebyl, "Teaching *Methodus Medendi* in the Renaissance." As Wear, *Knowledge & Practice*, 119, notes, individualized treatment was "mainly rhetoric."

81   Heseler, *Andreas Vesalius' First Public Anatomy at Bologna*, 224–225. I thank R. Allen Shotwell for this reference.

82   Stolberg, "Post-mortems," 72–73.

83   Bylebyl, "The Manifest and the Hidden." Stolberg, "Bedside."

Teaching in the local hospital of San Francesco, as well as in patients' homes, Da Monte taught students to use their senses to note external appearances, and so construct a description of the phenomena, or a *historia*.[84] Beginning in 1542, students and professors returned repeatedly to the same patients in the hospital next door, up to sixteen or seventeen times for a single patient. Students trained their senses and skills of observation. They learned uroscopy, the primary method for knowing the effects of the hidden internal causes of healthy and diseased bodies.[85] Professors and students compared urine from patients over time, which allowed them to establish the phenomena or characteristics of healthy urine, and the range of its states in diseases.

As Bylebyl showed so well, Da Monte self-consciously followed Galen in attending to the visible and tactile external signs of patients, including attention to uroscopy, pulse analysis, and palpation of the abdomen.[86] Like other physicians, he taught students to use their senses to track all the available signs and symptoms in order to make inferences to the hidden "defect" (*vitium*), "affection" (*affectio*), or "wound" or "lesion" (*laesio*), in some hidden internal organ. He called such local impairment of an organ or organs the "very essence and nature" of the disease. Like Galen, Da Monte and other physicians sought to identify the wounded function (*functio laesa*), and so the disease. As he told his students, "Let this be your rule, that always on your first visit you should immediately see which functions are damaged. For they will indicate the disease and they are signs which will not fail."[87]

Developing a rational method (*methodus*), Da Monte divided his students' attention along the categories of the animal, vital, and natural functions. He further subdivided these by their principal parts. Careful attention to one young patient revealed healthy functions for all of his external senses of sight, hearing, etc., along with his internal senses such as imagination and memory. He could move about, too, indicating healthy animal functions, and hence a healthy brain, in which they were seated. Similarly, a good pulse indicated a healthy vital heat from the heart, showing good vital functions. But the boy's legs and feet clearly showed emaciation, caused by deprivation of nourishment, contrasting with his swollen belly. Such an unhealthy process of nourishment pointed straight to a defect in the natural faculty, and thus in the liver, the chief organ of this faculty.

---

84   Bylebyl, "The Manifest and the Hidden," 43.

85   Stolberg, *Uroscopy*. Stolberg, "Bedside Teaching," 646.

86   Bylebyl, "The Manifest and the Hidden," 42–5, 50, 53.

87   Da Monte, *Consultationes*, trans. Bylebyl, in "The Manifest and the Hidden," 53.

Now, Da Monte continued, the liver could suffer from morbid coldness, and so produce unconcocted nutriment for the whole body. But this would cause ascites or swelling throughout the body, yet some of the boy's body parts showed emaciation. Thus there must be a blockage preventing nutriment from the liver to some parts. Da Monte tried palpation of the liver to confirm his diagnosis, but could not feel the inferred hardness through the swelling.[88] Throughout student accounts, palpation of the liver and pancreas, especially, were tactile means for knowing hidden disease states.[89] One student, Georg Handsch, studied with Gabriele Falloppio from 1550 to 1553 in Padua and recorded visits to thirty different hospital patients.[90]

Unfortunate patients ended their course of treatment in death; sometimes dissection followed. By 1578, students recorded that Paduan professors taught in the nearby hospital of San Francesco after lectures, so that they could "see the patients afflicted by various kinds of diseases, and so that they might apply the things which they had proposed in the public lecture in practice." The professors "demonstrated carefully those things about the patients which ought to be observed and customarily done by the skillful physician, training the listeners in all the patients."[91] When some women patients died in October, they opened their cadavers to "demonstrate to the listeners the affected places and the *fomites* [kindling] of diseases."[92] Complaints from "little old women" brought the dissection of the cadavers' excised wombs to a halt, and hospital administrators blocked the dissection of patients in the near future.[93]

When they could witness post-mortems, though, students eagerly noted the morbid appearances of the patients' cadavers, as Stolberg details. In the 1550s, students recorded Falloppio performing post-mortem dissections in the hospital, with students noting healthy and diseased anatomical states, such as inflamed membranes in pleuritic patients, abscesses in cerebral membranes, an enlarged spleen, and large stones in the pancreas or kidneys or other morbid obstructions.[94] Unlike most "public" anatomies, the bodies dissected in the hospital or private rooms were not generally those of criminals.[95] Though hospital patients were of lower status than many private patients, the families of the

---

88   Bylebyl, "The Manifest and the Hidden," 46, 55.

89   Stolberg, "Bedside Teaching," 650.

90   Stolberg, "Bedside Teaching," 656.

91   *Atti della nazione germanica*, Vol. 1, 138.

92   *Atti della nazione germanica*, Vol. 1, 143–144.

93   Cf. Klestinec, *Theaters of Anatomy*, 67.

94   Stolberg, "Post-mortems," 72–73.

95   Stolberg, "Teaching Anatomy," 65.

local patients must have allowed the post-mortem dissections. In one case in which they objected, local citizens came with swords to rescue the corpse![96]

The professor of anatomy and medicine, Falloppio, in particular, taught students to connect experiences with patients and the appearances in healthy and diseased cadavers. He discussed disease states in his public anatomies and experimented with the actions and uses of parts in clinical anatomies. For instance, he showed students the one-way action of valves from the small intestine into the colon by filling a sample set with water. He also made important anatomical discoveries, which did not appear in print until much later, such as demonstrating the lacteal vessels in dogs in the 1550s.[97] In northern Italy, at least, leading physicians of the mid-1500s combined methodical bedside teaching in hospitals with anatomical localization of disease states, and even anatomical research in public and clinical anatomies.

By the end of the sixteenth century, academic physicians increasingly sought to provide solid foundations for medical students' education by bridging the head-to-toe *practica* tradition and the demands of a philosophically-rooted, rational method in the Galenic tradition.[98] As early as 1539, Leonhart Fuchs at Tübingen provided an early textbook model of a humanist return to the original, rational Galenic theory of practice, part-for-part, and arranged from head to heel.[99] Heurnius' *New Method* updated and expanded beyond Fuchs' textbook, describing methods for precisely compounding remedies to cure the disorders of very specific parts and locations. In this, he likely followed both the Paduan model of teaching and the work of Jean Fernel, whose well-known medical textbook, *The Whole of Medicine* (*Universa Medicina*, with editions 1554–1679), also used a head-to-toe format for organizing his teachings on diseases and therapies.[100] Rather than follow the approach of Rhazes and the *practica* tradition and work through every disease of bodily locations and their cures, though, Fernel produced a rational pathology of principles and illustrative cases.[101]

---

96   Stolberg, "Teaching Anatomy," 65.

97   Stolberg, "Teaching Anatomy," 69.

98   Bylebyl, "Teaching *Methodus Medendi* in the Renaissance."

99   Fuchs, *De Medendis Singularum Humani Corporis Partium A Summo Capite ad Imos Usque Pedes*. Bylebyl, "Teaching *Methodus Medendi* in the Renaissance." Andrew Wear, "Explorations in Renaissance Writings," 121–2.

100   Johannes and Otto Heurnius used and commented on Fernel's *Universa Medicina*: Jean Fernel, *Universa Medicina...Nunc autem notis, observationibus, & remediis secretis Ioann. & Othonis HeurnI* (1656).

101   Bylebyl, "Teaching *Methodus Medendi* in the Renaissance," 167, 172, 174. Siraisi, "Disease and Symptom," 230–234.

Fernel, like Heurnius a few decades later, emphasized the different anatomical "seats" (*sedes*) of diseases. He did this in his extensive treatment of pathology, a separate medical area of study he marked out as "pathology" (*pathologia*) in his huge and hugely popular summaries of medical learning. Fernel summarized this study of diseases as the discussion of "the affects, the causes, and of the unhealthy signs, and finally of all things beyond nature which happen in the human body."[102] A disease is "an affect contrary to nature seated in the body."[103] Just as with Galen, for Fernel parts of the body were the sites for functions, and so for diseases as impaired functions: "Since indeed the individual part of the body is primarily and per se the worker of the functions, insofar as its constitution is whole and strong it completes its functions, and there is health; but when the part is weak and faulty, primarily and per se it overturns its functions, and this alone is considered disease."[104]

Fernel often organized diseases by their organ sites or "seats" (*sedes*), whether in part of an organ, a whole organ, or relations of organs or, in our terms, organ systems. Even some diseases experienced in the whole body such as fevers had specific "seats." Intermittent fevers, in particular, differentiated according to the rhythm of their heightened heat and their anatomical seats. They each developed from different morbid matter. Tertian fevers, with their crises every third day, found their material cause in yellow bile, seated in the gallbladder. Quartan fevers, reaching a crisis every fourth day, had their seat in the black bile, which had turned back toward the spleen and built up. Quotidian or daily fevers were seated perhaps in excessive phlegmy mucus which collected especially in the stomach and intestines. The region around the heart marked the primary seat of all, as well as regions around the stomach, diaphragm, liver, spleen, pancreas, and omentum. These lower parts of the belly are like the "public bilgewater of the body," collecting excess and morbid matter.[105] Sometimes Fernel placed more emphasis on faulty humors as causes of fevers, urging physicians to attend to humors first before faulty parts, but most often he located the seats and causes of diseases in the alteration and obstructions of specific anatomical parts.[106] To diagnose patients correctly, he instructed his readers to begin with a "damaged function, or abnormal excrement, or pain" and search for "the affected part."[107] Thus difficulty breathing should direct the physicians'

---

102 Fernel, *Pathologiae Libri VII* in *Medicina* (1554), 238.
103 Fernel, *Pathologiae Libri VII*, 1.
104 Fernel, *Pathologiae Liber VII*, 3.
105 Fernel, *Pathologiae Libri VII*, 16.
106 Fernel, *Pathologiae Libri VII*, 33, 40.
107 Fernel, *Pathologia* 2.8, trans. Nancy Siraisi, "Disease and Symptom," 233.

attention to the parts serving respiration in turn: the throat, trachea, lungs, diaphragm, pleura, etc.

A few times, as Stolberg has pointed out, Fernel followed up diagnoses with post-mortem dissections. For instance, he noted that epilepsia came in three sorts, depending on the part from which it was stirred up: the brain, the stomach, or another part. Post-mortem dissections revealed that patients who had epilepsy while alive later showed post-mortem abscesses in the brain, or corrupt sections of the meninges, rather than just the ventricles blocked by a phlegmy humor, as predicted by theory.[108] As we will see in the chapter seven, Fernel also made novel observations of the evidence of disease in the lungs of consumptive or phthisical patients.

From Galen to Fernel, Galenic medicine prized finding the impaired actions and functions of parts. After all, these constituted diseases. The pedagogical revival of Galenic methods in the sixteenth century, notably at Padua under Da Monte, increasingly emphasized students' experience of patients' body parts, through direct palpation or inspection or indirect inference from excreta. By the time Heurnius came to write and teach his lectures on the theory and practice of medicine, he had ample materials from ancient, medieval, and early modern sources—and his own practice—to build a rational, comprehensive system for effective teaching and Leiden students' own future practice.

3   Knowing Material and Other Causes of Diseases

Diseases, the causes of diseases, and the remedies for these lay at the heart of Galenic medicine. At Leiden and other early modern universities, professors taught students methods for reasoning from the signs and symptoms of diseases to their causes, and for matching the faculties of medicines to the alteration or evacuation of these causes. But how did they think about these causes? Did they fit with the four causes of Aristotelian philosophy? Did they agree with Aristotelian philosophers that one could have real knowledge only of universals, not particulars? How could they claim causal knowledge of individual patients and their cures? This brief section sketches answers to these questions, with the goal of setting out how professors taught students to think about causes. When we turn to evidence of actual bedside and hospital practice in future chapters, we will compare these theories and vocabularies of causes to the discussions of causes of diseases in living patients and their dead

---

108   Fernel, *Pathologiae Libri VII*, Bk. V, Ch. III, 72. Stolberg, "Post-mortems."

bodies. As we will see here, Galenic medicine consistently pushed physicians to attend to material causes, notably the qualities and powers of materials, most of all. Often, they even associated causes Aristotelians might see as more formal, such as qualities of heat, with corporeal and material causation.

Galen's categories of the causes of diseases aimed to exhaust all the possibilities, and produced contradictions and ambiguities that exhausted his readers. In general, he divided the causes of diseases into three main categories: imbalances or bad qualitative mixtures (*dyskrasiai*) of the simple parts, unnatural structures or compositions of the organic or compound parts, and dissolution of continuities of both types of parts.[109] There were obvious tensions in this scheme, for instance in his placement of bone fractures under dissolution of continuity rather than unnatural structure. Those three categories represented the more immediate causes of diseases. Galen added further layers by attending to the internal antecedent causes, such as the constriction of blood vessels prior to a nosebleed; external antecedent causes such the coldness of the air causing the blood vessels to constrict; and containing causes, which were much debated, but generally referred to the internal state co-incident with disease states, and acting as the grounds for a disease state.[110] By the early modern period, physicians engaged in heated debates over the categories, terms, natures, and possibilities of knowing all sorts of causes.[111] Yet Galen's works informed the early modern discussions deeply, and Galen shaped his categories primarily for the service of medical practice, as Ian Johnston has pointed out.[112]

One practical treatise, his *On the Affected Places*, is rich with causal claims. In passing, Galen defined causes in a commonsense way, noting that all humans consider a "cause" of a bodily affect to be "that which when it is touching us, we are affected, and when it is separated from us, the affect ceases."[113] Thus, fire is the cause of burning and a sword the cause of cutting. We perceive a variety of bodily effects by local contact with different substances: violent heating or cooling, a disturbance created by a bad temperament of a place, parts irritated to excretion, the distention of a containing part by windy spirits, wounds from violent impact, or erosion and biting away from humors. Most often, Galen emphasized qualitative causes and their effects on the temperaments of the parts. For instance, powerful heat causes excessive wakefulness,

109   Johnston, *Galen: On Diseases and Symptoms*, 81–125.
110   Johnston, *Galen: On Diseases and Symptoms*, 33–35. Maclean, *Logic, Signs, and Nature*, 262–265.
111   Siraisi, "Disease and Symptom." Maclean, *Logic, Signs, and Nature*, 146–147, 262–265.
112   Johnston, *Galen: On Diseases and Symptoms*, 117.
113   Galen, *De Affectorum Locorum Notitia*, 6v.

and strong cold causes excessive sleepiness.[114] Qualitative excesses of the ambient air can cause changes in the brain that send convulsions through the nerves to the muscles.[115] Of course, qualitative changes to the temperaments of organs, especially the principal organs, produce dangerously damaged faculties. The excess heat of an intempered liver causes it to burn the humors in it, producing overcooked, burnt blood which can be dark in color and a poor source of nutrition for the whole body.[116] Excesses or deficiencies of humors cause structural and qualitative changes. Excess or excessively hot yellow bile, by nature already relatively hot and dry, could wash, abrade, and ulcerate the intestines when ejected from the gallbladder, causing dysentery.[117] Moving throughout the body's vessels, excess heat carried by yellow bile can also cause putrefaction, generating fevers.[118] Different sorts of humors flowing into the lungs in excesses of quantity or quality cause predictable diseases, from excess heat producing inflammation then pneumonia and perhaps pleurisy, to cold phlegm building up, causing congestion, coughing, and inflammation as well.[119] Cold air can generate more phlegm, and cause the blood vessels in the lungs to harden, making their rupture more likely.

But Galen also described precise structural, anatomical changes and traumas as causes of diseases. In one striking example, he explained how excessive dilation of the pores of the kidneys, pores that help to filter the urine, could cause a thin bloody serum to pass out with the urine, and great thirst in the patient.[120] Galen also gave four case histories of patients with trauma injuries to their nerves, which produced symptoms including difficulty in phonation, total voicelessness, leg paralysis, and loss of feeling in the fingers.[121] In each case, Galen showed how impairments of the intercostal or recurrent laryngeal nerves, whether from inflammation, or from scraping or blows, or excessive cooling, produced the specific symptoms of each patient.

In contrast, sometimes neither his basic qualitative powers nor his attention to anatomical changes and actions could explain the causes of diseases. Famously, some unknown power in a rabid dog's saliva, even a tiny amount of it, caused rabies in people bitten by the dog, usually around six months after

---

114   Galen, *De Affectorum Locorum Notitia*, 23v.
115   Galen, *De Affectorum Locorum Notitia*, 30r.
116   Galen, *De Affectorum Locorum Notitia*, 60v.
117   Galen, *De Affectorum Locorum Notitia*, 6v.
118   Galen, *De Affectorum Locorum Notitia*, 58v.
119   Galen, *De Affectorum Locorum Notitia*, 49r–49v, 52–52v.
120   Galen, *De Affectorum Locorum Notitia*, 66r.
121   Galen, *De Affectorum Locorum Notitia*, 45v–46r.

the contact.[122] These examples of hidden structural changes, and especially of causes from the "total substance" rather than manifest qualities or actions, fit more loosely in his categories of disease causes, but played important roles in his medicine in this work and other texts.

Galen also set out three modes of instruction or teaching at the beginning of his *The Art of Medicine*, modes which later commentators sometimes con-flated or elaborated into modes of discovery. "There are three types of teaching [*didaskaliai*] [*doctrinae*] in all, each with its place in the order. First is that which derives from the notion of an end [*telos*], by analysis [*analysis*] [*resolu-tio*]. Second is that from the synthesis [*synthesis*] [*compositio*] of the findings of an analysis. Third is that from the *dialysis* [*dissolutio*] of a definition: and it is this which we shall now embark on."[123] In other works, Galen identified the process of "analysis" with reducing a problem to its basic shapes and elements, and "synthesis" with constructing a device to test a claim or theory.[124]

By the late 1300s and early 1400s, professors of medicine such as Jacopo (or Giacomo) da Forlì (d. 1414) at Bologna discussed analysis or "resolution" in terms of reasoning from symptoms to causes. At first, the phenomenon is com-prehended only confusedly, and then more distinctly, as the parts related to its causes and essence are each comprehended distinctly. At first, the physician understands the concept of "fever" in a patient confusedly. "[R]esolve, then, the fever into its causes; since any one exists either from the heating of a humor or of the *spiritus* or of the parts; and again [if] it exists from the heating of a humor, either of the blood, or of phlegm, etc.; finally you will come through the specific and distinct cause and knowledge."[125]

In the early modern period, the ongoing debates over the causes of diseases often tried to put Galen's categories and terms in conversation with Aristo-telian philosophy.[126] Aristotle had argued influentially that one could have true knowledge or science (*episteme, scientia*) only of universals, which do not change, and not of particulars, which change, come to be, and pass away. In the beginning of his *Metaphysics*, for example, he argued that experience was a kind of knowledge (*gnosis*) of particulars, but art (*techne*) and science (*episteme*) were knowledge of universals. As he put it, "art is produced when

122   Galen, *De Affectorum Locorum Notitia*, 71r.

123   Galen, *The Art of Medicine* K I.305, trans. Singer, in *Galen: Selected Works*, 345. The Latin interpolations are from Galen, *Claudii Galeni Pergameni Ars Medica*, trans. Akakia (1544), 1.

124   Tieleman, "Galen on the Seat of the Intellect," 267–268.

125   Da Forlì, *Expositio super tres libros Tegni Galeni*, a2. Randall, *The School of Padua*, 35–36. Of course, we need not agree with Randall's broader thesis.

126   For a brief overview of some of the relations and tensions, see Schmitt, "Aristotle Among the Physicians."

from many notions of experience a single universal judgement is formed with regard to like objects."[127]

One of his most telling examples came from medicine. To say that this or that remedy benefited Callias, and similarly Socrates, and others as individuals is a matter of experience. But, "to judge that it benefits all persons of a certain type, considered as a class, who suffer from this or that disease (e.g., phlegmatic or bilious when suffering from burning fever) is a matter of art."[128] Physicians practiced the art of medicine and could teach it, so they necessarily worked with universals. This meant they had universal causal knowledge or science (*episteme* or *scientia*). But wisdom (*sophia*) held a higher place, as contemplative knowledge of first principles and primary causes. In his *Nicomachean Ethics*, Aristotle similarly defined medicine as the "science of what pertains to health," but distinguished it from the nobler form of scientific knowledge of things that do not change and exist eternally.[129] Ideally, one would acquire this knowledge through the construction of syllogisms, which would provide demonstrative and certain conclusions.

Although Aristotle did not provide such syllogisms, and his followers struggled to construct sound syllogisms using universal propositions generated from the senses and intellect, demonstrative reasoning remained the ideal. The philosopher Rudolph Goclenius' *Philosophical Dictionary* of 1613, for instance, defined *scientia* most properly as "knowledge acquired by demonstration."[130] Goclenius gave many further distinctions and meanings, of course, for instance distinguishing contemplative *scientia* into its three branches of first philosophy, mathematics, and physics, and contrasting it with the different sort of "science" of civil prudence and art. Then there was *scientia* of "the that" (*to hoti*), when just the thing itself is known, and completed by induction; and *scientia* of "the reason why" (*to dioti*), or knowledge of the thing as such, through knowing its cause.[131] Further, Aristotle's four causes, discussed influentially in his *Physics*, the material, efficient, formal, and final causes, deeply shaped discussions of causes into the early modern period. By the late sixteenth century, though, as Robert Pasnau has shown, even Aristotelian natural philosophers increasingly shifted formal explanation to appear more like a material mode of explanation.[132]

---

127   Bayer, "Getting to Know Principles in *Posterior Analytics* II.19." Aristotle, *Metaphysics* I.1, 980b1, trans. Hugh Tredennick, Loeb, 5.

128   Aristotle, *Metaphysics* I.1, 981b26–982a4. Loeb, 8–9.

129   Aristotle, *Nichomachean Ethics*, trans. H. Rackham, 357, K X.1.

130   Goclenius, *Lexicon Philosophicum*, 1012–1013.

131   For the category of *historia*, see especially Pomata, "*Praxis Historialis*."

132   Pasnau, "Form, Substance, and Mechanism."

Early modern physicians often echoed these Aristotelian maxims, though they could just ignore them, and some eminent professors wrestled to fit them with Galen's Aristotelian-inspired, but more practical and materialist approach. Since physicians defined diseases in terms of impairments of the natural uses or functions of bodies, diseases could not have final causes—they hindered the final causes of parts and bodies. But the other four causes, and especially the material cause, at times merited consideration. Leonhart Fuchs included discussions of causes in his textbook *Institutes* of 1555 and explicitly followed Galen's categories from his books on diseases and symptoms, and seems to have been mostly unconcerned about Aristotelian distinctions.[133] For instance, he took it as "demonstrated" by Galen that the form of the body is not the soul, but rather the mixture or temperament of the four qualities hot, cold, wet, and dry.[134] Around the same time, Jean Fernel agreed that there was no *scientia* of singulars or particulars, but then mostly attended to individual diseases in his work on pathology.[135] He argued that the notion of "affect" or condition (*diathesis*) was broader for Galen than for Aristotle, so a disease could inhere in parts of bodily substances. But the *contents* of the body could not be diseases. Thus, humors, stones, and spirits could not be diseases themselves, but only the causes of diseases.[136] As Ian Maclean has pointed out, physicians often loosened the causal schemes of Galen and Aristotle, tacking on such categories as the accidental cause, the conserving cause, the preserving cause, the instrumental cause, the internal cause, the external cause, the helping cause, the wounding cause, and more.[137]

Teaching at Padua in the mid-1500s, Da Monte lectured extensively on medical method, and many of his students later published their notes. Like his exemplar, Galen, Da Monte understood the physician's primary task to be understanding and curing diseases through causal knowledge.[138] In this pursuit, Da Monte tried to reconcile Galenic and Aristotelian thinking about causation. He followed Galen closely, especially on the general scheme of all sorts of causes producing diseases defined as unnatural actions or impaired functions, and which produce the symptoms.[139] He agreed with Aristotle's *Ethics* that medicine was a factive art and the physician needed to know the reasons, causes, and natures of things, since all curative actions arose from the

---

133   Fuchs, *Institutiones*, 356–366.
134   Fuchs, *Institutiones*, 382–383.
135   Siraisi, "Disease and Symptom," 231.
136   Siraisi, "Disease and Symptom," 238–239.
137   Maclean, *Logic, Signs, and Nature*, 264.
138   Bylebyl, "Teaching *Methodus Medendi* in the Renaissance," 187.
139   Da Monte, *Opuscula*, 93.

natures of the parts and medicines.[140] To do this, though, the physician had to know universals, since all knowledge of causes and natures was of universals. Otherwise, physicians would be mere Empirics, curing particular patients only by particular phenomena, and thus by chance.

Da Monte also used the Aristotelian scheme of causes. He pointed to the material causes of diseases, or the matter from which the disease came about, as either corporeal or incorporeal. In putrid fevers, corrupt or putrid matter developed and settled, causing unnatural heat and fever. Incorporeal material causes are qualities, such as the general or "unbound" grades of heat in fevers. Knowing the cause of the putrid fever in the corrupt matter, the physician then ought to evacuate the matter. Incorporeal material causes such as excessive grades of heat ought to be countered by qualitative alteration, namely cooling. Formal causes, too, could be incorporeal and corporeal (which strained the Aristotelian notion of immaterial but always enmattered form). The form most simply is the disposition or condition beyond nature, by which the impaired operations come about. Incorporeal formal causes seem to blend into the incorporeal material causes, namely the grades of heat of fevers, as grades. Thus ephemeral fevers are distinguished in general by two grades of hotness, hectic (or chronic) fevers by four.[141] Efficient causes bring about things or states by composing or making them, but are outside of what they make.[142] Efficient causes also come in two kinds, the nature of the matter and the instrumental cause. In bodies, there are different natures such as those of the simple parts blood, flesh, and bone. There are also the instrumental causes, namely innate heat and *spiritus*, which perform a variety of services. Physicians, of course, also make things happen, and they deal with efficient causes with natures, such as food and drink, and instrumental efficient causes such as incisions and bloodletting.[143]

Yet, for all their claims to universal causal knowledge, physicians always cured *particular* patients. Thus, the central problem for Da Monte and other physicians invoking universal causal knowledge was how to relate the universal and the particular.[144] As always, the physician or philosopher started from the senses. Yet, "particulars are made manifest by the senses, causes, however, are not known by the senses, since they are universals, but are perceived only by the intellect."[145] The way of analysis or resolution proceeded

---

140   Da Monte, *Opuscula*, 99.
141   Da Monte, *Opuscula*, 104.
142   Da Monte, *Opuscula*, 101.
143   Da Monte, *Opuscula*, 108.
144   Cf. Bylebyl, "Teaching *Methodus Medendi* in the Renaissance," 179.
145   Da Monte, *Opuscula*, 112.

from the signs evident to senses through the intellect to the universal. The intellect compares the sign "conceived in the intellect… to the hidden causes, and makes an *analogismus*, which is a certain relation of the particular to the universal, and concludes to the particular, and there is a demonstration from the sign. Therefore that which is represented to the intellect, when there is a particular appearing in the individual, and while the affect is apprehended by the intellect, it compares it to the cause recognized already by the intellect, under the mode of the universal."[146] For example, we know the nature of fire from many perceptions, memories, and experience of fire. We know fire's properties and why it emits smoke. So when we see or smell smoke, we recognize smoke as the sign of a hidden fire.

Galenic explanatory principles acted like our prior knowledge of the nature of fire. We know the causal principles of the hot, cold, wet, and dry, the nature of bodily organs and their functions, the properties of the six non-naturals, and the temperaments and faculties of medicines.[147] When we come to individuals, we learn their own idiosyncratic temperaments, and the temperaments of their principal organs, and all the other causes that might affect their bodily conditions, from the air to food to exercise, contagion, and the influence of the stars and planets. Thus, we come to know the particular nature of any given patient, the patient's disease, its causes, and the specific proper remedies "under a universal mode."[148]

At Leiden, Heurnius taught a similar Galenic rational method, and at times called it the method of "analysis," or reasoning from signs and symptoms back to hidden causes.[149] In investigating diseases, he taught, physicians should "illuminate the causes of diseases: which are internal or external; which indeed have proceeded from those things which are accustomed to call forth diseases, such as air, method of life, and we will note which causes are accustomed to excite which diseases; and whether this disease will respond to such a cause; we will pay attention to helps and harms; and which kinds of diseases commonly flowed about."[150] As noted in greater detail below, Heurnius' list of sixteen indications attempted to isolate possible causal relations one by one, beginning with the disease and the part occupied by the disease. The non-naturals (the air, sleep and waking, motion and rest, excretion and retention, food and drink, the passions of the soul) often acted as antecedent causes of the more proximate buildup or alteration of matter inside the body into morbid states.

---

146   Da Monte, *Opuscula*, 112. Cf. p. 44.
147   Cf. Bylebyl, "Teaching *Methodus Medendi* in the Renaissance," 180.
148   Da Monte, *Opuscula*, 100.
149   Johannes Heurnius, *Nova Ratio*, 478.
150   Johannes Heurnius, *Nova Ratio*, 478.

Galen's method of division, practiced elaborately by Da Monte, also characterized Heurnius' methodical search for causes. Following Galen, Heurnius divided the body into the containing parts, the contained, and those making it move.[151] For Heurnius, these are the organs and simple parts, the humors and fluids, and the *spiritus*, respectively. Humors often cause diseases by erring and changing parts qualitatively or structurally so they cannot perform their natural functions. Humors and other fluids are faulty in terms of their motions, qualities, and quantities.[152] Changes to humors often acted as the "proximate causes" of diseases.

When he taught students how to reason through their encounters with specific patients, he aimed especially to identify and treat proximate causes, since such causes mostly closely brought about the diseases. Like Galen and Da Monte, he emphasized material causes. Throughout his book, he stressed preternatural or contranatural qualitative alterations to patients' organ temperaments as the main causes of diseases. He also used a broader causal scheme of formal, efficient or instrumental, and material causes. As he put it in his *Institutes*, "With the diseased part recognized, we will investigate the formal, efficient, and instrumental cause of the disease, and especially the material cause, its hearth."[153] Formal causes were those that changed the size, shape, or innate quality of a part, such as swelling from inflammation due to extravasation of blood, or excessive drying or hardening of a part.[154] The efficient cause "births, increases, constitutes, fosters," or increases an effect.

But the material cause is usually the proximate cause when it settles in a body part, its "hearth," and produces disease there. Thus, Heurnius taught his students to start with the internal causes first, and especially the proximate cause, and then consider the external causes. For instance, a phlegmy matter builds up and drains from the head, causing catarrh; or settles in the joints and limbs, causing arthritis; or a similar matter collects in the lungs, causing inflammation and asthma.[155] Of course, there are usually other causes involved, beyond the proximate material or qualitative cause. For instance, the arthritis that follows from the buildup of matter in the joints could not occur unless the vessels and ducts bearing this matter were loose. In this case, the looseness

---

151   The original Hippocratic source is *Epidemics* 6.8, section 7, meaning more "bodies that restrain or stimulate, or are restrained." Hippocrates, *Epidemics 2, 4–7*, ed. and trans. Smith, 264–265. For Galen, see Petit, "Hippocrates in the Pseudo-Galenic *Introduction*, 350.

152   Johannes Heurnius, *Nova Ratio*, 523.

153   Johannes Heurnius, *Institutiones*, 542.

154   Johannes Heurnius, *Nova Ratio*, 709, 710.

155   Johannes Heurnius, *Nova Ratio*, 710.

itself is a "cause without which" the disease would not come about.[156] From the morbid matter as the proximate cause we can then run long chains through intermediate to the most remote causes. Thus the proximate cause of inflammation of the membranes of the ribs is a humor causing a swelling there. Congestion collected that humor there, or otherwise caused it to flow to the part, which in turn came about due to weakness of the side, due to faulty nutrition or an injury, another disease state, pain in the part (pain often attracts fluid), or external cold.

Heurnius admitted that there might also be occult or hidden causes, such as poisons, pestilence, and contagion.[157] But he strongly objected to thinking these causes were more divine, or that Hippocrates and Galen did not know about them. After all, he pointed out, the work *On the Sacred Disease* by "Hippocrates" denied that there was anything more divine in epilepsy than in any other disease. But Hippocrates, and by proxy Heurnius, argued that all things were divine since nothing happened without "divine nature," and it was certainly licit to refer every disease to the wrath of God, especially unusual malignant qualities of the air.[158] After all, these changes to the air caused most epidemic diseases. Yet physicians, ancient and early modern, "prudently" confined themselves to natural causes. From all the many causes together, especially the material, proximate cause and the part occupied by the disease, the true Galenic-Hippocratic physician derived the curative indications.

4   Teaching Students to Treat the Faulty Part

Carrying on the methods of his *alma mater* Padua, Johannes Heurnius took the localization of diseases further. Drawing extensively from ancient sources, especially Galen's works, he constructed a comprehensive rational method for curing each sort of qualitative or structural variation in each part, and almost always passed over notions of the general mixture of the humors. Theories of qualities and quantities informed the practical instructions for making medicines in the *New Method*. This massive work ran to over five hundred double-columned pages in the 1590 quarto edition.[159] Heurnius treated in exhaustive detail everything from medicinal weights and measures to ingredients and operations for making medicines, medicinal recipes "proven by

---

156   Johannes Heurnius, *Nova Ratio*, 711–712.
157   Johannes Heurnius, *Nova Ratio*, 713.
158   Johannes Heurnius, *Nova Ratio*, 713.
159   Johannes Heurnius, *Nova Ratio* (1590).

use" for different qualitative diseases of the different parts of the body, the true method of healing from signs and indications, and tips for questioning and examining patients. Medicines and sick body parts combined naturally. For Galen and his Renaissance physicians, the proper, rational way of curing (*methodus medendi*) and the philosophical schemes of the qualities and faculties of drugs joined and reinforced one another.

Physicians had to know first the capacities for causing bodily effects—the faculties—of the simple medicines or medicinal simples, as we saw in chapter four. Chicory, for example, cooled without harming the stomach. It also showed mild astringent effects and helped obstructions in the eyes.[160] Since chicory did this on its own, it was a common medical "simple." Combining simples allowed the learned, precise physician to fine-tune the elemental qualities and powers of a drug mixture, for instance blunting the violent purgative power of scammony or hellebore with roses or anise, or tempering opium with crocus.

Heurnius structured his book as a systematic overview of practical medicine, united by his new method. In the front matter, he cut a small harvest from recent humanist scholarship to provide precise weights and measures for ancient through early modern standards. Extensive conversion tables allowed for easier translation of recipes into common measures and so into everyday practice. In the first major section, he described the methods, operations, apparatus, and examples of making medicines, including chymical apparatus and techniques, as we saw in the previous chapter. The second section laid out accepted medicines proven by use, drawn mostly from ancient, medieval, and early modern sources. Scholarly skills and his reverence for ancient "Asclepian" medicine drew him especially to medicines approved by Hippocrates, Dioscorides, and Galen, as well as later writers such as Oribasius and Avicenna. These appear arranged systematically from head to toe by major body parts, with a short aside on the four major humors, and then by their actions (e.g., purgatives). The third, final section described Heurnius' rational method for practice by a set of "indications" or determinative signs, which ought to pinpoint the disease and its properties by careful consideration of all possible causes from the perceived effects (the impairment in a specific function or action, perceptible qualitative changes, the pain of the patient, etc.). This section also included short practical guides for treating two or more diseases at once, and tips for questioning patients and conducting consultations.

Heurnius even brought the method in the *New Method* (with five editions from 1587 to 1650) into his influential textbook of medical theory, the *Institutes*

---

160   Johannes Heurnius, *Institutiones*, 464. Johannes Heurnius, *Nova Ratio*, 339.

of Medicine (Institutiones Medicinae), which appeared in at least seven editions from 1592 through 1666 and formed the core of Leiden theoretical medicine pedagogy through the 1640s.[161] Heurnius concentrated on the "seats" of diseases, and spent little time considering the body's general temperament. In fact, Heurnius rarely referred to the whole sick patient, thinking instead of each "sick part" (*pars aegra*). Again and again, he taught that the physician ought to direct his mind to "the part occupied by the disease, the disease, and its cause."[162]

As he summarized his method in his textbook *Institutes*, students in their consultations with patients should always locate the *seat* of the disease: "Indeed sometimes the seat of the disease [*sedes morbi*] is known from one symptom, and disease and its cause are recognized...and again we move from the symptoms to the disease and its cause, and then it should come about in discussion, that we run back from cause and disease to the symptoms."[163] Heurnius stressed localization by parts: "See whether there is a fault in many parts or in one. Note its position, order, figure, process, recess, and temperament, and the part greatly exposed to the cause and disease."[164]

Faulty parts took the primary place, with whole-body temperaments considered later and of much lesser importance, if at all. In fact, the number of diseases matched the number of ways organs or parts could go wrong. After all, diseases just were changes in the parts which injured their proper actions. "Diseases, as we said, dwell in the parts. However many ways therefore those become faulty, there are just so many diseases."[165] If the part alone is troubled, Heurnius asserted, "the total temperament can be passed over: for it will be enough to reveal the nature of the part."[166] In his lengthy articulation of the proper method of healing (*methodus medendi*), Heurnius barely mentioned diagnosing and treating according to the temperament of the whole body.[167] Moreover, the temperament of the body properly refers to the tempering action of the elements in the process of generation, and follows most of all from the qualitative mixtures of the heart and the liver.[168] In other works, he continued this line of localization, arguing in his work on the diseases of the

---

161   Johannes Heurnius, *Institutiones Medicinae* (1592). Lindeboom, *Dutch Medical Biography*, col. 858.

162   Johannes Heurnius, *Institutiones*, 534.

163   Johannes Heurnius, *Institutiones*, 538.

164   Johannes Heurnius, *Institutiones*, 540.

165   Johannes Heurnius, *Institutiones*, 516.

166   Johannes Heurnius, *Institutiones*, 537.

167   Johannes Heurnius, *Nova Ratio*, 620–622.

168   Johannes Heurnius, *Institutiones* (1638), 47, 542.

head that the part also determined the type of remedy to be used, and "sets the bounds of its efficacy."[169]

How did students learn to recognize a disease? The senses of the patient and physician perceived the bodily changes of diseases. They attended to the symptoms, sometimes singly, usually many taken together. Symptoms were any change or "affect beyond nature, near the disease and near the cause of the disease."[170] Here, likely for the benefit of beginning students, he passed over the Renaissance confusion over the distinctions between the causes, symptoms, and signs of diseases.[171] Like Galen and the Paduan Galenist Da Monte, Heurnius envisioned a causal line from the cause to the disease, and from the disease to the signs. Thus, as Galen put it, a sign or symptom is an "affect of the body, beyond nature, which follows the disease as a shadow follows the body."[172]

These morbific causes, especially excesses of hot, cold, dry, and wet qualities, often traveled to organs and impaired their temperaments due to the humors. The humors, then, often contained the causes of diseases (and were called the "containing causes"): "The morbific causes, as I said, dwell in the humors."[173] When a humor putrefied and generated heat, causing a type of "putrid fever" (categorized by the fever and discharge of some stinking, apparently rotten substance), then the putrefied humor is the containing cause. Remove the cause, and the disease ceases.

External and antecedent causes of diseases frequently assaulted healthy bodies. Changes in humors, which changed organs to cause diseases, often resulted from external causes. The air, food, drink, motion, rest, sleep, waking, excretion, retention, and the passions of the soul (*animus*), often called the "non-naturals," could also be *antecedent* causes of disease. For example, the excessive summer heat caused fevers, and winter's cold caused the congelation of phlegm and blockages of vessels.

Heurnius recommended making inquiries about patients' non-naturals in his instructions for bedside practice. First, of course, the physician should carefully examine the nature of the disease and of the sick patient, and the strength of the rest of the indications himself, before taking the patient's own narrative or history.[174] After assessing and asking about the function of the

---

169   Johannes Heurnius, *De morbis*, Preface.

170   Johannes Heurnius, *Institutiones*, 244.

171   Maclean, *Logic, Signs, and Nature*, 282. Siraisi, "Disease and Symptom."

172   Galen, *De Symptomatum Differentiis*, 39. Da Monte, *In Nonum Librum Rhasis ... Expositio*, 67v. Heurnius, *Nova Ratio*, 599.

173   Johannes Heurnius, *Institutiones*, 492, 237–238.

174   Johannes Heurnius, *Nova Ratio*, 685.

patient's powers, from the temperaments and faculties of the brain, stomach, and liver, inspecting the face and excrements, and the pulse, the physician should turn to the non-naturals.[175] A similar approach structured Heurnius' guide for conducting consultations with other physicians, beginning with the disease, then the patient, then the non-naturals.[176] After this, the physician ought to concentrate on the natural powers of the patient, and most of all on the preternaturals, the disease, the symptoms, and the morbific cause. All of this aimed at knowing and treating the cause of the disease, with the faculties, temperament, and structure of the sick part or parts foremost.

Food and drink, vital for life and health, presented constant dangers of excess qualitative and quantitative changes in bodies. Too much or too little food, or a meal at the wrong time, and especially foods too hot and too cold, caused diseases. Daily experience from Hippocrates on showed that roasting and boiling produced the most salubrious foods. Similarly, pure fountainwater was best, then rainwater, especially when filtered and cooked first. As Heurnius and other humanists knew, the Roman architect Vitruvius had already shown that water from lead pipes carried the "pernicious power" of lead, causing diseases such as dysentery. Swamp water often created pestilent environs, where people suffered from epidemic fevers. Wine often produced diseases, since people over-indulged, from Alexander the Great (as Heurnius noted) to Leiden students in the early 1600s. Heurnius followed local custom in generously doubling the amounts which generated different states. Galen's opponent Asclepiades had often recommended wine (Roman elites welcomed his ministrations), and taught a handy aphorism: the first glass reaches thirst, the second to desire and love, the third to drunkenness, and the fourth to madness. Heurnius revised this maxim for Leiden: "We have it a little looser: the first drink to thirst, the second to happiness, the third to desire, the fourth to sleep, the fifth to drunkenness, the sixth to wrath, the seventh to quarrels, and the eighth to madness."[177]

Exercise, the "violent motion of the body," helped to excrete what ought to be excreted. Hippocrates, after all, had argued that retaining things that ought to be excreted—mucus, bile, urine, etc.—was the most efficacious cause of diseases. Playing ball games and speedy walking were the best, Heurnius recommended. In contrast, the exertions of sexual activity had no good effects, especially for youth such as Leiden students.[178]

---

175   Johannes Heurnius, *Nova Ratio*, 685–687.
176   Johannes Heurnius, *Nova Ratio*, 688–691.
177   Johannes Heurnius, *Institutiones*, 221.
178   Johannes Heurnius, *Institutiones*, 228.

How did students and professors know which parts were faulty, and what their faults were? At times, Heurnius wrote, one can recognize a disease from a single symptom, but usually clusters of symptoms following from the injured function or action and part were more reliable. Heurnius listed each step in the rational method. Curing could come about "aptly and from the law of method" if one followed a series: identify the affect against nature (that is, the disease, the cause of the disease, and the symptoms); the "part occupied by the disease"; the temperament of the sick patient; the powers (air, age, custom, nature, and sex); and the art (brevity or length, arrival, order, remedies, the heavens).[179] The disease occupying the part remained foremost.

Renaissance physicians spun increasingly elaborate webs of disease signs and their contested significations.[180] Here, we will concentrate on the most important signs for practice, or "indications." These are signs that point out what is to be done, or more sure guides to treatment. Physicians from at least the late 1400s on had emphasized the "curative indications" as essential for rational, methodical practice, and hailed Galen's *Method of Medicine* (*Methodus Medendi*) as the exemplar. As Bylebyl has shown, influential teachers such as Giovanni Michele Savonarola, Leonhart Fuchs, Jean Fernel, and Da Monte all emphasized the Galenic method of curative indications.[181] Teaching at Padua in the 1400s, Savonarola included "the disease, its quality, quantity, location, periodicity, and symptoms," as well as the "temperament, age, occupation, sex, region, habitude, customs, and repletion" of the patient, and the state of the air and season.[182] Da Monte, also teaching at Padua, but a century later, incorporated the curative indications into his threefold method. First, the physician followed Galen's recommended method of division, which related each individual disease to its broader class, and distinguished diseases by their anatomical seats and pathways. Next, the physicians followed the relevant signs indicating all aspects of the disease, such as its location, matter, humor, quality, pathways, and source, in order to determine the lowest, most particular species of the disease. Finally, the physician gathered all of this detailed causal analysis together to consider the cure that properly took into account all of the causes and conditions of the disease, patient, and environment. The disease and its cause(s) were foremost, but the physician also had to consider all the other causal relations, such as the temperament of the patient, the

---

179   Johannes Heurnius, *Nova Ratio*, 466.
180   Maclean, *Logic, Signs, and Nature*, ch. 8.
181   Bylebyl, "Teaching *Methodus Medendi* in the Renaissance," 161–168, 171, 176.
182   Bylebyl, "Teaching *Methodus Medendi* in the Renaissance," 161.

KNOWING AND TREATING THE DISEASED BODY

temperaments of the patient's organs, the air, and the other six non-naturals.[183] Without this approach, the physician would be a mere Empiric, correlating diseases and remedies.

For Heurnius, reasoning with indications also meant that the physician followed a rational method of perceiving signs and reasoning to root causes. By identifying all the specific qualitative intemperances of the affected parts, the physician could compound a drug that would target and alter the parts as needed. The affect or change beyond nature is knowable from the altered perceptible accidents of the part, the excrements, or the wounded action of the part. Further combining diagnosis and therapy into his method, Heurnius provided an ordered method of *sixteen* indications which expanded on the brief method summarized above.[184] For each indication, he walked students through the proper principles or methods for identifying these crucial signs for diagnosis and therapy, and described concrete examples.

But Heurnius, ever the pedagogue, distilled down the most important "founders and leaders" from among the list of sixteen, to four that should be used "in every curing, and in all diseases." In easy-to-read small caps, he picked out "THE AFFECT CONTRARY TO NATURE, that is, the disease, the cause of the disease, and the symptoms...THE PART OCCUPIED BY THE DISEASE... THE TEMPERAMENT of the sick patient...THE POWERS: air, age, custom, nature, and sex... THE ART: brevity, as of time, when it comes, order, remedies, the heavens."[185]

---

183   Bylebyl, "Teaching *Methodus Medendi* in the Renaissance," 187–188.

184   Johannes Heurnius, *Nova Ratio*, 465–466, lists: 1. From the affect itself, that is, from the disease, the cause of the disease, or the pressing symptom. 2. From the temperament of the whole body of the sick patient. 3. From the part occupied by the disease. 4. From the powers of the sick patient. 5. From the ambient air. 6. From age. 7. From daily custom. 8. From the particular nature of the one who is occupied. 9. From exercise. 10. From the length or brevity of the disease. 12. From the four times of the disease, namely, beginning, increase, height, and decline. 13. From the particular paroxysms of the diseases. 14. From the ordained functions of nature. 15. From the powers of medicines. 16. From the influx of the stars. Cf. Johannes Heurnius, *Institutiones*, 485. Compare the earlier list from Ferrier, *Vera medendi methodus*, 20–21: From the nature of the disease, and its magnitude, together with its causes, and consideration of the pressing symptoms. From the temperament of the whole body. From the temperament, formation, position, faculty, dignity and necessity, and acuity or feebleness of the sense of the affected part. From the powers of the sick. From the ambient air considered in the state of the heavens, in its region, in the place of habitation, and time of year. Those which have insufficient principals, from age. From the property of nature. From sex. From the custom and art of life. From the length or brevity of the disease. From the times of the disease. From particular onsets. From the manifest functions of nature. After these, from the faculties of the medicines. Maclean, *Logic, Signs, and Nature*, 310, gives a different list from a later edition.

185   Johannes Heurnius, *Nova Ratio*, 466.

Across his text and teaching, Heurnius practiced what he preached and concentrated on these, especially the first three.

Like Galen, Heurnius encouraged his students to begin with the primary
qualities first: "those accidents perceived by touch (hot, cold, moist, etc.)."[186]
Firstly, these changes are perceived by touch, especially excess heat or cold.
If a patient feels a flaming heat around the mouth of the stomach, one should
suspect a hot affect there. This is further confirmed by signs such as burnt
excrements, foul belching, or a breath smelling of fried eggs.[187] But the real
change could be in the neighboring parts, so we should check the excrements
and wounded actions. If the patient's appetite languishes, and he feels hurt by
taking hot things, the affect should be lessened by cold remedies. If there is a
bitter taste in the patient's mouth, nausea, or vomiting, there is likely too much
bile somewhere, and the hot matter should be expelled.

Of course, in this practical medicine course and his theory course, the
Institutes, Heurnius presented a rationalized method which did not dwell on
the ambiguities and uncertainty of actual medical practice with ever-varied
patients. Although Heurnius emphasized the greater certainty that came with
his carefully-localized method of tracking qualitative and structural impairments, physicians and critics of Renaissance medicine often emphasized its
uncertainty. Medicine, though an art and, in part, a science, rarely rose to
universal truths in practice. A common saying shared among physicians and
their critics alike was the assertion that the conjectural nature of medicine
arose from the uncertainty of the signs.[188] Even indications, supposedly more
certain than other signs, came in for criticism.[189]

Heurnius acknowledged the complexity of diagnosis, and the frequent necessity of making inferences from many signs taken together. Differential diagnosis
also depended on ruling out possible competing diseases and causes of symptoms and signs. Symptoms unique to a part "very manifestly reveal the sick
part," as when disgust toward food speaks of weakness of the stomach. Similarly,
a watery, bloody discharge from the "bottom," resembling water used to wash
recently butchered meat, indicates an impaired liver (though one should also
rule out hemorrhoids and check for swelling of the liver to confirm).[190] A ruddy
jaw, combined with the patient coughing up foam, indicates inflammation of
the lung. Yet a ruddy jaw alone could also follow merely from the patient's florid
nature or be sign of an oncoming crisis or turning point of a disease.

---

186   Johannes Heurnius, *Nova Ratio*, 467.
187   Johannes Heurnius, *Nova Ratio*, 467.
188   Maclean, *Logic, Signs, and Nature*, 291. Siraisi, "Disease and Symptom."
189   Maclean, *Logic, Signs, and Nature*, 306–310.
190   Johannes Heurnius, *Nova Ratio*, 477.

Different parts correlated with distinct diseases. Many parts "oppressed by a disease" generated characteristic fluid excrements, which often flowed to specific other parts. These fluxes could pinpoint the sick part, too. There are also diseases "specific to each part," given the different properties and faculties of the parts. Ligaments and lungs do not feel pain like other parts, worms are frequent causes of worn-out intestines, and kidneys and bladders are often injured by stones.[191]

Here, as elsewhere, Heurnius glossed Galen's *On the Affected Places*, often without attribution. Heurnius took the vivid example of bloody excreta caused by a liver intemperance directly from Galen's text, though he combined elements from across the work for the differential diagnosis of inflammation of the lung.[192] Galen had supplied similar, but more detailed, diagnostic lists for specific signs for different parts. For example, he also mentioned that the lungs and ligaments do not feel pain, and that kidneys and bladders suffer injuries from stones, but so does the large bowel.[193] Galen also re-emphasized the fundamental place of temperament: "the essence of each of the primary organs consists in the temperament of the four qualities," and this temperament produces their faculties.[194] Throughout his text, Heurnius also followed Galen's general summary, that the physician knows the injured part primarily from a few types of causes: the violent cooling and heating of the part, an intemperance in the whole body or in one place, the passage of something through continuous parts, forceful excretion, from a vaporous flatus arising and distending the part, from a violent impact, and from erosion or biting away of a part.[195] Heurnius even paraphrased directly from Galen's text. For instance Heurnius noted that the "afflicted part" is known from many signs, but most powerfully from the excrements, and even more from pains.[196] Galen concluded that the beginning of the method for finding the affected "seat" came from the impaired action, since no part is affected without such impairment.[197] He pointed especially to pain, swelling, and most of all to the injured action as indicating the affected part, the "seat" of the disease, and, like Heurnius later, added the excrements as a lesser but noteworthy source of signs for localization.

Throughout his teaching on signs, as across his remarks on temperaments or mixtures, Heurnius also relied on Galen's method from *The Art of Medicine*, especially the scheme of tracking the signs of localized qualitative affects. Even

---

191   Johannes Heurnius, *Nova Ratio*, 478.
192   Galen, *De Affectorum Locorum Notitia*, 60v, 49r–49v.
193   Galen, *De Affectorum Locorum Notitia*, 10r.
194   Galen, *De Affectorum Locorum Notitia*, 60v.
195   Galen, *De Affectorum Locorum Notitia*, 6v.
196   Johannes Heurnius, *Nova Ratio*, 478.
197   Galen, *De Affectorum Locorum Notitia*, 7r–7v.

in that short summary, Galen's attempt to draw signs "from the excellence or otherwise of the bodily functions, and individually from the individual functions" fell into thickets of complexity.[198] There were signs of incipient disease, which might still belong to the category of "normal," signs of the neutral state in which bodies are neither diseased nor fully healthy, signs which are both "neither" and morbid, signs which indicate future health and present disease, and many more. The varied individual mixtures of the principal parts, the simple parts, the organic parts, and the humors changed, with corresponding changes of health, disease, and the wide latitude of the "neither" state.[199]

But Heurnius tried to capture the complexity of localized qualitative and structural affects with a straightforward scheme. He moved quickly from attention to the sixteen indications and simple affects to higher-order qualitative changes. If the patient shows no signs in the primary qualities of hot, dry, cold, and wet, the physician should proceed to the secondary qualities such as softness, hardness, swelling, roughness, and lightness in the various places, as perceived by touch. The signs of each swelling should be noted: its size and number, as well as if it is accompanied by pain, inflammation, or pulsation. The excrements, again, can tell of wounded actions among the internal organs of the body.[200]

Pain often indicated the location and type of the disease. *Pace* Foucault, Heurnius never urged students to inquire of patients, "What is wrong with you?" but instead taught his students to ask, "Where does it hurt?"[201] Pain, included under the sense of touch, appears as an especially reliable index: "thirdly we will ask whether he is disturbed by *some pain* in *some part*, or whether it is poured into the *whole body*: for where there is *pain*, there most often *the disease* resides."[202] Varied pain is due to the different parts and the different morbid matter involved. Diseased membranes produce pointlike pain; nerves a pain more like lacerations. Important organs such as the liver, lungs, and spleen give a weighty pain, and flesh a looser spread of pain. The different types of morbid matter also produce different sorts of pain. Hot and cold matter localized in a part of the opposite temperament produces a biting pain. Cold matter applied to a cold part causes a stupefying pain like a toothache. Too much matter in a place causes a painful compression. Acrid matter, eating away at a part, makes

---

198   Galen, *Art of Medicine*, 372.
199   Galen, *Art of Medicine*, 370, 346–351.
200   Johannes Heurnius, *Nova Ratio*, 468.
201   Foucault, *Birth of the Clinic*, xviii.
202   Johannes Heurnius, *Nova Ratio*, 468: "nam ubi *dolor*, ibi plerumque habitat *morbus*." Heurnius, *Institutiones*, 486–7. Italics in original.

an ulcerous pain. Pain suggests its origin in a diseased organ, at least as an index. For instance, if there is pain deep in the region below the heart and to the patient's right, the liver is injured, not the spleen.[203]

Sight notes changes of color, especially of expelled humors in and around a part. Morbid changes in the venous blood, black bile, yellow bile, or phlegm indicate diseases affecting the organs that produce them. If a part is too ruddy, that indicates excess blood; too white, phlegm; too befouled, black bile; too yellow, yellow bile. Following good Hippocratic tradition, the student should observe carefully the changes in the face, especially around the eyes, tongue, and nose.[204]

Taste and smell played lesser roles, and hearing almost none, as in earlier Galenic medicine.[205] A bitter flavor the patient tastes from bile poured into the stomach requires purgation. A salty flavor indicates a salty phlegm. Smells either came from the whole body, as a stinking sweat does, or from a part, as sour fumes from the stomach indicate either uncooked matter or an affect or disease of the spleen.

Inevitably, early modern physicians came to the excrements, especially urine. Discharges from the body revealed signs of the processes of coction hidden inside (the cooking of food into nutriment by the stomach, liver, and other parts), or the excess and deficiency of humors and matter from other causes. As Heurnius instructed his students, physicians asked about and examined urine, feces, menstrual flow, blood from hemorrhoids, mucus from the nose, and sweat.[206] Students should look for spots of blood where they should not appear, changes in the apparent humoral amounts, and even the appearance of bits of cartilage or flesh. Then they should consider the qualities of the excrements, their amounts, timing, and mode of excretion. For example, Heurnius taught, if feces mixed thoroughly with blood appeared, with pain around the belly button, and ongoing pain, then that will indicate an ulcer, likely in the upper intestine.[207]

Across this period, examination of the urine, especially by visual uroscopy, was often the primary form of diagnosis. Students learned the smells, color changes, inclusions, precipitates, and other characteristics of morbid urine. A whole industry flourished, with jobs for the carriers of urine from patients

203   Johannes Heurnius, *Nova Ratio*, 470.
204   Johannes Heurnius, *Institutiones*, 470.
205   Bylebyl, "The Manifest and the Hidden," 47.
206   Johannes Heurnius, *Institutiones*, 406, 227. Bylebyl, "The Manifest and the Hidden." Stolberg, "Bedside Teaching."
207   Johannes Heurnius, *Nova Ratio*, 471.

to physicians, who shuttled flasks to and fro in wicker coverings. As Michael
Stolberg argues, the rise of anatomy as the marker of academic physicians'
expertise gradually displaced uroscopy as the central social signifier, but uroscopy persisted well into the nineteenth century in some regions, such as southern Germany.[208] Physicians increasingly displayed skeletons and anatomical
parts as tokens of their knowledge, and sought anatomical training, but patients
demanded uroscopy and long learned tradition provided rich resources for its
practice.[209]

With the seat of the disease, the "sick part," identified, students could then
consider whether it communicated any morbid matter or quality to neighboring parts. Disease could thus be communicated by "sympathy" or "contagion" in
very material terms, as a humor or vapor moving within the body. By sympathy
a disease could affect parts similar in temperament and structure, participating in a similar work or action, or parts connected by vessels.[210] For instance, a
blow to the head that uncovers the meninges and exposes that membrane to
the air changes it, and also affects the other membranes in the body, causing
the stomach to vomit bile. A broken humerus injures the action of the muscles
there. Local trauma wounds could spread morbid matter to different organs,
affecting their proper actions and functions. As Hippocrates taught, fracturing
a heel bone requires great force, which injures the attached parts such as the
tendons and nerves, and morbid matter travels through veins and arteries to
the heart, causing fever, or through the nerves to the brain, causing delirium.[211]

Fluxes, or the movement of morbid matter from one part of the body to
another, played important roles in Heurnius' pathology. Here he explicitly followed Galen and Fernel, arguing that disorders of a single quality or humor, or
"simple intemperances" are rare.[212] Instead, students should pay most attention
to why morbid matter flows, and why into one part rather than another, "for on
this many causes of diseases depend." Here he also joined the widespread discourse of illness shared by patients and physicians which Michael Stolberg has
studied, especially patients' records throughout the sixteenth through eighteenth centuries. As Stolberg puts it, "In the overwhelming majority of cases,
disease was not explained by an excess of one of the four natural humors but
by more or less specific, harmful, or corrupt morbid matter."[213] Heurnius' text-

---

208   Stolberg, *Uroscopy*, 24–28.
209   Stolberg, *Uroscopy*, 151. Klestinec, *Theaters of Anatomy*. Guerrini, *Courtiers' Anatomists*,
       ch. 1.
210   Johannes Heurnius, *Nova Ratio*, 473.
211   Johannes Heurnius, *Institutiones*, 195.
212   Johannes Heurnius, *Institutiones*, 234.
213   Stolberg, *Experiencing Illness*, 95.

book and core courses at Leiden surely strengthened this emphasis on local movements of morbid matter, reaching thousands of students and readers.

When morbid matter moved to a different part with a different function, an "epigenesis" occurred. "Epigenesis" for Heurnius was not the gradual development of the parts of the body in generation, as William Harvey would coin the definition in 1651.[214] Instead, he used it as a general Greek term for the development of a disease from another disease. Movement of the morbid matter from one part to another causes epigenesis. This is worse when the "more noble" parts, the ruling parts of the brain, heart, and liver become diseased. If the morbid matter moves from a "more noble" part to a less-noble one, such as from the brain to the lung, this is diadosis. If from a less noble to a more noble part, as Hippocrates teaches in the *Aphorisms*, then that is the more dangerous "metastasis."[215] In either sort of movement of morbid matter, a different disease appears when the morbid matter impairs a different part with its own vital actions and functions.

Contagious diseases, too, worked by transferring little material bits from body to body. Here, Heurnius and his colleagues followed Fracastoro's terminology of contagion and seeds of disease without adopting his atomism.[216] Other physicians in the sixteenth century also adopted theories of material contagion, especially for the venereal French Disease. Lecturing at Padua in the 1550s, Gabriele Falloppio encouraged his students to use a moistened strip of linen to prevent "pustulent corpuscles" from reaching and lodging in their genitals.[217] For contagious transmission, incorporeal qualities could do the job, but more often physicians invoked corporeal, material things such as humors, spirits, or vapors. Plague killed by a poisonous vapor, which caused death without obvious signs of putrefaction. Like many other diseases, plague could develop from unusual changes of the surrounding air, which affect the air and spirits of our bodies. Thus different diseases and cures acted more strongly at different times of the year. Or so Hippocrates, Galen, and Avicenna taught.[218]

Students touched the patients to take the pulse and feel swellings. Learning to take the pulse, as Galen taught at great length in multiple treatises, took long experience and practice. Each patient had her or his own healthy pulse rhythm, strength, frequency, and other variations in the three dimensions of the arterial coats over time.[219] Uroscopy and feeling the pulse appear as the

---

214 Harvey, *Exercitationes de Generatione Animalium*, 251–252.
215 Johannes Heurnius, *Nova Ratio*, 474. He cites *Aphorisms*, 5.7.
216 Nutton, "Reception of Fracastoro's Theory," 203, 213.
217 Ragland, "'Making Trials,'" 515.
218 Johannes Heurnius, *Institutiones*, 200–213.
219 Bylebyl, "Disputation and Description."

most-discussed methods of diagnosis in Heurnius' *Institutes* course on the theory of medicine.

For students who may have nodded off during lecture, Heurnius summarized his method of therapy toward the end. The emphasis on purgation comes through clearly:

> First, they set up a diet serving nature and fighting the disease. Second, they wash out the gut with a gentle remedy, or suppository, rarely a clyster. Third, if blood is to be emitted, they open a vein, and they draw it out. Fourth, with a mild decoction they cut the supply of the morbific matter. Fifth, they prepare obstinate matter for expulsion. Sixth, they purge strongly. Seventh, they apply these things for revulsion so far: they bring into use urine-producing drugs, sweat-producing drugs, rubbings, and little cucurbits [for cupping]. Eighth, they draw toward the neighboring [parts]. Ninth, they drain out by warming, burning-plasters, and cauteries, by which the containing cause is moved away. Tenth, they dissipate the remaining matter; and strengthen the part. Eleventh, let them restore the powers with pleasing nourishment.[220]

As we saw in detail in the previous chapter, the senses of taste and touch also picked out the right qualities of ingredients for making medicines. Heurnius and others at Leiden thought that tasting the medical simples of drugs and the compound medicines delivered flavors which were an "index" of their primary qualities. This practice was an instance of medical "reason" rather than "experience," since the flavors acted only as indexes of the elemental qualities, with sensation mediated through reason to point to their elemental qualities of hot, cold, dry, and wet.[221]

Heurnius strongly endorsed chymical practices, and gave his own recommendations for the most effective remedies. But, like most of his colleagues and healers across Europe, he remained well-assured of the effectiveness of the remedies proven by long use in the "Asclepian" tradition. He joined his voice once again to Galen's: "Assuredly, says Galen, whoever condemns the already-explored remedies, always trying new remedies, acts disgracefully. These now are sacred, on account of their greater agreeableness according to use."[222]

---

220   Johannes Heurnius, *Institutiones*, 533.
221   See chapter four. Cf. Saskia Klerk, "The Trouble with Opium."
222   Johannes Heurnius, *Institutiones*, 548.

In summary, then, training in diagnosis depended on students learning to use their senses to track the signs of material changes in bodies, and especially in different organs. In Heurnius' textbooks and teaching, diseases are primarily function- or action-specific localized disorders or changes—*affectiones*, *pathemata*—of individual organs or a few parts, rather than general disorders of the body's humoral balance. Feeling the pulse to sense the activity of the chief vital faculty of the heart and arteries, and inspecting the urine to make inferences about the chief faculty of nutrition formed the two main, Galenic, techniques of identifying disease states. But students also learned to detect changes in patients' faces, sweat, skin, heat, and breathing, and even palpable changes in their abdomens and other body parts. Patient narratives held relatively little weight, except to indicate the important place and type of pain, which revealed local concentrations of morbid matter and diseased organs.

It is also important to stress again the localization of disease in the terms Heurnius sketched in his courses and texts on practical medicine. These followed closely on the foundations built in his teaching of medical theory, described in chapter three. Disease comes about through a specific part or organ, which has changed in specific ways perceptible to sight and touch (and sometimes taste), with a specific wounded action, and curable by targeted remedies. There is no obvious sense of Foucault's "pathological species inserting itself wherever possible," but the body itself becoming ill, in specific parts and ways.[223] There is no possible room for the *same* disease to move from one part to another in Heurnius' teaching, the mainstay of Leiden medical pedagogy for five decades.[224] Despite recent objections by historians, widespread representations of early modern pathology still give an impoverished portrayal of sixteenth- and seventeenth-century medicine, and present disease states primarily in terms of a total "humoral imbalance, that is, from a general state of disequilibrium."[225]

Yet the localization of diseases, and the language of "seats of diseases" extends back to antiquity, as Adrian Wilson demonstrated using the case of pleurisy.[226] Historians such as Andrew Wear and Michael Stolberg have recently pointed out that in physicians' practical medicine and patients' experiences, localization triumphed over general humoral imbalances and treatments designed for a patient's bodily temperament.[227] And one did not have to await Descartes

223   Foucault, *Birth of the Clinic*, 136.
224   *Contra* Foucault, *Birth of the Clinic*, 10.
225   Lindemann, *Medicine*, 13, cf. 18.
226   Wilson, "On the History of Disease-Concepts."
227   Wear, *Knowledge & Practice*, 117–148. Stolberg, "Post-mortems."

to understand disease in terms of the local malfunctioning of physical parts. Years before Descartes's 1637 *Discourse* and his 1662 *De homine*, Paduan professor of medicine Santorio Santorio even insisted that the body resembled a clock, which stopped working if one wheel malfunctioned.[228]

The primacy of training the senses to detect localized diseases, and then make targeted therapies, in early modern medicine is put in its pedagogical and intellectual context by attending to Heurnius' lectures and textbooks, which came into use across Europe, and formed the core of medical instruction at Leiden University's popular medical school until at least 1648.[229] As the next section details, students learned this approach well, replicating and defending specific localized definitions, diagnoses, and treatments in their disputations.

5   Localizing Diseases in Students' Disputations

Early medical disputations varied in length and quality, but they required scholarly work from the students and followed detailed structures. Students followed Heurnius' emphasis on the localization of disease in their definitions, differentiation, diagnosis, and treatment of diseases. In most cases, they addressed a single disease in a disputation, and began with the definition of the disease. Students could give at least a nod toward familiarity with Greek, such as when Nicolaus Mulieris noted, "pleurisy has its name from *pleura*, which in Greek means the side or rib."[230] Similarly, ulceration of the kidneys, like pleuritis and many other diseases, takes its definition from "the affect and the affected part."[231] More than any other criterion, the part or parts of the body injured by a disease state (usually some sort of morbid matter) defined the categories, characteristics, and treatment of that disease.

Even more whole-body diseases such as cholera and fever found locations, especially around the mouth of the stomach and in the excessive heat of the heart, respectively.[232] Jaundice appeared as a characteristic yellowing of the whole body, but students and professors seated it especially in the skin, liver,

---

228   Siraisi, *Avicenna in the Renaissance*, 351.

229   Resoluties van Curatoren 1648, in Molhuysen, *Bronnen*, vol. 3, 14. As Harm Beukers notes, Heurnius' *Institutiones* "formed the basis of medical tuition by his successors." Beukers, "Studying Medicine in Leiden in the 1630s."

230   Quoted in Kroon, *Bijdragen*, 38.

231   Henricus Florentius, respondent, *Disputatio Medica de Exulceratione Renum* (Leiden, 1611).

232   Nicolavs Petreivs, respondent, *Disputatio inauguralis de cholera hvmida* (Leiden, 1614); Diodorus Schvttivs, respondent, *Theses Medicae de Natura Febris* (Leiden, 1616).

and spleen.[233] Melancholy, like epilepsy and convulsions, is primarily an affect of the brain.

Even the early disputations concentrated on medical practice. They recounted the pathological details expected in patients' bodies, described procedures for interventions such as bloodletting or draining morbid matter, and detailed the diagnostic and prognostic signs from a patient's urine and pulse.[234] Most disputations spent more time on curing (*curatio*) than any other theme, with diagnosis a close second. In nearly every case, purgation or removal of the morbid matter was the therapeutic goal. For ulcerated kidneys, the site of pain indicated the location of the disease, and the pain as well as passed purulent matter acted as signs of the inflammation, then the erosion and putrefaction of parts of the kidneys. The physician had to avoid strong medicines, which would cause more violent flows or fluxes of humors and possibly injure the kidneys further.[235] Instead, first the acrimony (*acrimonia*) of the humors, which ate away at the kidneys, needed blunting through cooling, soothing medicines, such as those from melon seeds, cucumbers, and syrup of violets. Vomiting could help to purge the morbid, rotting matter lodged in the kidneys, but better still would be the patient passing out the "pustulent matter." Passing blood indicated greater danger, and bloodletting from the usual cubital vein in the arm was then urgently necessary. With the morbid matter removed, gentle washing with honeyed wine or syrup of roses should further soothe the injured parts.

Student discussions of diseases with more general symptoms followed a similar structure. Dropsy, a swelling of the belly or even the whole body, found its seat in the liver, as Galen taught, whose action went beyond nature in creating an excess of useless rather than nourishing blood. In the abdomen, this produced an excess of water. Here, as on other questions, disputes among ancient or modern authors allowed the students room for their own resolutions and suggestions: "How this water pervades into the cavity of the Abdomen the Neoterics battle among themselves; some say that it is carried through hidden ducts, others through manifest ducts. We think that both are possible."[236] The weakened liver, apparently failing in its task to concoct the nutritive, venous blood, should receive strengthening, easily-digestible food, medicine promoting excretion, and perhaps even direct surgical drainage of the fluid through paracentesis, but only if the patient's vitality remained constant. As

---

233   Theodorus Vlaxcq, respondent, *Theses medicae de ictero* (Leiden, 1616).

234   Schlegelmilch, "Andreas Hiltebrands Protokoll," 64–67.

235   Henricus Florentius, respondent, *Disputatio Medica de Exulceratione Renum* (Leiden, 1611).

236   Menelaus Vinshemius, *Disputatio Inauguralis de Hydrope* (Leiden, 1612).

with other diseases, the emotions or "passions" of the patient affected their bodily functioning, so strong passions, especially fear and grief, ought to be avoided. Quotations from Hippocrates and Galen, or at least citations, pointed the way through the thickets of signs, symptoms, variations, and treatments.

The fact that this localization appears even in the timeworn pedagogical practice of student disputations further emphasizes its everyday importance to the Galenic medicine of the time. Already in the late sixteenth century Heurnius had developed an influential new scheme of practical medicine, drawing on precedents from Galen, the *practica* tradition, Fernel, and Renaissance anatomists. To this he occasionally added post-mortem dissections, which revealed the hidden causes of the diseases in the bodies of patients.[237] In the medical practice and teaching of Johannes Heurnius, Petrus Paaw, and Johannes's son Otto Heurnius, post-mortem dissections became essential practices for determining the identity and causes of diseases.

6   Conclusions

The different ways body parts became disordered or impaired constituted the diseases of bodies. Canonical Galenic sources emphasized the sensory localization of disease. As Galen defined diseases, "a disease is an affect of the body, primarily impeding some action," so "one must always begin from the organ of the injured action."[238] Medieval and early modern university professors often followed Galen in categorizing diseases by their parts of the body, noting which part was the "seat of the disease" or the "sick part." Humors mattered as morbific causes, building up, moving about, and altering organs and parts in ways that impaired their temperaments and structures, and so injured their faculties and actions. But humors most often were not the seats of diseases or the sick parts, and whole-body imbalances of humors caused very few diseases. Anatomy mattered at every stage of diagnosis and therapy, from finding the precise seat of a disease by location and characteristics of the different pains that matched different simple parts, to the practice of bloodletting along direct vascular routes connected to the morbid locations.

Using Galen's method as an exemplar and his language and examples as shared discourse, professors sought to construct a rational practice and reason securely from signs back to diseases and the causes of diseases. They emphasized first the disease, the part occupied by the disease, and the causes

---

237   Johannes Heurnius, *De morbis pectoris Liber*, 16, 100.
238   Galen, *De Symptomatum Differentiis*, 39 and Galen, *De Affectorum Locorum Notitia*, 6r.

of the disease. Physicians such as Da Monte at Padua, Fuchs at Tübingen, Jean Fernel in Paris, and Johannes Heurnius at Leiden all followed Galen's method. They drew extensively on Galen's *Method of Medicine, The Art of Medicine,* and *On the Affected Places* most of all. Heurnius, for example, knew the latter work so well he slipped between explicit citations and uncited quotations and paraphrases throughout his books. Dividing up functions and morbid impairments by hierarchies of faculties and parts allowed physicians to reason back to the impairments, all from perceptible signs. Especially important were the curative "indications," which pointed to the causes of diseases and the causal contexts necessary to administer the proper treatments. Heurnius taught in detail a system of sixteen indications ranging across, inter alia, the disease, its cause, and the pressing symptom to the temperament of the patient, the part occupied by the disease, the ambient air, the non-naturals, the course of the disease, and the powers of medicines.[239] With this method of "analysis" or "resolution," physicians could interpret signs through the principles of Galenic medicine to track down the causes of diseases and identify the proper causal powers of treatments. Otherwise, in their view they would be mere Empirics, curing not by reason but only by chance.

Touch and sight dominated the perception of the signs of diseases and indications for treatment. As in other Galenic sources from ancient Rome on, taking the pulse by touch and performing uroscopy by sight allowed physicians to sense indexes of the vital and nutritive faculties, chiefly residing in the heart and arteries, and the liver, respectively. For example, sight detected colors in the excrements which indicated faulty processes of concoction of food, such as dark or "burnt" urine. But the use of the senses extended well beyond these core techniques. Sight noted changes of color in the skin, eyes, tongue, and other visible parts, indicating too much red blood, yellow bile, or white phlegm in a part. Putrid smells pointed to putrefaction, as throughout nature, but more specific odors could point to more specific diseases, such as when a patient's breath indicated excessive heat of the stomach by the odor of fried eggs. Palpable changes to abdomens, such as a hardness in the region of the

---

239   Johannes Heurnius, *Nova Ratio*, 465–466, lists: 1. From the affect itself, that is, from the disease, the cause of the disease, or the pressing symptom. 2. From the temperament of the whole body of the sick patient. 3. From the part occupied by the disease. 4. From the powers of the sick patient. 5. From the ambient air. 6. From age. 7. From daily custom. 8. From the particular nature of the one who is occupied. 9. From exercise. 10. From the length or brevity of the disease. 12. From the four times of the disease, namely, beginning, increase, height, and decline. 13. From the particular paroxysms of the diseases. 14. From the ordained functions of nature. 15. From the powers of medicines. 16. From the influx of the stars. Cf. Johannes Heurnius, *Institutiones*, 485.

liver or spleen, pointed to morbid swellings or dessications of organs. Patients' reports of pain, by type and location, presented generally reliable indicators of the sick part and its injury. As we will see in the next chapters, the Galenic-Hippocratic commitment to learning from the senses is shockingly demonstrated in their up-close bodily engagement with disgusting phenomena in the "massacres and cadavers" they viewed with "an unwilling spirit."[240]

In their courses on practical medicine, students learned to target specific organ intemperances with precisely-weighed and compounded ingredients. Humanist scholarship empowered Heurnius and his fellows to convert ancient units from Greek and Latin texts into contemporary measures. They targeted each intemperate organ with the faculties of different ingredients: For example, if the increased heat of the liver was due to bile rather than to a simple intemperance of the organ, the physician would cool the openings from which the bile flows, using plants such as Venus's hair, but avoiding sweet, bitter, or salty plants. If there was pain, the physician would also add a drachm of opium, in a syrup of absinth, to alleviate the pain and the bitter taste of the opium.

Even formal disputations, the ultimate rituals of scholarship for students becoming physicians, trained students to emphasize diseases as local impairments, and concentrate on practical advice for treating them. Most disputations discussed a single disease, seated in a specific part of the body. Students brought their philological and logical learning to bear, giving definitions and quotations from ancient and recent sources, and then assessing them for consistency and accuracy. But they aimed more at practical medicine, and usually spent more time explaining the treatment for their chosen disease than they did discoursing on definitions, causes, diagnosis, or prognosis. As we will see in the next chapter, this scholarly training in a rational method of diagnosing and treating sick parts of bodies mutually reinforced the frequent practice of public and private anatomies.

---

240   Johannes Heurnius, *Modus*, 580.

Disease Displayed in Public and Private Anatomies

1595, 16 Jan. With Drs. Trelcatius, Heurnius, and Trutius present
... I opened a young girl of eleven years, who was believed to be
enchanted, since she had been seized by marvelous symptoms for
eight years. In this one, the Heart within the Pericardium was swimming in poisonous water, the color of which was green and as if you
had seen sea water. The cause of death was the pancreas, which had
swollen up in a marvelous manner, and was very tightly attached
to the hollow part of the liver, and so scirrhous that we thought it
was a stone when we touched it. Dissected, it was observed to have
a white color throughout the interior, scarcely otherwise than if it
had drawn in excessively hardened white phlegm; diminished, she
was wholly snuffed out by the hectic fever.[1]

∴

Anatomies arrested everyone's attention. They exposed the hidden geography
of bodies, healthy and diseased, human and animal.[2] In 1591, professors cancelled classes for three days to observe a public anatomy, held in the old ex-con-
vent, the Faliede Begijnekerk. Across the Rapenburg canal from the Academy
Building and the garden, this site was requisitioned by the Curators for anatomical demonstrations, the surgeons' guild examinations, the library, and the
fencing school.[3] In 1604 and 1611, public anatomies stopped classes for a week.[4]
Special events such as this usually took place on the Wednesdays or Saturdays
which were expected to be free from scheduled lectures. Professors, students,
administrators, and townspeople attended the public anatomies held in the
theater toward the end of 1595, after its construction in 1593. Importantly,

---

1   Paaw, *Observationes*, 20.
2   Jean Fernel famously argued that anatomy should be learned thoroughly as a foundation for
    medicine, just as knowledge of geography gives support to history. Fernel, *Physiologia*, trans.
    Forrester, 178–179.
3   Bronchorst, *Diarium*, 27. Huisman, *Finger of God*, 22.
4   Kroon, *Bijdragen*, 52.

professors and students also attended some of the private or clinical anatomies held as post-mortems in the city hospital or private homes.

But did all of this pomp, erudition, spectacle, and expense really matter for medical practice? What was the main point of performing anatomical dissections? Professors, students, and university administrators celebrated anatomical events across Europe, but what did students observe there, and why did they want to? And why should the professors go through the trouble of petitioning the Curators of the university for expenses, sending out anatomy servants to fetch bodies, handling diseased bodies, and carefully recording the morbid and healthy evidence found in them?

In short, professors and students eagerly practiced the often-repulsive study of anatomy in healthy and especially diseased bodies because understanding the body's parts in health and disease was best achieved by using the senses of sight and touch (and, alas, smell) to gain experience directly. As we have seen, the theoretical and practical teaching at Leiden defined diseases in terms of affects or conditions that injured the function of the body's parts. Dissections of diseased parts—which also occurred in the public anatomy theater—were practices by which students and professors could observe the parts and their perceptibly diseased or damaged states, and so confirm or disconfirm prior diagnoses by the evidence of the senses. Reasoning with this sensory-perceptible evidence, and the principles of Galenic medicine, physicians, surgeons, and students followed the causal links from signs or effects back to hidden proximate causes of diseases. In dissections, they directly sensed the swellings, hardenings, corruptions, blockages, erosions, and other processes that changed and impaired organs and simple parts.

Once again, we will begin with the professors. Johannes Heurnius' publications render novel evidence of his anatomical activity, which included a keen interest in post-mortem dissections and at least some vivisections. This evidence fits beautifully with the central importance of the anatomical localization of diseases in Heurnius' core medical theory and practice courses. Taken together, it presents a clear picture of decades of medical teaching by an important early modern medical faculty which combined anatomical and clinical teaching in theory and practice.

Early Leiden anatomy centers on Petrus Paaw (1564–1617).[5] Shortly after the university hired Paaw as a lower-rank "extraordinary" professor in October 1589, he performed his first public anatomy on the body of a woman,

---

5   Kroon, *Bijdragen*, 97–100. Huisman, *Finger of God*, 20–31. Houtzager, "Het Leids Anatomisch Onderzoek."

Jannetgen Jorisdochter van Deventer, in December of the same year.[6] He continued anatomizing for nearly three decades, and oversaw the construction of a temporary theater in the Faliede Begijnekerk, and a new, larger one there in 1593. Paaw had started his own anatomical education in Leiden as a medical student, when professor Gerardus Bontius "presented an anatomy in 1582."[7] In his major anatomical work of 1615, Paaw reminded his readers of his "Very Famous" Preceptor, Bontius, who "practiced this art first in this Academy, and with the highest praise." Under Bontius, Paaw explained, he learned the clinical necessity of anatomy. Bontius taught, for example, that the pressure of the fluids of dropsical patients causes the organs to rub together, making them rough. It is also possible that Paaw learned about post-mortem pathological dissections from another Leiden professor, Rembertus Dodonaeus. Although Dodonaeus only taught at Leiden for just over two years, from late 1582 to early 1584, he included short reports of post-mortem dissections in his *Rare Examples of Medical Observations* before he took up his teaching post.[8] Paaw next studied anatomy in cadavers at Paris and then took his degree at the University of Rostock, and may have encountered public anatomies there. In Italy, he attended some of the anatomical lectures of Girolamo Fabrici (Hieronymus Fabricius) in Padua, as well as several private anatomies.[9]

Historians have provided accounts of Paaw's material and intellectual culture in terms of the institutional records of the university and some of the prints adorning the anatomy spaces, but have not examined his own writings.[10] Here, I give close readings of unstudied published anatomical treatises and a set of thirty-three post-mortem dissection reports (and one anatomy of a rabbit) by Paaw. These sources have been left out of even recent histories entirely, which has made it difficult for historians to grasp the pedagogical and practical aims of Paaw's anatomical practice.[11] In the next chapter, I examine the range of evidence from the thirty post-mortems performed and recorded by Otto Heurnius decades later, in which he continued and extended Paaw's practice with even more detailed reports and patients from clinical teaching in the hospital, though he apparently did not perform the dissections himself. Relying on institutional sources, previous histories have missed the medical,

---

6   Huisman, *Finger of God*, 22.

7   Paaw, *Primitiae Anatomicae*, 130. *Pace* Huisman, *Finger of God*, 19, who dates the beginning of Bontius's anatomical teaching to 1584 and Kroon, *Bijdragen*, 92, who dates it to 1587.

8   Dodonaeus, *Medicinalium Observationum exempla rara*, 2, 43, 69, 105. Stolberg, "Post-mortems," 76–77.

9   Huisman, *Finger of God*, 32–34.

10   Esp. Huisman, *Finger of God*, 21–43.

11   *Pace* Huisman, *Finger of God*.

practical purposes of Paaw's anatomical practice, as well as the frequent presence of students and other professors at the "private" post-mortem dissections. Since he embraced similar Galenic understandings of disease as those of his colleague Johannes Heurnius, Paaw performed anatomies in order to understand healthy and diseased bodies. This first-hand knowledge of body parts and morbid matter and lesions attracted students and followed the theories of disease and practice taught in lectures.

In his dissections, Paaw modeled for students the right way to see and touch the bodies: he noted the shape, color, texture, and other changes of the organs perceptible to sight and touch. He paid close attention to the membranes containing and dividing the parts, and any changes or perforations in those. And he followed the primacy of fluxes of humors or buildup of morbid matter in disease theory at the time. He carefully described and traced the presence, movements, and even quantitative amounts of pus and other morbid fluids. Morbid fluxes were so important that Paaw often took the trouble to measure their amounts in pints and pounds. Paaw's practices persisted among later professors. All of these ways of seeing and touching, these practiced forms of observing states of disease and health, appear in the later clinical anatomies of Otto Heurnius. Students frequently attended the post-mortem dissections of Otto Heurnius. In his diary, they are recorded as witnesses for eight out of the thirty cases.

The histories of post-mortem dissections from Paaw's diary, drawn from published manuscripts preserved by his students, extend and re-frame the concentration on moralizing, philosophical anatomy emphasized in current scholarship. Throughout his works, Paaw most often described the good of anatomy in terms of its necessity for medical *practice*. As also taught in the courses on practical medicine, Paaw directed students to the phenomena of dissected bodies detectable by the senses. His post-mortem notes are limited almost entirely to descriptions of the observable details of the cadavers. Personal histories and whole-body temperaments played little-to-no role in his accounts of the causes and progress of the diseases. This near-exclusive focus on the phenomena of the dissected bodies departed from the form of some earlier post-mortem reports, such as those published by Antonio Benivieni in 1507, which included information on the identities and lives of the patients.[12]

Paaw's dissections also show a great range in the social status of the people whose bodies he dissected. Patients varied, from unnamed poor men from the hospital to the daughter of the governor and the body of Johannes Heurnius himself.

---

12   Benivieni, *De Abditis Nonnullis ac Mirandis Morborum et Sanationum Causis*, trans. Charles Singer.

The danger of shame, apparently, was not in dissection as such but in *public* dissection or display. Paaw's post-mortem dissections in the hospital or private homes gave students opportunities for anatomical observations in the spring, summer, and fall, when there generally were no public anatomies in the theater. Nineteen of the twenty-seven autopsies listing a month occurred in months from April through November. This evidence demonstrates regular, frequent private anatomies beyond the winter months, which historians, and even Paaw's own publications, closely associate with anatomical practice. No doubt, in the winter months the cold weather allowed professors and surgeons greater leisure and flexibility in their tours of dead bodies. But they dissected readily in the spring, summer, and fall, too.

Post-mortem dissections became increasingly popular in northern Europe around this time, with the practice possibly migrating from flourishing traditions further south. As Katharine Park has demonstrated, post-mortem dissections were quite common in late-medieval and Renaissance Italy.[13] The use of autopsies to detect incorruption and other signs of sanctity in the bodies of possible saints continued well into the early modern period, as Bradford Bouley recently describes.[14] Anatomists in other Catholic territories also performed postmortems, even to reach innovative medical conclusions. In the middle of the 1500s, a series of post-mortems in Spain allowed physicians purportedly to isolate the organ at fault in the French disease.[15] In the Low Countries, the famous physician Pieter van Foreest performed a number of autopsies for hospital patients, and even the post-mortem autopsy and embalming of the body of Prince William the Silent in 1584, even though the Prince had died from an assassin's bullet.[16] The evidence from the Leiden practices of Paaw and Otto Heurnius demonstrate the regular performance of autopsies there from 1590 to 1641. In France, Andreas Vesalius likely performed the post-mortem autopsy of Henry II in 1559.[17] Autopsies and embalming were common for French kings and aristocrats in France and England, with eminent figures such as Ambroise Paré writing instructions for their proper performance.[18] England, as David Harley and Andrew Wear have shown, presents a similar history, with the dissection of Henry, Prince of Wales, in 1612 setting a high bar for the social

---

13   Park, *Secrets of Women*. Park, "The Criminal and the Saintly Body."

14   Bouley, *Pious Postmortems*.

15   Skaarup, *Anatomy and Anatomists in Early Modern Spain*. I thank R. Allen Shotwell for this reference.

16   Houtzager, "Enkele medici rond de prins van Oranje en jet postmortale onderzoek van de prins." Santing, "Spreken vanuit het graf."

17   Zanello *et al.*, "The death of Henry II, King of France (1519–1559)."

18   Harley, "Political Post-Mortems." 1–28, 7.

acceptability of such anatomical, medical practices.[19] Post-mortem pathological dissections followed several high-profile cases of aristocratic deaths, from
the later 1500s through the dissection of John Pym, an English Parliamentary
leader, in 1643. Eight physicians signed the official autopsy report, as well as
surgeons and an apothecary, and hundreds or even over a thousand people
viewed the body.[20] Just as in sixteenth-century medical controversies and later
experimental philosophy, expert testimony of perceptible details appears in
reports as the means for resolving controversies.

Autopsies for private patients soon followed the well-publicized dissections
of aristocratic bodies, with perhaps the earliest in England that of the scholar
Isaac Casaubon in 1614. William Harvey performed autopsies not only on the
cadavers of his sister, father, and other relations, but also on a number of aristocrats' bodies, from 1620.[21] Learning the causes of death for kings and princes
could reveal murderous actions and change the power of political factions. But
merchants, scholars, and common folks wanted to know why their loved ones
had died, too. Physicians, professors, and students wanted to know the hidden
causes of disease and death.

1   Anatomy Serving the Practice of Physicians and Surgeons

Professors and students understood medical practice as the primary aim of
anatomical teaching, with practical learning the aim of public and private
anatomies. This point stands out in the programmatic statements from the
anatomists and professors of the core medical lecture courses. In 1615, Petrus
Paaw published his major anatomical work, *Anatomical First-Fruits on the
Bones of the Human Body (Primitiae Anatomicae)*. This publication helped to
earn him a raise, and to express his main goal for practicing anatomy:

> I myself estimated the profit of this business [*existimavi creditum
> negotii*], that I would prepare not theoretical, but practical physicians,
> that is, not those who would be able to set up an unfinished enumeration
> and cutting out of the parts of the human body with Herophilus, but who
> would thoroughly understand the affects and diseases of the individual
> parts of the whole body, and of those what is required for their curing.[22]

---

19   Andrew Wear, *Knowledge & Practice*, 147. Harley, "Political Post-Mortems."
20   Harley, "Political Post-Mortems," 13–14.
21   Harley, "Political Post-Mortems," 11.
22   Molhuysen, *Bronnen*, Vol. 1, 58. Paaw, *Primitiae Anatomicae*, unpag. preface.

Paaw used mercantile language to describe the value of the "business" of anatomy in producing practical physicians who would understand the changes and diseases of the parts of the body, and how to cure them. He may have echoed here the common speech of local merchants or his powerful uncle, Reinier Paaw (or Pauw), a regent in Amsterdam who became one of the richest people in the city in part through his involvement in the Dutch East Indies Company.[23] The point was not an erudite enumeration of parts alongside the ancient Alexandrian anatomist Herophilus. Rather, he aimed at practical, sensory instruction informed by book learning. Paaw and his later colleagues likely also used an extensive set of individual bones, which by 1620 Otto Heurnius set on thirteen shelves and some baskets, in the medical lecture room of the main university building, the Academy Building.[24] Otto also brought skeletons from the anatomy theater into the lecture room for these osteology lessons, and in the summer would bring bones from the auditorium to the anatomy theater as needed to illuminate a structure.

Paaw dissected frequently, cutting and displaying human as well as animal bodies. A 1625 publication celebrating the erudition and innovation of the Leiden faculty praised Paaw's "consummate skill" in the art of anatomy, and noted that in twenty years Paaw had "publicly dissected sixty human bodies of both sexes, as well as various animals."[25] He clearly dissected far more often than just those sixty public anatomies, roughly three a year. Paaw performed frequent private anatomies as well as dissections of dead and living animals, but held back the grisly details about the latter. "Therefore no winter slipped away for us, in which I did not dissect some human subjects, either two, or three, or indeed frequently four; but about the various examinations and living dissections of brutes, and about the fetal pups, I may say nothing."[26] It is striking that Paaw refrained from narrating these violent histories, since Galen himself was the prince of vivisections as well as medicine, and seemingly felt no such compunctions. Images of Galen dissecting live pigs adorned his collected works, and in his book *On Anatomical Procedures* he coolly recounted a stunning range of surgical mutilations. At one point he claimed that open-heart vivisections presented no problems: "It is surely more than likely that a non-rational brute, being less sensitive than a human being, will suffer nothing from such a wound."[27]

---

23   Cook, *Matters of Exchange*, 112.

24   Barge, *De Oudste Inventaris*, 71–74.

25   Meursius, *Athenae Batavae*, 35.

26   Paaw, *Primitiae Anatomicae*, *ijv.

27   Galen, *On Anatomical Procedures*, trans. Singer (1956), 192.

Like Galen, Paaw noted the necessity of seeing for oneself to learn anatomy, or *autopsia*. He strengthened students' autoptic learning with anatomical lecturing. Ultimately, students studied anatomy and Paaw taught it for medical practice: "[E]ither because the students themselves demanded something of this discipline from me, or out of zeal for the inviting public good [*bonum publicum*], I seized the opportunity to unite together some of the above [listed book projects]. I explicated: Hippocrates on wounds (book of the head); Galen on the Bones, Celsus on Wounds, Fractures, Luxations, Caries, and similar treatises, and any understanding and every use of these depends on Anatomical teaching."[28] Paaw explained that the "chief contemplation of the physician is turned toward the action of the parts."[29] After all, the proper actions of the parts constituted health; their impaired actions, disease.

Since Paaw, Heurnius, and other Galenic physicians defined health in terms of the natural disposition of a body's parts completing actions and functions, disease must be any affect or change contrary to nature wounding the parts. Anatomy mattered a great deal for proper diagnosis and therapy. Even the shapes of the bones were crucially important. For instance, the lungs often became faulty in their actions due a faulty shape of the ribs.

Of course, some real knowledge of anatomy was vital for the surgeons. Galen made the point centuries before, arguing in *On Anatomical Procedures* that anyone cutting bodies for therapy needed to know the complex structures and locations of essential nerves, tendons, and vessels.[30] Paaw gave his students more examples, from his own experience. For instance, surgeons cutting between the ribs to drain pus built up around the lungs in an empyema needed to know how to avoid the networks of blood vessels and nerves ramifying below the skin.[31]

At Leiden, the close relation of anatomy to medical practice is also apparent in the social and intellectual blending of local physicians and surgeons. Surgeons and academically-trained physicians mixed frequently at Leiden, as they did in Paris and other cities with medical schools.[32] After 1590, the physicians performed their public anatomies in the same building the surgeons used for dissections and examinations, the old Faliede Begijnekerk, which soon also housed the library and fencing school. From at least 1637 to 1669, the local surgeons' guild held examinations in the anatomy room in the Caecilia

---

28   Paaw, *Primitiae Anatomicae*, *iijr.
29   Paaw, *Primitiae Anatomicae*, 4.
30   Galen, *On Anatomical Procedures*, trans. Singer (1956), 60, 81.
31   Paaw, *Primitiae Anatomicae*, 120.
32   Guerrini, *Courtiers' Anatomists*, ch. 1. De Moulin, *History of Surgery*, 160–163.

Hospital.[33] Even before this, Paaw noted dissecting with at least three different surgeons: Joannes Simon, Mr. Cornelius, and Mr. Meleman. In the 1630s
Johannes's son Otto Heurnius worked regularly with Joannes Camphusius, the
official or "ordinary" surgeon of the hospital, of the "Republic of Leiden," and
of the Academic Practical College, through which the university instituted formal bedside, clinical teaching in the local municipal hospital.[34] Otto praised
Camphusius's learning and relied on his skill in removing morbid parts, such
as putrefaction in bones. His father, Johannes, learned from surgeons, too, for
instance passing on to Paaw and students the proper procedure for restoring
displaced bones in the wrist.[35]

Otto Heurnius himself combined surgical skill and teaching with academic
theoretical and practical medicine. He appears celebrated in the university records as "Professor of Anatomy and of Surgery" in 1623 and "Doctor of
Medicine and ordinary professor of practical Medicine and Surgery" in 1634
and into the 1650s.[36] His colleague, Adrianus Valckenburg (Falcoburgius),
who had presented anatomical dissections joined Otto as an extraordinary
professor of surgery in 1624, and an ordinary professor in 1629, as well as teaching through "some dissections and demonstrations" in the anatomy theater.[37]
Otto's research and teaching in surgery continued a Leiden tradition. Earlier,
Paaw's planned publications in 1615 had included two dedicated works on
wounds of the head and chest, as well as treatises on wounds, ulcers, fractures,
dislocations, contusions, structural injuries to bones, and various surgical
ailments of the skin.[38]

The sites of anatomy foregrounded surgical works and specimens, too.
In the anatomy theater, eight different books of surgery by authors such as
Tagliacozzi, Van Foreest, and Fabricius or Fabrizi, took their places besides
the works of Hippocrates, Falloppio, Cardano, Platter, Fabricius Hildanus,
Colombo, Riolan, Bauhin, Van Foreest, and Johannes Heurnius.[39] Looking to
the back of the anatomy theater, students could see over two hundred different types of surgical instruments, some of which professors and dissecting
surgeons used to cut, probe, and retract body parts.[40] The importance of surgery for wound care remained pressing. In his public anatomies and osteology

33   Huisman, *Finger of God*, 168–171
34   Otto Heurnius, *Historiae*, 9, 10, 11.
35   Paaw, *Primitiae Anatomicae*, 158.
36   Molhuysen, *Bronnen*, 2, 111, 191. Molhuysen, *Bronnen*, 3, 66.
37   Molhuysen, *Bronnen*, 2, 117, 145.
38   Paaw, *Primitiae anatomicae*, "Praefatio."
39   Barge, *De Oudste Inventaris*, 58–61.
40   Barge, *De Oudste Inventaris*, 46–50.

lectures, Paaw used the skull of an "Ethiopian servant," killed in the siege of Haarlem in 1572, to demonstrate the structure of the interior of the skull and the dangers of head wounds.[41]

Anatomy developed knowledge through one's own senses, even of disgusting phenomena, and so stood superior to other means for knowing bodies such as books or lectures. Earlier, in his 1592 guide for students, Johannes Heurnius had insisted on following Galen to the study of anatomy in order to know the parts and their actions and uses, as well as how to cut veins, arteries, and nerves.[42] Anatomy also appears alongside botany as disciplines necessary to learn from sense perception, not books: "While the young man is occupied with philosophy, he should learn anatomy and botany together, for these are thoroughly learned by sense alone and imagination [the internal sense of image-formation from the senses]....Thus through massacres and cadavers we proceed to the pleasant gardens of medicine: and *bearing an unwilling spirit* we gaze on dissections."[43] Even though Heurnius and his students felt some repugnance at the gory sights of dissections, only these "massacres and cadavers" allowed students to learn properly. Thorough knowledge of anatomy, like knowledge of botany, came only from sensory experience of many particulars. Particularly, bodies of live and dead animals, and human cadavers.

Decades after the publications of Paaw and Heurnius, Albert Kyper's guide for students expressed very similar practical goals for the study of anatomy. It helped students to learn the parts of the body and train for manual practice: "In the winter times you should not neglect Anatomical demonstrations ... so that you will be among the preparations, by which you will more diligently contemplate the parts, and especially you will be able more directly to learn the manual practice of this art."[44] Kyper presented post-mortem dissections as even more important than the public anatomies. After praising the institution of frequent bedside clinical teaching at Utrecht and Leiden in 1636, he advised the students to listen to their professors Otto Heurnius and Ewaldus Screvelius and observe their actions in the hospital, especially the outcomes and the effects of the medicines prescribed.

Anatomical post mortems revealed diseases and their causes, according to Kyper: "neglect nothing, so that you will be involved in the opening of cadavers, and inquiring after diseases, and the causes of them and of death."[45] Only in

---

41   Paaw, *Primitiae Anatomicae*, 28.
42   Heurnius, *Modus*, 596.
43   Heurnius, *Modus*, 580. Italics in original.
44   Kyper, *Methodus*, 288
45   Kyper, *Methodus*, 257.

this way could students avoid becoming unlearned, unskilled physicians who tested their medicinal recipes (*experimenta*) through deaths, killing patients out of their ignorance. Across several decades, and sources from their lectures and textbooks to the official course listing and university announcements, Leiden professors trumpeted a consistent program of investigating the causes of diseases and death through post-mortem dissections.

The Leiden professors' consistent declarations of the central use of anatomy for medical practice continued a long tradition. In early sixteenth-century Italy, the anatomists Alessandro Benedetti and Jacopo Berengario also proclaimed the necessity of anatomy for proper understanding and treatment of the body parts.[46] Berengario drew the lines in the introduction to his massive commentary on Mondino's classic anatomy text:

> And that anatomy is necessary for the Physician is clear, since the sicknesses of the interior members cannot be known without it...from the wounded operations the sicknesses are known, and the wounded operations are known by having knowledge of the operations of the members, and such knowledge cannot be had except through good anatomy. Therefore anatomy is necessary, and not only in knowing sicknesses, but indeed also in curing and even preserving and conserving bodies in health.[47]

This approach continued, as we have already seen, in the work of eminent academic physicians such as Fernel and Falloppio. Students of professors such as Falloppio carried on this strong interest in pathological anatomy. For example, Volcher Coiter (1534–1576), a Groningen-born Dutch anatomist and physician, studied at Padua with Falloppio in later 1550s, as well as Bologna, where Ulisse Aldrovandi inspired his interest in sequential chick dissections to reveal embryological development and Coiter received his doctorate in medicine in 1562.[48] Coiter edited and published students' notes on Falloppio's lectures on the simple parts, along with some of his own fine studies and lifelike engravings of animal skeletons.[49] In his major work of 1573, Coiter followed the Galenic model of using anatomical knowledge to understand the "causes of human actions, which are according to nature, and the causes of the affects,

46   Lind, *Studies in Pre-Vesalian Anatomy*, 82.

47   Berengario, *Commentaria*, 5v.

48   Schullian, "Coiter, Volcher," in *Complete Dictionary of Scientific Biography*, vol. 3, 342–343. Murphy, *A New Order*, ch. 3.

49   Coiter, *Lectiones Gabrielis Fallopii de Partibus Similaribus Humani Corporis*.

which come beyond nature."[50] He explicitly recommended his anatomical and surgical *observationes* as a model for knowing diseases by anatomy, or knowing "by the judgment of our senses the concealed diseases."[51] Only by dissection can we gain such understanding of diseases. "If only the Magistrates and common folk everywhere would provide abundant bodies for opening to true Physicians and Surgeons, versed in dissections (I do not mean here the arrogant and unskilled barbers who demonstrate the bladder for the stomach, worms for nerves, and the lungs for the liver, and who tell tales of monstrous things to the common folk as well as to certain credulous doctors) for the investigation of unknown diseases and their causes."[52] As Hannah Murphy points out, Coiter put into practice this interest in pathological dissections, from at least his early dissections of phthisic patients' bodies with professor Girolamo Cardano in Bologna in 1563, to his autopsy of the body of professor of medicine Johannes Peregrinus in 1566, and a number of other cadavers in German lands in the later 1560s and 1570s.[53] He occasionally put his findings into pathological series, for instance connecting the inflammation and putrid abscesses in the brain of a woman in Amberg in 1567 with the appearances of other dissected brains.

In sum then, physicians across Europe, often connected by networks of education, recognized the necessity of dissections of diseased and healthy bodies for revealing to the senses the causes and conditions of diseases, diseases understood as impaired functions of the organs and parts. Anatomy alone offered this knowledge through the reliable and necessary means of the senses and judgment, both trained by repeated observation and practice along with the best philosophical theory of qualities and causation.

2   Piety and Decorum

Anatomical practice also served religious, moral, and social goods. As many historians have pointed out, anatomy's moral message—you, too, will die—and religious appreciation for the handiwork of God appeared in the banners

---

50   Coiter, *Externarum...tabulae*, 88.
51   Coiter, *Externarum...tabulae*, 106.
52   Coiter, *Externarum...tabulae*, 106. Cf. Murphy, *A New Order*, 86–87.
53   Siraisi, *The Clock and the Mirror*, 113–118. Murphy, *A New Order*, 81, 85–88. Given the widespread attempt to connect anatomy and therapy from Galen to all sorts of physicians across early modern Europe, including Coiter's teachers at Bologna, it is not clear how his connection of anatomy and therapy was supposedly unusual in this regard or "transcended established categories of medicine." *Pace* Murphy, *A New Order*, 70, cf. 17, 80, 88.

and art adorning the anatomy theater.[54] But this was not the primary message of the writings of the anatomists. Pious, moral teaching was of course present here and there in the publications of the anatomists, but it was not nearly as frequent or as prominent as the value of anatomy for understanding the healthy and diseased parts of the body. Paaw intoned that "after the winter took away the summer heat," he turned from teaching about plants to human bodies. There, he worked "extravagantly," out of a certain piety for "that divine temple," or because he could consider God himself greater in the formation of the human body, where the "lessons of his wisdom, power, and goodness appear more clearly."[55] These pious, lofty ideals certain informed Paaw's practice and presentation of his work. But in his publications and post-mortem notes, he spent far more effort and attention on the value of anatomy for training students to understand the diseased and healthy parts of bodies.

What did the public anatomies look like and who attended? Eyewitness reports give us a good idea of the social arrangements and ideals of these events. They appear, at least in ideal form, as sober, egalitarian events in which all are invited to "observe rightly" and so learn about human nature. In his vernacular *Description of the City of Leiden*, originally published in 1614, J. J. Orlers recounts his stop in the theater. He notes that in the very cold winter months the professors "walk through the whole Body," and only the "Professor who does the Cutting" has a place next to the dissection table at the center of the theater.[56] In the first row, the best place for seeing, come the other professors and any officials, then the surgeons and students studying medicine. Then, farthest out, those who have the desire to see such things. Paaw anatomized many different bodies of men, women, and animals "to the ineffable advantage and profit of those who have seen, understood, and observed rightly."[57] As in the Paduan anatomies beautifully described by Cynthia Klestinec, seeing well and seeing rightly acted as norms for the practice of observing an anatomy.[58] Students wanted clear sight lines and sober, proper behavior from those present, even the common folk.

Scholarly decorum held sway in Leiden, at least in the ideals of the public anatomy demonstration, but of a sort more fitting the young republic. An idealized portrait of Paaw in "the Anatomical act," accompanied by a didactic poem, appeared in print in 1615, distributed with copies of Paaw's major anatomical

54   E.g., Lunsingh Scheurleer, "Un Amphithéâtre." Huisman, *Finger of God*.
55   Paaw, *Primitiae Anatomicae*, *ijv.
56   Orlers, *Beschrijvinge der Stadt Leyden*, 208.
57   Orlers, *Beschrijvinge der Stadt Leyden*, 210.
58   Klestinec, *Theaters of Anatomy*, 111–121.

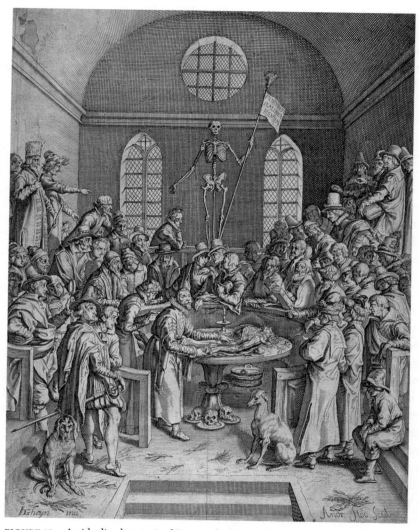

FIGURE 12   An idealized portrait of Paaw and other professors in the performance of a
public anatomy in the theater. Engraving by Andries Stock after a drawing
by Jacques de Gheyn II, 1615.
COURTESY, WELLCOME COLLECTION, 247571. CREDIT: CC BY.

work, *Primitiae Anatomicae*.[59] The artist Andreas Stoc (or Andries Stock) made
the illustration, after the work of Jacques de Gheyn II (see Figure 5.2). Petrus
Scriverius, a scholar trained by Scaliger and friends with the Leiden professor
of poetry, Greek, and politics, Daniel Heinsius, wrote the moralizing poem.

---

59   Paaw, *Primitiae Anatomicae*.

Scriverius' poem, like the illustration, emphasized Paaw actively "dissecting and speaking at length." Audience members had to remain still and sober to hear and see rightly. One might guess rowdy common folk would mob the anatomies. Not so, claimed Scriverius: "The crowd which the Library rejects, and the Mathematician drives away, you perhaps think adores these games... this sordid crowd and the torch of the common man do nothing to the stomach of Paaw, nor does he seek those who are stupid and boorish."[60] All may come, especially the spirited, but only as proper citizens: "This is the republic, but a wee one, of Paaw. / Here reigns the decorum of the Lynx of Batavia / Venerable in ruling, in teaching." The poem depicted "Great Scaliger" sitting with the scholar and librarian Janus Dousa, alongside the Stoic philosopher Justus Lipsius. This was impossible in reality, since Scaliger replaced Lipsius in 1593, after Lipsius left in 1591, and all three died before 1610.

The engraving changed the actual architecture of the theater, too, from six rows of observation benches to two, and altered the placement of the windows and the shape of the ceiling.[61] But the illustration retained the ideals of the poem, which portrayed an audience of great scholars, "thoroughly mixed with the people," all listening and seeing intently. On the left, a young man even appears to use a magnifying glass; others are watching or talking calmly, as Paaw, who "treats and receives all together," invites the viewer in. Everyone should learn the message of mortality, per the sign of the skeleton, "Death, the ultimate boundary-line of things." As Scriverius put it, "Here, learn to die, Traveler, and to / Know before all things, that you may learn, learn, what you are."[62]

These republican, scholarly, discursive ideals likely held good in practice. Students in Leiden, as well as Padua and elsewhere, paid money and time to learn about healthy and diseased bodies in person. If anything, as Scriverius' poem suggests, these were not carnivalesque episodes of transgression but well-ordered lectures with moral, religious, philosophical, and mostly medical themes. The spatial arrangement of the events constrained how well students and other audience members could see and hear, but they came to see, hear, and learn. These anatomies reinforced social relations and values, reproducing a sober republic for learning the ultimate lessons of human nature. They also fused together the two Paduan models of practical teaching in private dissections with Fabricius' practice of philosophical anatomies, and infused them with Dutch republican virtues.[63]

---

60   Scriverius, "In Theatrum Anatomicum" (1615), in Kroon, *Bijdragen*, 50–51.
61   Swan, *Art, Science, and Witchcraft*, 60
62   Scriverius, "In Theatrum Anatomicum" (1615) in Kroon, *Bijdragen*, 50–51.
63   Klestinec, *Theaters of Anatomy*.

While the nature of life and the afterlife was a greater good, most of the time and effort in dissections aimed at educating the students for medical practice. As we will see in the next sections, Paaw's anatomical practice, recorded in his own diary of dissections, shows that students learned not only about mortality and the parts of healthy bodies, but in public, private, and hospital anatomies alike observed the causes and signs of diseases in anatomical lesions.

3   Disease Displayed in Public and Private Anatomies

On 12 August 1601, the day after professor Johannes Heurnius died, Petrus Paaw dissected his friend's body to learn about his disease and death. He opened the bladder, and found seven stones, each about the size of a walnut and weighing two drachms, coming to about two ounces total. He kept those stones in a case at the north end of the anatomy theater, and later six of them lay alongside an Egyptian mummy, a large kidney stone, two vertebrae from a rhinoceros, old toadstools, a thunder-stone, and other wonders—the seventh was apparently lost to theft.[64] From Paaw's skeletons of a man and a woman—"Adam" and "Eve"—with a tree in between, as well as the moralizing messages of human mortality and finitude, it is clear that Paaw and Otto Heurnius sought to teach religious and pious messages. In collecting the prized Egyptian mummy, other relics from ancient Egypt, and especially Egyptian hieroglyphs and Chinese writing, they also participated in the project to recover the ancient, original names of things.[65]

Yet Paaw, Otto Heurnius, and the other keepers of the collection *primarily* used their items to teach students about diseases and their concomitant morbid anatomical states. For instance, after the great humanist historian Isaac Casaubon died in 1614, Paaw managed to ship from London to Leiden his diseased, distended bladder. As in the case of Lipsius, Casaubon's immovable dedication to scholarly study had given him too much strength to resist his body's natural complaints, and greatly exacerbated a congenital defect.[66] The collection included other morbid specimens, such as two sets of diseased bones, and kidney and bladder stones, such as a great dark one taken from a cadaver in 1602.[67] Otto Heurnius, at least, used bones from the anatomy theater in the winter osteology course held in the medical lecture room of the Academy Building.[68]

64   Barge, *De Oudste Inventaris*, 41. Blancken, *Catalogus Antiquarum, et Novarum Rerum*, 10. Sandifort, *Mvsevm Anatomicvm Academiae Lvgdvno-Batavae*, Vol. 1, 283.
65   Jorink, *Reading the Book of Nature*, 283–289.
66   Pattison, *Isaac Casaubon*, 417.
67   Barge, *De Oudste Inventaris*, 38, 41–2; Sloane MS 3528 3v, 4r, 6r.
68   Barge, *De Oudste Inventaris*, 39, 74.

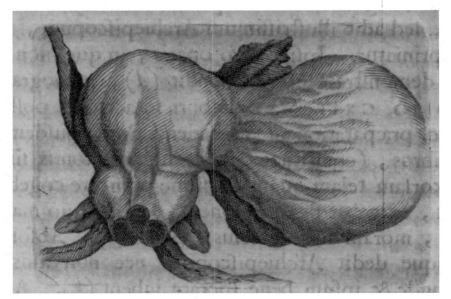

FIGURE 13   Illustration of Isaac Casaubon's bladder, displayed in the Leiden anatomical
theater. *Isaaci Casauboni Epistolae* (Rotterdam, 1709), 60.
COURTESY, STAATLICHE BIBLIOTHEK PASSAU, S NV/A MHG (B) 2, P. 60,
URN:NBN:DE:BVB:12-BSB11348335-6.

Earlier in the same year, 1601, Paaw had privately dissected Christophorus Raphelingius, the eldest son of the famous printer and Leiden professor of Arabic, Franciscus Raphelingius (1539–1597). There, the problem was equally obvious. When
opened, his abdomen poured out an abundance of "corrupt yellow water," and the
liver was scirrhous, yellowed, and hardened.[69] His gallbladder was turgid, and was
revealed to contain a black, filthy, stinking blood. The intestines and mesentery
were yellowish, tinged with a burnt color. If students could get close enough, this
is what they would learn to see. Anatomists such as Paaw emphasized how carefully and diligently (*diligenter*) they did their work. Such diligent practice offended
the senses, but Paaw modeled focusing his senses and cultivating manual and sensory skill in distinguishing the body's parts, as well as morbid matter and lesions.

Paaw's own accounts recount some of his public and private anatomies. His
Anatomical Observations provide us with his narratives of thirty-four dissections he performed from 1590 to 1602. They show that Paaw regularly practiced
post-mortem dissections to determine the cause of death and learn about diseases, and often demonstrated and taught his method and findings to students.
In 1596, for example, he performed *six* dissections: two public dissections in
the theater and four post-mortem autopsies. Printed by Thomas Bartholin in

---

69   Paaw, *Observationes*, 30.

1657 along with other selections of the more rare anatomical histories, these records come directly from Paaw's own hand.[70] Bartholin had studied at Leiden around 1640, and greatly expanded on the family tradition of anatomical expertise and publications. Bartholin reported in his preface to the reader that Petrus's son Johannes Paaw retained several pages of Paaw's *observationes*, and Bartholin acquired others from a relative of a student who had borrowed them. Yet, despite their provenance, rich detail, and long chronological coverage, these records and Paaw's other major Latin anatomical works have not been used in even recent histories of Paaw's anatomical practice.[71]

Paaw's post-mortem *observationes* represent a small part of a wider trend in Renaissance medicine toward the study and knowledge of particulars, a history recently mapped by Gianna Pomata.[72] Moving from individual bodies with their organ temperaments, healthy balance of humors, and disease histories to *general* knowledge of healthy organ action and function, or disease states in general, was not a simple epistemic transition. As Nancy Siraisi has argued, physicians hotly debated concepts of diseases, symptoms, signs, and causes, and the relevance of post-mortem lesions was not clear or universally accepted.[73] Yet early modern physicians, especially in hospital settings, *did* make attempts to connect particular bodies and disease narratives into larger "series" and categories.[74] Paaw's records give us an invaluable window onto how one anatomist around 1600 did so in a pedagogical setting.

In his 1615 *Primitiae Anatomicae*, Paaw promised the university Curators twenty-one forthcoming books, should God grant him the time. He listed these works—ranging from a lengthy treatise on anatomical method, to a study of the spinal cord, spices, fevers, crises, wounds of the head, the plague, surgical methods, and even the whole of medicine in question-and-answer form. From this list, Paaw appears like other ambitious, apparently "bookish" Leiden professors, winning favor from the Curators and scholars abroad for his learned publications. After all, Johannes Heurnius had received acclaim and a silver dish from the Curators for his 1587 *New Method of the Practice of Medicine*.

Paaw also engaged in anatomical research, and used his expertise and observations to critique and expand on the work of other anatomists. He also used his public, private, and clinical anatomies to pursue research agendas shaped by his book learning. He critiqued and confirmed other anatomists' claims in his

---

70   Paaw, *Observationes*, printed with Bartholin, *Historiarum Anatomicarum Rariorum*.
71   Huisman, *Finger of God*.
72   Pomata, "*Praxis Historialis.*" Pomata, "Observation Rising."
73   Siraisi, "Disease and Symptom." See also chapter seven.
74   De Renzi, "Seats and Series." See also chapter seven.

dissections of diseased patients, and remarked on disease states found in the bodies anatomized in public dissections in the university theater built in 1593.

Like other anatomists, Paaw also aimed to innovate. Long practice with a range of animal and human bodies allowed him to establish some novel claims by 1615. For example, following the work of the Paduan physician Gabriele Falloppio, Paaw argued against Vesalius and Berengario that there were three characteristic little bones in the inner ear, not just two. His own comparative practice allowed him to conclude that sometimes bull calves had a fourth, like a sesame seed, joined to the others, but only in those that had lived for a long time.[75]

His anatomical practice included whole-body anatomies in the public theater, as is known, but also clinical post-mortems in the Leiden hospital, private rooms in Leiden and other cities, and even the Amsterdam hospital. His practice in the anatomy theater and his published anatomy works were broadly comparative. Like his teacher Fabrici, he compared parts of different animals and human bodies in different stages of development, but in a far less systematic and exhaustive manner.[76] He took advantage of chance opportunities, such as two dissections of human bodies in the early stages of development which drew very large crowds, and added dissections of rabbits, sheep, dogs, and oxen as needed.

Paaw's anatomical practice across the anatomy theater, hospital, and private post-mortems shows several unifying characteristics. First, Paaw often performed his own dissections; cutting, touching, and observing the bodies himself. Second, he relied primarily on his senses of sight and touch, with occasional offensive deliverances about corrupted parts from his sense of smell. Third, Paaw took careful measurements of things, from the dimensions of a six-month-old fetus and the bones of a man's head to the amount of morbid watery fluid or pus flowing from diseased organs. A hydropsical woman produced two urns of yellowish water, another 56 pints; pus from one man's lung weighed twenty pounds, from another's liver it filled up half a pot. Fourth, Paaw attended closely to visible and tactile structural changes, noting ruptures or changes in membranes enclosing organs. This may have been because he understood membranes as the first formed divisions of the body.[77] He trained his attention especially on the organs since those performed many of the vital actions, and affects of those organs injuring their actions constituted diseases. Fifth, Paaw named the expert witnesses at hand to attest to the credibility of his findings in

75   Paaw, *Primitiae Anatomicae*, 55.
76   Cunningham, "Fabricius and the 'Aristotle Project.'" Siraisi, "Historia, actio, utilitas."
77   Paaw, *Primitiae Anatomicae*, 3.

each particular dissection. He named not only his fellow academic physicians such as Johannes Heurnius and Gerardus Bontius, but also local surgeons who had expert skill with bodies. Finally, Paaw readily relied on his own expertise in dissection and diagnosis to confirm or disconfirm suspected causes, or point out marvelous and monstrous variations.

We can see many of these themes well-illustrated in a record of an early dissection:

> 25 July 1591 I opened (with Dr. Heurnius and Dr. Exaltus present) a boy of around 10 years. Some years before death this one had complained continually about pain in the left part of his abdomen, and the whole belly, and he was saying variously the Middle, here the Liver, there the Spleen, third the Kidneys were at fault. I discovered the stomach to be very thin, so much that there was no part of all the intestines, which did not exceed it by mass: although natural, this was a fault of the first conformation. Moreover all the intestines were distended in a marvelous way, and as if inflated, because the stomach was never correctly concocting, and transmitted semi-concocted [things] to the intestines, which there, converted into flatus, were attested by the continual pains, almost colic pains. I discovered the glandular body of the pancreas so very hard and dried out, that when I first touched it I thought that I perceived a huge stone. The left kidney of this boy was clearly and wholly consumed by pus: for the whole of it was strewn with abscesses, thus indeed, so that as soon as I pressed harder with a finger, the abscess ruptured and a festering substance came out. Moreover, by the same dissection, a great quantity of semiconcocted stuff flowed out (not at all bloodless). Beyond this, I discovered a huge and irregular white stone in that same kidney, from which filth all that festering undoubtedly was born. The opposing right kidney was so wasted, as it could scarcely be found, and it had not reached its natural shape or substance, and appeared very spongy and flaccid to the touch.[78]

Paaw's close description almost revels in the sights and tactile qualities of the dissected cadaver, and the unnatural affects of its parts. This was the sort of thing fellow professors and students crowded around to see. This was disease displayed.

---

78   Paaw, *Observationes*, 8–9.

In the private anatomies, his diary records students present in at least three instances, across eight years. This provides good evidence that students regularly attended these post-mortem dissections to identify and observe diseases inside bodies first-hand. Paaw's diary records students present at *observationes* from 1598 and 1602. The first post-mortem *observatio* actually recording student attendance, in 1598, likely occurred in the university theater or the hospital, since Paaw opened the body of a Danish university student. Drs. Bontius and Heurnius also attended as named witnesses. Paaw easily identified the characteristic internal lesions of inflammation of the liver: ulcers in two places, conglomeration of the parenchyma of the liver separating it from the covering membrane, and a conspicuous cavity which poured out "half a pot" of foul pus.[79]

In 1602, Paaw recorded anatomizing the body of a hydropsical woman with students and Dr. Trelcatius and his son present, in the "forum boarium." Mentioned twice in his record of anatomies, this was likely the Latin name, in humanist spirit borrowed from ancient Rome, of the ox and pig market on the northwest side of town.[80] This is a curious location, but perhaps that was the nearest spot with the necessary equipment allowed by relatives of the deceased. And, after all, the Leiden surgeons guild performed their public dissections over the Waag, the place for official weighing and measuring of commercial goods.[81] As we will discuss below, Paaw had performed an earlier post-mortem in the same place eight years earlier, in 1594. In the 1602 history, several dozen pints of thick water poured from her belly, as expected given her hydropsy. The spleen, kidneys, and liver were totally consumed, and much of the internal uterus changed into "a matter like honey," which poured out of it. Yet the woman had only been thirty-four years old.[82]

Beyond the anatomy theater, students likely attended many more dissections for the purpose of learning about diseases through cadavers. These are recorded as "public" dissections, often performed in hospitals. Students learned about more than just the organs and parts implicated in the fatal diseases, though, since Paaw seized the chances to note anatomical variations and continue his research projects on the bones and muscles of the head and face, as well as the spinal cord and nerves. He gave "public" dissections in 1591, and twice in 1593—one listed as dissected in the Leiden St. Catharine hospital with two named surgeons present (Mr. Johannes Simon and Mr. Albertus), the other

79   Paaw, *Observationes*, 29.
80   See the map by Blaeu, Figure 1.1. Paaw, *Observationes*, 18, 31.
81   Cook, *Matters of Exchange*, 113.
82   Paaw, *Observationes*, 31.

just "publicly dissected...in the hospital."[83] In 1592, he recorded a lengthy narrative of his description of an anatomy of a pregnant woman and her unborn fetus of six months. This drew a large audience, including Drs. Heurnius, Exaltus, and Arly, as well as "other spectators."[84] Another dissection held "publicly," a suicide by knife wound in the abdomen, gives no name or date due to the shame of the act, though it is placed in sequence between dissections from 1593 and before those from 1594.[85] Again, Paaw took the chance to dissect not only the abdomen, but the muscles of the face, and the bones of the head, noting shapes and measuring dimensions. He also spent some time revealing the nerves of the body, and especially the spinal cord and its seven major nerves to the brain. In 1594, he was called to dissect "publicly" a body in the hospital of Amsterdam.[86] In this case, likely performed just after the undated one above, Paaw again took the opportunity to go well beyond the dissection of the diseased, hydropsical abdomen and dissect the muscles of the face and head. Paaw took every chance offered to dissect bodies for his research on the anatomy of the muscles of the head, the bones, and the spinal cord.

Wherever he dissected, in the theater, private homes, hospitals, or the ox and pig market, Paaw showed an interest in finding and recording anatomical variations. In February of 1595, he "publicly" dissected a "masculine cadaver" which had interesting variations, with two ducts coming from the gallbladder, one leading to the stomach, and a portal vein with not one but three trunks.[87] The cause of death appeared clearly in the thick, melancholic matter nearly as hard as stones obstructing the interior ducts of the lungs. Two other public dissections in the late winter of 1595 and early 1596 also showed interesting variations, with a kidney lacking an emulgent vein, another doubled gallbladder duct, and "tendon-like filaments" in the abdomen.[88] Just a week after the second dissection, he publicly dissected an infant "monster" who had survived only twenty-four hours.[89] In front of a packed theater, Paaw noted features across the whole body, critiqued recent work by other anatomists, and pointed to signs of disease as well as preternatural anatomical variations. A second public anatomy in 1596 of a man strangled in nearby Delft also gave Paaw the chance to demonstrate the anatomy of diseases.[90] He noted odd fibers, a rotten right kidney, and eroded, speckled intestines in the unnamed man's body. Another

---

83   Paaw, *Observationes*, 19, 14, 15.
84   Paaw, *Observationes*, 12.
85   Paaw, *Observationes*, 18.
86   Paaw, *Observationes*, 19.
87   Paaw, *Observationes*, 21.
88   Paaw, *Observationes*, 22.
89   Paaw, *Observationes*, 22.
90   Paaw, *Observationes*, 25.

public anatomy in 1598 listed four clear variations: a divided pectoral muscle, a conjunction of veins of the stomach and liver, missing third and fourth nerves of the brain and spinal cord, and no spermatic arteries.[91] Even Paaw's practice of public anatomies went well beyond moralizing demonstrations of the normal, healthy parts of human bodies. Students learned about variations and diseases in public anatomies as well those done in private homes, hospitals, or the "forum boarium."

Animal bodies across a range of species provided ready complements and comparisons for human bodies. As Tim Huisman has noted, Paaw frequently used animals to demonstrate anatomical structures, and from 1598 on used a shed for drying their bones for display in the theater.[92] He compared these directly with human bodies in his public anatomies. In 1615, he bought animal parts—an ox's heart, liver, and eyes, as well as a sheep with young—to demonstrate alongside the dissection of a human body fetched from Delft.[93] A dissection of a rabbit from 1593 shows his comparative method in practice. Before students, Paaw noted the many parts that agreed among rabbits, humans, and dogs. Humans and rabbits shared similar stomachs, kidneys, livers, spleens, gallbladders, pancreases, hearts, lungs, and aortas. He pointed out the differences: rabbits lacked an omentum, and had a suspending ligament for the liver like humans, but unlike dogs. Rabbits possess "an especially vast intestinal colon" or "cecum," and to show it to students Paaw dissected the rabbit.[94] Since a rabbit's cecum is marvelously large, about ten times the size of its stomach, Paaw's dissection here is a striking case of an anatomy teacher using comparative dissection to teach nature's marvelous healthy variations.

For Paaw, anatomical practice, from the theater to private homes and beyond, served to make students into practical physicians by demonstrating the states of healthy and diseased parts of bodies to their senses. In his programmatic statements and the record of his actual practice, Paaw brought to life this method of knowing the dead.

4 Generation and Murder

How do humans come into the world? What forces their souls to leave it? The two framing events of every human life seized the attention and expertise of physicians, surgeons, and students. Paaw opened up the anatomical sites of

---

91 Paaw, *Observationes*, 29.

92 Huisman, *Finger of God*, 38.

93 Molhuysen, *Bronnen*, II, Bijlagen no 468, 75.

94 Paaw, *Observationes*, 16.

generation to his colleagues and students, demonstrating his participation in weighty questions beyond his research on bones and muscles. He also used even public anatomies to produce new pathological knowledge, correlating their phenomena with evidence from private anatomies. He tracked carefully the qualities and quantities of morbid fluids, such as a yolk-like liquid he found in different bodies. Dissecting to evidence of poisons could provide evidence of murder against suspects, and rebut accusations of witchcraft. In his own language, the bodies of the dead displayed evidence that could confirm or disconfirm the diagnoses and prognoses of learned physicians.

The secrets of generation, for the most part hidden inside women's bodies, had long attracted speculation and anatomical interest. As Katharine Park shows, the origins of a sustained tradition of human dissection in the late 1400s appear in response to women's secrets of sanctity and generation.[95] In 1592 and again in 1596, Paaw's public anatomies of the early stages of human generation drew large crowds. Drs. Heurnius, Exaltus, and Arly acted as witnesses alongside Paaw, as well as "other spectators."[96] For the first, Paaw wrote the longest history among all his *observationes*. He detailed the uterus, especially noting its color, in which it resembled those of virgins or women not pregnant. Here, he again drew on comparisons among many individual cases to establish norms according to health and age. Most of the text described the fetus, precisely noting its position head-down and toward the right. He described the folds of limbs necessary for the cramped quarters, and measured the body: length, two and a half palms or eight digits, with the umbilical cord six palms or twenty-four digits. Paaw demonstrated the lack of sutures knitting together the bones of the skull, unlike those of adults, and found healthy organs throughout the chest and abdomen. He weighed in on a longstanding debate about whether and how the fetus urinates by compressing the bladder, much like Berengario did nearly a century earlier.[97] Urine exited the penis, but Paaw found no trace of the urachus, the link that connected the bladder to the umbilical cord earlier in development.

What had caused the mother to die? Paaw noted she was an asthmatic, and found an unnatural color and some filaments in the lungs. In the right ventricle of the heart he found a phlegmy substance, slippery to the touch, like the yolk of an egg. He connected the appearance of this morbid substance to the previous anatomy performed two months earlier. Then, in the ventricles of a hydropsical woman also dissected publicly, he found a similar "sticky, phlegmy

95   Park, *Secrets of Women*.
96   Paaw, *Observationes*, 13.
97   Ragland, "'Making Trials,'" 520.

substance" like egg yolk.[98] Strikingly, Paaw also referenced the pathological nature of this substance in his major published work on anatomy, *Primitiae Anatomicae*, in 1615. Pointing out that there is much else still to be discovered in anatomy, though not purported bones in the heart, as some claimed, he referenced his repeated encounter with this yolk-like substance in the ventricles of the heart. It was this, he suggested, that "suddenly snuffed out" the woman "by an unexpected death."[99] Evidence from multiple post-mortem dissections allowed Paaw to suggest seemingly new general pathological substances, such as this yolk-like liquid in the heart. He highlighted the importance of this evidence and novel thinking by including it in his major published work.

Four years later Paaw again dissected a body close to its origins. A day-old infant brought a great crowd of spectators, including Drs. Scaliger, Heurnius, Merlua, Bontius, and Arly, as well as, no doubt, many students. Earlier, the crowd had turned up to peer into the secrets of a healthy generation. This "infant monster" also drew a large crowd. Paaw noted and dissected a large "mass" or tumor of the occipitus. Cinched within the skin, it had two membranes, one from the dura mater, one from the pia mater. Within the tumor, blood vessels ran this way and that, and its origin in the cerebrum caused corruption within, collapsing the front of the skull. Also marvelous, the testes remained inside, in the places where the "testes of women" resided.[100]

Importantly, Paaw used this opportunity to test a recent anatomist's claim and to continue his research on the urachus. In 1596, he used the dissection of this day-old infant to confirm Costanzo Varolio's report that the umbilical arteries extended from the umbilical cord to the trunk of aortal artery, a bit above the lumbar vertebrae. Varolio had recently published these claims in 1591, showing that Paaw kept up with the anatomical research literature.[101] He also dissected the urachus again, and found it solid and not a vessel for fetal urine. It must function as "nothing but a ligament," then, holding up the bladder.[102] Two years later, a post-mortem in the hospital of a young man who died of lung disease gave Paaw the chance to dissect to the portal vein of the liver, and confirm the teachings of Vesalius and Colombo on the single root, against the opinions of "some others." Paaw even referenced the 1555 edition of Vesalius' *Fabrica* directly: "see the thing pictured on 458."[103] Clearly, Paaw's interest in anatomical

---

98   Paaw, *Observationes*, 11.

99   Paaw, *Primitiae Anatomicae*, 145.

100   Paaw, *Observationes*, 22.

101   Varolio, *Anatomiae*, 106.

102   Paaw, *Observationes*, 23.

103   Paaw, *Observationes*, 15. Vesalius, *Fabrica* (1555), 458.

research combined his book learning and his practice of dissection. Rather than hand on a stale, static anatomy from Galen's books, Paaw sought to evaluate the best of more recent anatomists' work with his own dissections.

Poisonings and witchcraft spurred people to call for the dissector's knife and the physician's expertise. In Paaw, they had both. Paaw's diary records five cases of suspected poisoning or bewitchment. This naturalization of superstition was likely part of the academic culture of the university. In January of 1594, the faculty debated the trial-by-water method for witches, and concluded that "floating on water was not an indication of Witches."[104] Johannes Heurnius took the lead, arguing for a two-pronged naturalism: there were no natural causes for why water would so abhor witches to hold them up, and that any women whose hands and feet were bound could still float due to the buildup of "winds" or airs throughout their looser bodies, especially their lungs, wombs, and intestines.[105] Air held in the lungs alone, especially larger lungs, allows even dead bodies to float (as pirates well knew, since they cut out lungs to ensure bodies would never rise). Their naturalizing opinion, written up in large part by Heurnius, followed similar arguments by the Dutch physician Johan Wier decades earlier. On the recommendation of the faculty of medicine and philosophy, the court of Holland and Zeeland banned the water test and other torture for confessions of witchcraft.[106]

At just that time, people in Leiden and neighboring cities called on Paaw to identify the causes of death in uncertain cases or cases with high stakes. Paaw used his skill and expertise to reduce two cases of suspected witchcraft to instances of poisoning. All together, we have two tragic cases of infants, two men, and one woman. Working through these in chronological order shows Paaw going beyond particular cases to construct case series, and find characteristic lesions among the members of the series.

The editor of Paaw's manuscript, Thomas Bartholin, placed two of these autopsies together, in a series, as a single *observatio*, "Observation 12." On 21 June 1594, with Drs. Johannes Heurnius and Trelcatius present, Paaw dissected the body of a one-year-old girl who had "labored under a bewitchment from which she was said to have died." As in the case of a later 1602 anatomy at which students are recorded as present, Paaw performed this dissection in the "forum boarium."[107] He noted that the abdomen had swollen greatly, and purplish spots appeared on and around the clavicles. The organs and parts of the

---

104   Johannes Heurnius, *Opera omnia*, Vol. 2 (1658), 132.

105   Heurnius, *Opera omnia*, Vol. 2, 133. Cf. Molhuysen, *Bronnen*, 1, 289–91.

106   Swan, *Art, Science, and Witchcraft*, 157.

107   Paaw, *Observationes*, 18, 31.

chest appeared whole. But the liver was whitish, "which was conspicuous from the very cold intemperance." Significantly, the upper orifice of the stomach was eroded in two places, "just as has been seen prominently when poison is given to someone." By making a post-mortem dissection, Paaw used his expertise to naturalize suspected witchcraft, turning a "curse" into heinous poisoning.[108]

The second case came less than five months later, in a private dissection in November. The legal stakes were clearer, notable from the named witnesses of Paaw's colleagues Johannes Heurnius, Gerardus Bontius, the surgeon Mr. Johannes Simonis, and the prefect of the hospital, Mr. Albertus. Paaw anatomized Mr. Jacobus van Werchhorst in't Koorteijnde in the patient's private dwelling. He had been "handed over" to the hospital prefect, Mr. Albertus, to cure him of "venereal plague," likely the French Disease. Yet when he seemed restored to health and began thinking about leaving, "suddenly he began to exclaim that poison had been given to him to drink, and a little later was seized by frenzy and some hours later died." By order of the magistrate, Paaw dissected the targeted organs, the esophagus and stomach. Again, they found the upper orifice of the stomach eroded and eaten away, and even the whole internal "membrane" of the stomach appeared eroded, so that it could be broken by the touch of a finger. Inside, the stomach was purple or black. Paaw concluded, "without a doubt he had consumed some corrosive, caustic drug."[109]

The next year, on 16 January 1595, Paaw dissected the body of a young girl of eleven years in a private home. She had been believed to be bewitched for eight years, since she "had been seized by marvelous symptoms." Paaw found a variety of disease states, and pinpointed the cause of death. Poisonous water, "green and as if you had seen sea water," surrounded the heart in the pericardium. But clearly "the cause of death was the pancreas, which had swollen up in a marvelous manner, and was very tightly attached to the hollow part of the liver, and so scirrhous that we thought it was a stone when we touched it." Once dissected, the pancreas showed a white color throughout, very likely because it had "drawn in excessively hardened white phlegm."[110] The movement of humors was important to Paaw's reconstruction of the cause of death, but not in a vague or general way. Only the localization of a morbid humor in an organ, an organ visibly changed and from its healthy state, could qualify as the right sort of impairment of the body's healthy actions and functions, resulting in death.

---

108   Paaw, *Observationes*, 18.
109   Paaw, *Observationes*, 19.
110   Paaw, *Observationes*, 20.

In the heat of August in 1596, Paaw dissected the body of another infant, this one only ten months old. Perhaps incited by the confirmed case of poisoning from the summer of two years earlier, people attributed this early death to vile poison. Once again, Paaw found the organs inside the chest healthy and whole. The liver, though, was unnaturally pallid, and the gallbladder distended with a limpid liquid. Lacking the distinctive corrosion of caustic poison, this body did not indicate poisoning to Paaw.[111]

Less than three weeks later, it seems Johannes Heurnius' reputation came into question in another case of suspected poisoning. On 14 September, "at the request of Dr. Trelcatius," the city physician, Paaw dissected a fifty-year-old man "to whom Dr. Heurnius had provided medicine." He found visual indications of inflammation of the liver, which was conspicuous for its burnt color. Puncturing its membrane revealed that the whole of its matter—the parenchyma— had wasted away in putrefaction, and a large amount of pus poured out. Paaw emphasized this liver wasted by disease, as well as elements from the patient's history, to confirm that the man had suffered a continual fever. He found evidence of this fever, "which had consumed the native juice of the heart," in the dissected heart. It was clearly contracted "in the manner of a pear," and flaccid, by touch much like a lung rather than a tough, springy heart.[112] No doubt this evidence cleared Heurnius of any wrongdoing.

A final case of suspected poisoning came to the opposite conclusion, and with emphasis. The anatomical observation, dated 13 December 1596, is worth inspecting in detail. With Drs. Trelcatius and Heurnius present, Paaw opened the body of a woman of seventy years, "who was said to have been stung by a poisoner, which very thing the autopsy confirmed."[113] Paaw went beyond his usual dissection of the stomach and esophagus, the usual places to find lesions from ingested poison, to include the heart. He found it swollen, with a huge aneurysm in the vessel coming from the vena cava to the right auricle. A hardened, yellow material had collected in the right auricle, and a flood of hardened black blood poured out of the ventricles and the vena cava when he cut them open. In fact, all the veins of the body were full of hardened blood, which "gave us the suspicion that a very cold poison had been administered to her, which had extinguished the heat and congealed the blood." Nor was this hardening of the blood due to the body lying dead for some time: "It is a marvel that in the living body the blood can harden: the dissection occurred in the second hour after noon, when she had died that same day in the seventh

---

111   Paaw, *Observationes*, 23.

112   Paaw, *Observationes*, 24.

113   Paaw, *Observationes*, 25.

hour of the morning." Only something violently strong could cause the blood everywhere to congeal in this way. Paaw noted that they did not even need to dissect the head, since they could already see the effects of the power of the poison there. The lips were swollen, and the eyelids so distended that they pushed back the eyes into the orbits. The terrible "malignity and acrimony" of the poison even ate away at the skin of the face in various places, leaking yellow discharge.[114] Early modern people faced threats from daily diseases and murderous neighbors. Through post-mortem dissections and long experience sensing and knowing healthy and morbid bodies, physicians could cut down to the causes of natural and criminal deaths.

5   Cutting to the Causes of Disease and Death

In sum, Paaw and his colleagues routinely relied on post-mortem dissections to "confirm" (*confirmare*) or disconfirm suspected causes of disease and death.[115] Paaw took obvious lesions and other clearly perceptible deviations from healthy states as the evidence of disease and poisoning. He relied primarily on his sense of sight, noting color changes, changes in size, and alterations in the connections of organs to other parts. Touch played an important role, as it did for other anatomists. Touch revealed organs and parts changing in hardness or softness, or becoming fragile and wasted. At times, touch could reveal the properties of fluids, such as the "slippery" yolk-like liquid he found in the hearts of two women's bodies.

Pedagogy shaped how Paaw and his students imagined and detected evidence of disease processes. Medical theory played strong and explicit roles in shaping his attention to the movement of humors, especially pus, as well as the localized anatomical changes and sites of disease. Repeatedly, he found the causes of death in specific organs, such as the pancreas, the heart, the lungs, and liver. Qualitative thinking inclined him to suspect a cold poison was responsible for congealed blood or the whitening of a liver. This trained way of thinking also implicitly directed Paaw's attention to the divisions between organs and their membranes, since Galenic and Hippocratic tradition took organs as the active units of bodies. Practicing and teaching a very Galenic medicine, Paaw moved toward greater differentiation of the types of materials making up organs, membranes, and other parts. This was not the tissue theory

114   Paaw, *Observationes*, 26.
115   E.g., Paaw, *Observationes*, 25, 30.

of physicians around 1800, but it was far more than an understanding of the body's structural parts as mere containers for humors.

As we have seen, Paaw also took advantage of bodies to dissect other parts beyond those targeted by the known or suspected disease states.[116] He also used post-mortem private and clinical anatomies to follow up lines of research. As mentioned above, he took advantage of several bodies to investigate the muscles and bones of the head as well as the nerves and spinal cord. In two patients, one who died of lung disease and the other a suicide from an abdominal knife wound, Paaw turned to research the spinal cord and its connections to the brain. This likely fed into his planned book *On the Spinal Cord*, which he advertised to the university Curators in 1615.[117] Even private dissections gave university anatomists the chance to advance their own research and publication interests.

For Paaw, anatomical dissections, whether public, private, or clinical gave him vital opportunities to test the claims of other anatomists, such as the structure and function of the fetal urachus or blood vessels. Each sort also gave him the chance to view diseased parts of the body, and compare evidence from across particular cadavers. He connected the yolk-like liquid found in a public anatomy with a similar substance found in a private or clinical anatomy a few months earlier. The evidence from dissected bodies trumped prior diagnoses. Each post-mortem could confirm or disconfirm suspected causes of death, from poison to disease.

Faced with finding the hidden causes in patients' bodies, living and dead, physicians and surgeons at Leiden used their senses to locate material evidence of morbid changes. As Galen urged in his works and Johannes Heurnius taught across his courses, as discussed in previous chapters, Paaw attended to the evident material causes of diseases. When patients were alive, professors and students could sense some of the qualitative and structural alterations that caused impairments of the parts. By touch, they could sense the grades of heat and pulse rhythms characteristic of different fevers. Sight revealed the discoloration of jaundice in the eyes and skin, as well as the emaciation and curved nails of wasting diseases such as consumption or phthisis. Together with the tactile evidence of a swollen liver, sight also grasped the importance of bloody discharge, indicating a liver disease. Smell could perceive other signs, such as the rotten breath of consumptive patients or the peculiar odors of excrements. But for the most part the primary qualitative changes of organs in terms of their hot, cold, wet, and dry

---

116   *Pace* Huisman, *Finger of God*, 143.
117   Paaw, *Primitiae Anatomicae*, preface.

temperaments remained hidden from direct sensation. Reasoning or "analysis" from signs to causes remained the most common path to the causes of diseases.

Dissecting dead bodies allowed the physicians, surgeons, and students to see, touch, and even measure quantitatively the unnatural changes of diseases and death. Of course, they had to read the phenomena of the dissected cadavers through the language and concepts of Galenic theory. The eleven-year-old girl had lived for years as if bewitched, but the post-mortem dissection of her cadaver revealed the "cause of death" in a swollen, hardened pancreas.[118] The white color found throughout the interior of the pancreas suggested a proximate cause in the hardening of white phlegm. Similarly, Paaw identified an excessively hardened spleen as the cause of death in the body of the boy from Amsterdam.[119] He reasoned from the smallness and thinness of the stomach in another boy to its weak faculty of concoction, and from there explained the inflation of the intestines by their reception of only semi-concocted matter.[120] No doubt, too, the purulent abscesses and stones in the lungs of a consumptive patient formed from the concretion of a phlegmy, rotten humor.[121] Poisons caused violent erosion of the mouth or esophagus and stomach.

The dead bodies of patients could not longer speak to help reveal their pains and impaired parts. But with Paaw as the learned, experienced interpreter, dead bodies spoke in languages familiar to physicians trained in Galenic-Hippocratic medicine. From the anatomy theater to private homes and other dissection sites, bodies could speak new things in Galenic language. Through Paaw, they often had the final say.

6   Conclusions

How did public and private anatomies combine with lectures, textbooks, and disputation practice to train students in recognizing and understanding diseases? And how did students' bookish training fit with the actual practices of public and private anatomies, when they finally witnessed the hidden phenomena of bodies? In short, they directed their senses to the perceptible signs and evidence of diseased parts. Their courses in theoretical and especially practical medicine extended the system of qualities and temperaments to

---

118   Paaw, *Observationes*, 20.
119   Paaw, *Observationes*, 21.
120   Paaw, *Observationes*, 8–9.
121   Paaw, *Observationes*, 15.

describe morbid changes of patients' body parts. Public and private dissections revealed perceptible evidence of these diseased states and their development in a range of bodies. They read bedside signs and post-mortem dissection evidence through the language and concepts of Galenic medicine, as systematized and taught by their professors. Professors also collected and displayed examples of disease states in the university's collections of bones, professor Heurnius' kidney stones, and other specimens, such as the scholar Isaac Casaubon's diseased bladder.

As with all knowledge, understanding of healthy and sick parts began in the senses. Professors, students, and surgeons then read the phenomena of living and dead bodies through the terms and theories of Galenic medicine. Despite the "massacres and cadavers" necessary for the sensory practice of anatomy, students sat close to the disgusting dissection tables and listened carefully to the professors' accounts of the perceptible evidence and its meaning for the proper diagnosis, pathological understanding, and treatment of the diseases finally revealed in their hidden seats. Anatomy professor Petrus Paaw modeled close sensory and bodily engagement with cadavers by often performing his own dissections. He cut, probed, touched, and observed dead bodies himself, rather than relying on surgeons. His senses of sight and touch picked out changes in color and structure, discerning the green color, "as if you had seen seawater," of the poisonous fluid surrounding the heart of a young girl.[122] A violent change of color of the pancreas to white, and a stone-like hardness to the touch revealed its morbid changes as the cause of death. His color palette extended to include categories such as yellowish, white, yolk-like, slate-colored, yellow tending white, pallid blue, purplish black, reddish, and burnt. Touch identified healthy and diseased membranes, and found organs swollen, hardened, softened, and even consumed by pus into corrupt fluid, and perceived the properties of fluids such as the sticky, yolk-like substance clogging the hearts of two women.

The proximate causes of diseases and death that Paaw identified in the bodies he dissected consisted mostly in obvious alterations to organs he could identify by sight and touch. They could not always reach directly to the fundamental qualities of hot, cold, wet, and dry, in room-temperature cadavers, of course. Paaw and his colleagues did note morbidly dry or wet parts. They also made inferences to the action of excessive hot or cold intemperances when they saw blackened or "burnt" parts, or congealed substances. Similarly, they connected a whitish liver to the supposed cold intemperance of the disease, just as everyday experience showed body parts turning white in the cold winter. They inferred stories of changes of organs and humors in these terms, as in their conclusion that the white concretions in a patients' pancreas formed from the solidification of a humor.

---

122   Paaw, *Observationes*, 20.

Across public and private anatomies, Paaw's practice remained strikingly consistent. Whether he performed the dissections in the theater, private homes, or even the "forum boarium," Paaw looked for signs of diseased parts and anatomical variations, touched organs and membranes, tested other anatomists' claims, measured fluids, pursued his research projects, and made connections in the morbid appearances across cases, at times making suggestions about novel causes of diseases. He waded into longstanding controversies during these anatomies, giving confirmations or critiques of other anatomists' accounts, based on his own expertise. Experience with many cases of generation allowed Paaw to have a sense of the norms of maternal and fetal anatomy. Even in clear cases of knife wounds or other clear local sites of the cause of death, Paaw dissected well beyond the causes of death to follow his research on the bones, the muscles of the head and face, and the spinal cord and nerves.

Like other physicians, Paaw persistently naturalized and materialized causation, with his senses populating the pool of potential causes. Private anatomies of bodies in cases of suspected death by witchcraft allowed anatomists to naturalize the causes of death. This was part of a broader university push to identify natural causes, for example in their recommendation against using the water test for accused witches, since internal gases, not demonic powers, generally caused floating. Eroded lesions revealed in cadavers' digestive tracts proved death by corrosive poison rather than by magic. Professor Johannes Heurnius stood accused of poisoning a patient, but the body revealed to Paaw a pus-filled and wasted liver and flaccid heart, and no corroded lesions, showing death by long disease rather than by a toxin. Another private anatomy "confirmed" suspected death by poisoning. Violently congealed blood in the ventricles and vena cava, corroborated by swollen lips and eyelids, pointed to the power of poison. Even in these very particular anatomies, demanded by legal authorities for evidence of guilt or innocence, Paaw dissected throughout the bodies to test and discover new knowledge.

Later, by the mid-seventeenth century, Leiden professors and students routinely combined anatomical post-mortems, experiments on live animals, chymical investigations, and clinical testing to make discoveries and test traditional and novel claims.[123] But even well before that period of the efflorescence of experiment across Europe, medical professors and students drew on their training and traditional practices to make discoveries and test claims. The next chapter illustrates some of this gradual innovation in anatomy, pathology, and therapy.

---

123   Ragland, "Experimental Clinical Medicine" and the forthcoming second volume.

Innovation and Clinical Anatomies

The Professor, with both the ordinary city doctors ... with the students, together with a good surgeon, will visit the sick persons in the public hospitals, and examine the nature of their internal diseases, as well as all their external accidents, and debate their cures and surgical operations, prescribing medicines according to the order of the hospital, and, also, will open all the dead bodies of the foreign or unbefriended persons there and show the causes of death to the students.

–Resolution of the Curators and Burgomasters of Leiden University, 13 May 1636[1]

• • •

With the recent sabbath day elapsed, in the public Hospital in individual weeks the protegees of Asclepius and the Practical Professor of Medicine come together, so that they may inquire into the nature of diseases, their causes and remedies, and I was present for the dissection of a human cadaver. We were occupied in the investigation of the hidden cause of death, but truly from the more principal parts, which were preternatural, we found none, for which reason the cause was referred to the spirits or humors.

–THOMAS BARTHOLIN, Leiden student, 1638[2]

.:.

On January 7th, 1639, Leiden professor of anatomy and medicine Otto Heurnius demonstrated the cause of death in a patient's body in the anatomy room of the city hospital. David Jarvis, a man of twenty-eight from Scotland, had lain in the city hospital for the poor, suffering the characteristic symptoms of phthisis: coughing up blood and pus, his body burning with fever and wasting

---

1 Molhuysen, *Bronnen*, 3, 312*.

2 Thomas Bartholin to Ole Worm, 3 October 1638, in *Olai Wormii...Epistolae*, Vol. 2, 653.

away. Like millions of others in the early modern world, Jarvis had died from phthisis, tabes, or consumption (the Greek, Latin, and English names, which all meant "wasting"). After Jarvis died, Otto and his surgeon followed the official hospital teaching program: they dissected Jarvis' emaciated body the next day and revealed the causes of his death. In the lungs, Otto and his surgeon showed the students the "cause of death seated in the lungs, namely that the whole parenchyma was filled with tiny tubercles from a crude viscous matter."[3] These tubercles or "swellings" (*tubercula*) filled the substance or parenchyma of the lungs, blocking and compressing them.

Otto matched the observed symptoms from Jarvis' bedside with his body's final hidden states through an inference to the progression of the disease. Unable to breathe out the excess heat from the heart, the lungs overheated, producing putrefaction and pus which created these tubercular swellings and ate away at the lungs, making ulcers. The liver overheated, too, and its change in temperament impaired its faculty of making nutritive blood, so the lungs and all the rest of the body began to waste away, starved of proper nourishment. As the ulcers ate away at the lungs "like a wild beast," they produced blood which Jarvis spat up from his hospital bed. His whole body overheated in a "hectic" or chronic fever. Repeated experiences with other living and dead patients' bodies confirmed this pedagogical correlation of symptoms and post-mortem evidence. Another phthisic cadaver from 1637 also displayed the ulcers, abscesses, and pus at the root of the symptoms of the patient, his dead lungs "marbled with dark and pale droplets."[4] Like other physicians of his time, Otto took careful note of the visible appearances of the organs, membranes, fibers, and fluids he found in the dead bodies he dissected, building up his own diary and memory with their usual and unusual variations.

Clinical anatomies connected the regular observation of hospital patients' symptoms, treatment, and progression with the sense-perceptible evidence of the seats and proximate causes of disease in interior organs. Professors and students could infer and imagine these interior seats and causes while the patients lived, but could only confirm, directly sense, and so really *know* them after post-mortem dissections put them on display. Regular clinical instruction in the hospital and routine post-mortem dissections to seek the causes of disease and death were not rare or marginal at Leiden. They were the prized and official practices which brought together living patients and diseased organs, giving flesh to the methods and theories learned in the lecture hall and private chambers. Students' direct sensation and regular experience of professors treating

3   Otto Heurnius, *Historiae*, 22.
4   Otto Heurnius, *Historiae*, 10.

many patients and dissecting their diseased cadavers modeled the best practical medicine. It also constituted the best means for sensing and experiencing first-hand what diseases really were, through actual diagnosis, treatment, and the final testimony of restored health or the revealed evidence of death.

Early modern students and professors recognized the importance of regular hospital observation and instruction *combined* with frequent post-mortem dissections of patients. These "clinical anatomies" provided the Leiden students and professors with the regular experience of multiple patients suffering from a given disease, often in close temporal and experiential proximity. This practice yielded an understanding of the common symptoms and progress of a disease, as well as their variations. Clinical anatomies of patients, especially those who had suffered from phthisis or consumption—a notoriously fatal disease—gave professors and students visible evidence of the seats, causes, and progress of disease. In the case of phthisis, they found the purulent ulcers of the lungs which Hippocratic and Galenic healers had long suspected as the origins of patients' expectorated pus. They also increasingly recognized the importance of swellings, or tubercles, in the lungs, which appeared in a range of sizes, as well as the open ulcers eroding the lungs and producing pus. Seeing the ulcers and tubercles of the lungs across many patients' dissected bodies generated the necessary breadth of experience for gradual innovation in pathology.

Leiden medical scholars innovated in other ways, too. First, they performed anatomical experiments, including dissections of living animals such as frogs, in order to work toward a resolution of the ongoing ancient-to-early-modern debates over the pulse. Did the heart and arteries contract and dilate simultaneously, as Galen most often argued, or in sequence, as his opponent Erasistratus claimed? Leiden anatomists seem to have joined in the pattern of using experiments to attempt to resolve controversies. In this they followed a fellow Dutch anatomist, Volcher Coiter, who had trained in Italy and worked in Germany, although they did not imitate his unusually rich, first-person historical narratives of his dissection experiments on living animals.

Second, they founded the first successful program of hospital bedside teaching for university students in northern Europe. The goals of the Leiden program and its rival at Utrecht University were substantially the same: the demonstration of medical teaching in the healthy and diseased bodies of patients, and the formation of students into practical physicians. Combining regular bedside teaching with the observation of the sick or injured parts revealed in post-mortem dissections stands out as a primary goal emphasized by all the medical faculty and the official requirements for the "Academic Practical College." This early clinical teaching tested students by showing them the signs of patients and asking for the recommended diagnoses, prognoses, and treatments. Pedagogical practice then tested these recommendations by observing the course of a patient's progress and, God willing, cure, or by revealing the evidence of diseases and causes in the patient's dissected cadaver.

In searching for these causes, Otto and his colleagues followed good Galenic tradition in looking first to the organs and simple parts, especially the principal parts (the heart, brain, and liver). In these the chief causes of death usually occurred, and deadly diseases had their anatomical seats. Only after checking these chief vital organs did professors and students turn to the humors or the material but insensible spirits. Note the sequence in the 1638 report from student Thomas Bartholin: "We were occupied in the investigation of the hidden cause of death, but truly from the more principal parts, which were preternatural, we found none, for which reason the cause was referred to the spirits or humors."[5]

This program allowed Otto's practice of clinical anatomies to flourish. Students' eagerness to learn by their senses, first-hand, the phenomena of diseased bodies sent them crowding around the dissecting table in the anatomy room of the hospital. In some cases, they drew a little too close, such as when pus from an incised morbid liver spattered those standing nearby. But with these clear morbid appearances of organs, Otto and the students could make direct inferences to their altered actions and temperaments, and their impaired faculties. Visible swollen nodules or tubercles blocking airways in the lungs would have impaired their cooling function while the patient was alive, making the liver overheat and produce poorly-concocted venous blood, causing the liver and other organs to waste away, and corrupt pus to build up from the putrefying heat and impaired faculties. These morbid impairments of the lungs matched patients' characteristic symptoms of difficulty breathing and coughing up pus and blood. In their clinical anatomies, professors limited their inferences and imaginations to the evidence of the senses. On other cases which lacked clear evidence of diseased organs, they could find no causes or infer any reasons.

Third, in their program of hospital teaching, professors tried new remedies for new diseases, including some picked up from the Dutch imperial invasion of the New World. In 1637, seven years after the establishment of an imperial headquarters for the WIC (West Indische Compagnie), a soldier from the colony in Brazil returned with flea-like parasites in his feet. Professors and surgeons had to cut out the gangrenous portions and then try to concoct an imitation of

---

5   Bartholin to Worm, in *Epistolae*, 653.

the effective indigenous remedy, the "oil of Couroq." They used the indigenous ingredients at hand, especially Peruvian bark (guiacum or *quina* or *cinchona*).

As in other cases from the hospital, Otto took care to set down his recipes for remedies in detail, since students prized this practical knowledge. And, as his father, Johannes, had argued at length in his works and courses, the precise amounts and preparation methods of ingredients were crucial for the targeted application of their powers to the sick parts. In the hospital, from the bedside to the anatomy room, students learned from their own senses the appearances and nature of diseases, as well as how to treat them.

Within their long traditions of learning and practice, students and faculty at Leiden aimed to innovate and produce new knowledge. We have already seen innovation in research and teaching at Leiden, from Cluyt's and Clusius' studies of new plants to Johannes Heurnius' new method of practical medicine, as well as Paaw's ambitious plans for new books on anatomy and his search for new pathological substances in cadavers. To show the growth of innovation through experimentation and the combination of hospital teaching and clinical anatomies, this chapter begins with the earliest documented anatomical experiments over the pulse. As with other anatomical and medical experiments of the time, scholars performed them and wrote about them in order to engage and resolve an ongoing controversy.[6] This work in Leiden, of course, appeared in the context of the rise of anatomical practice and innovations across Europe. This renaissance of anatomy, and especially the new discoveries of Gaspare Aselli and William Harvey, inspired Leiden students in the early 1630s to critique older anatomical knowledge and practices and to begin to accept and extend new knowledge. These innovations in healthy anatomy helped to frame the production of new knowledge in pathological anatomy. In many cases, students increasingly led the way by eyeing or embracing more radical innovations, and more quickly, than their gradualist professors.

Next, I turn to clinical teaching and anatomical practices. I argue that bedside teaching very probably occurred even earlier than the 1636 establishment of the official program in the hospital. This earliest Leiden bedside teaching probably continued the pedagogical model from Padua of students accompanying professors on private visits. I describe the pedagogical reasons and context for the founding of the 1636 program, especially the primary goals of gaining practical experience at patients' bedsides and then finding the causes of death in dissected cadavers. The chapter then expands to analyze Otto Heurnius' practice of clinical anatomies in detail, drawing from his own diary of

---

6   Ragland, "'Making Trials.'"

observations of thirty cases. It concludes with a close study of the history of the diagnosis, pathology, and treatment of phthisis in influential sources from the ancient Hippocratics to early modern Leiden. I show that Leiden pedagogical practices, especially clinical anatomies, allowed a Leiden student-turned-professor, Franciscus Sylvius, to construct a new theory of phthisis or consumption based on the presence and development of tubercles. His new theory extended previous findings, and gained praise into the next century for its emphasis on tubercular formation and effects, as discovered through the correlation of post-mortem dissections and patients' symptoms. This attention to change and continuity over time highlights the vitality of these long traditions, and the innovative contributions of Leiden university's early hospital teaching to them.

1 The Pulse Controversy and Anatomical Innovation

Before we examine innovation in clinical anatomies, we must get a better sense of some of the broader innovations and debates in anatomy that shaped Leiden anatomy. Anatomical, even experimental, innovation gradually broke out from the university anatomical practices into the lecture halls. In the sixteenth and early seventeenth centuries, anatomists increasingly gained reputations and created controversies for their innovative claims about structures or actions of body parts.[7] By the end of the 1500s and the early 1600s, Leiden professors and students accepted and debated these novel claims, and critiqued anatomical practices near and far. These debates and innovations grew from and elaborated ancient disputes about the pulse, blood, and heart. Student notes from lectures in the early 1630s show that professors used the senses and reason to examine and then temporarily reject influential new doctrines such as the circulation of the blood.

In the late 1400s and early 1500s, the professor and surgeon Berengario da Carpi had relied on his own experience in dissections and surgeries to identify new structures, from the cartilage in the throat to structures of the skull, and to write a treatise on head wounds and skull fractures. He also questioned Galen's claims to the existence of the *rete mirabile*, a network of blood vessels at the base of the brain, in humans, and experimented with kidneys and fetal urination structures.[8] A few decades later in the 1530s to the 1560s, Vesalius relied on his

---

7 E.g., Shotwell, "Revival of Vivisection." French, *Dissection and Vivisection*. French, *Harvey's Natural Philosophy*. Bertoloni Meli, *Mechanism, Experiment*. Guerrini, *Courtiers' Anatomists*.
8 French, "Berengario de Carpi." Ragland, "'Making Trials.'"

remarkable skill in dissection of human and animal bodies to critique Galen's errors and identify a host of new structures.[9] For instance, he rejected the existence of the *rete mirabile* and the five-lobed liver in humans, corrected Galen on the bones of the jaw and the longest bones of the body, and distinguished many muscles. Anatomists such as Colombo critiqued Vesalius (who criticized him harshly back) for his own anatomical errors, and announced the vivisectional observation of the pulmonary transit of the blood. Of course, Falloppio then attacked Colombo, alleging that Colombo had gained in reputation for stealing the priority of discoveries from him. From the middle of the sixteenth century, anatomists eagerly used their own experience to gain renown and credit for critiques of other anatomists and to generate new knowledge.[10] Following the lines of anatomical texts, pedagogy, and the pulse of the arteries, this stance flowed into Leiden as well. After all, professors such as Paaw read the latest anatomical works, and taught from new treatises, such as Colombo's 1559 *De re anatomica*.

In one telling instance, Johannes Heurnius' lectures on medical theory waded into ongoing debates over the pulse by appealing to experimental vivisections of frogs. Those vivisections likely formed some of Paaw's "living dissections of brutes" which he did not deem proper to describe. The controversy over the heart's action and pulse reached across Europe in time and space. Renaissance physicians disagreed vehemently over the action of the heart and the pulse—did the heart and arteries contract and dilate simultaneously, or in alternating sequence? Like so many others, by at least 1592 Heurnius argued for simultaneity based on personal experience. Place a hand over a heart and the other hand at a wrist, Galen's favored site for taking the pulse, and you will find simultaneous action from the vital faculty shared by the heart and arteries, Heurnius urged his students. The clincher came from frogs, though: "in frogs dissected alive, this is discerned with the eyes."[11]

In this way, Heurnius taught students to use personal experience and vivisectional evidence to resolve a centuries-old, vigorous debate, rather than depend on textual authority or rational argument. By the 1640s, Leiden professors would perform elaborate experiments to confirm the opposite conclusion. Following Harvey, they proved that the heart and arteries alternate in systole and diastole (as the heart empties it pushes blood into the arteries).[12] But experimentation on live animals could still play an important adjudicatory

---

9   O'Malley, *Andreas Vesalius of Brussels*.
10   E.g., Shotwell, "Revival of Vivisection." Ragland, "'Making Trials.'"
11   Johannes Heurnius, *Institutiones*, 336. Cf. Johannes Heurnius, *Institutiones* (1592), 355.
12   Schouten, *Walaeus*. Ragland, "Mechanism."

role for Heurnius, even in his lectures on medical theory. Experiments producing phenomena open to the senses could resolve learned debates.

Once again, ancient writings and a commentary tradition on them framed the debate. The ancient Alexandrian anatomists Herophilus and Erasistratus had originated this debate, and generated a controversy carried forward by Galen and his readers into the early modern period. Renaissance anatomists ascribed another position to Erasistratus, Galen's rival and target for misrepresentation, whom he claimed combined anatomical skill with wavering support for Nature's wondrous *techne* and foresight.[13] According to Galen's *On Anatomical Procedures*, a favorite text of Vesalius, in Erasistratus' view the contraction of the heart pushes the *pneuma* into the passive arteries, dilating them, and then the heart dilates, drawing *pneuma* in from the lungs as the arteries passively contract. Thus, the heart and arteries contract and dilate in sequence rather than at the same time. Aristotle provided another view, in which the concoction and ebullition of the blood in the ventricles of the heart cause its motions, with the heart itself passively dilating and contracting as the blood continually enters, heats up, and boils over.[14]

Galen's own position remained ambiguous, despite his obvious rejection of Erasistratus' claim that the contents of the arteries carry the pulse, rather than their coats. In his influential works on diagnosing by the patient's pulse, Galen opposed Erasistratus on the sequence of motions. He argued that the arteries and heart dilate and contract simultaneously, no doubt due to a shared faculty.[15] He also divided the phases of the pulse into "dilation" (*diastole*) and "contraction" (*systole*) of the arteries and heart, with the "systole" phase not perceptible in the arteries by touch, which produced a tactile "interval" between active "diastole" phases. In *On Anatomical Procedures*, he detailed an experiment from Erasistratus which he claimed actually refuted Erasistratus' own position: uncover a main artery in the limb of a living animal, cut out a section, and tie the cut ends to the ends of a tube. The blood or *pneuma* should continue through the tube, as Erasistratus claimed. But Galen averred that the pulse cannot be detected below the tube, and thus must be carried by the arteries themselves.[16] Galen also described methods for exposing the living heart to the direct sensation of sight and touch, but then left the true motion

---

13 Von Staden, "Teleology and Mechanism."
14 Aristotle, *On Breath*, 479b28–480a11.
15 Bylebyl, "Disputation and Description," 228–229. Cf. Galen, *On Anatomical Procedures*, Bk. VII, Chs. 4, 8, 14, Singer trans., 176, 184, 194. Galen, *On the Pulse for Beginners*, Kviii, 453, trans. Singer, in *Galen: Selected Works*, 325–326.
16 Galen, *On Anatomical Procedures*, Bk. VII, Ch. 16, trans. Singer, 199.

of the heart and arteries in doubt. Anatomical tests, then, did not settle the matter neatly. Yet Galen's example and the ongoing controversy provoked further trials or experiments from Renaissance anatomists. Naturally, their opponents performed further trials in response, generating a self-catalyzing cycle of a controversy provoking trials, which generated new claims, which in turn elicited further trials and claims.

In later European academic medicine, as Jerome Bylebyl has shown, textual, rational, and experiential considerations pushed physicians and scholars to accept the Erasistratean alternation of motions, with the arteries dilating as the heart contracts.[17] In the later middle ages, scholars ascribed an anonymous Greek *Compendium of Pulses* to Galen, which argued for the sequential, asynchronous contraction and dilation of the heart and arteries. These two contradictory opinions of "Galen" caused consternation and controversy, but in the 1300s and 1400s nearly all commentators sided with the alternation view of the *Compendium*. After all, it seemed to have anatomical evidence and reason on its side—material expelled out of the heart needed arteries to take it in through their dilation.

Anatomists adopted experimental tests again in the 1500s, often emulating and then elaborating on Galen's sophisticated procedures. Vesalius and other anatomists attempted to replicate Galen's tube-in-artery procedure, but did not reach a consensus on the sequence or cause of the motions of the heart and arteries.[18] Humanist scholarship debunked the assumed Galenic authorship of the *Compendium*, casting its asynchronous theory as Erasistratean. Some, such as Leone Rogano (d. 1558), included vivisectional support for their own views, for instance noting that even a heart completely emptied of blood continues to beat for a time, against Aristotle's ebullition account. Yet leading figures such as Jean Fernel and Vesalius (at least in his early work such as the 1539 *Letter on Venesection*), taught alternation models. Fernel's *Physiologia* described the contracting heart impelling vital spirits into the arteries, dilating them. Vesalius relied on the anatomist's *autopsia*, which first confirmed the alternation model. Later, in lectures to students he encouraged an apparently agnostic *autopsia*: "feel yourself with your own hands and trust them."[19] Even more sophisticated procedures such as opening the thorax and periodically re-inflating the lungs did not clearly resolve the matter in his 1543 *Fabrica*.

The next generation of anatomists critiqued their predecessors, and extended their anatomical procedures and tests. Realdo Colombo's 1559 *De re*

---

17   Bylebyl, "Disputation and Description."
18   Shotwell, "Revival of Vivisection." Bylebyl, "Disputation and Description."
19   Quotation in Bylebyl, "Disputation and Description," 235.

anatomica confidently asserted the power of vivisectional *autopsia* to confirm the vigorous contraction of the heart—expelling blood and spirit in systole, and the alternation of the dilation and contraction of the heart and arteries. Other writers, such as Falloppio, were more explicit in exploring accounts in which the arteries moved only passively like an "inflated glove," as the heart pushed spirit or blood into them and then drew it back, likely on the model of Erasistratus.[20]

Students from the Low Countries such as Heurnius and Paaw learned anatomy in the midst of these controversies played out largely in universities in Italy. Volcher Coiter, born in Groningen, educated in Italy, and later working in German lands, dissected a strikingly wide variety of animals. He anatomized frogs, lizards, snakes, fish, eels, pikes, bats, tortoises, hedgehogs, vipers, and especially cats.[21] Instead of writing in terms of prospective procedures like most anatomists from Galen on (e.g., "If you do this, you will see that"), Coiter described what *he had seen* in a variety of dissections and vivisections. He presented singular events, coordinated with other, similar events, as warrants for general knowledge of the movements of "the" heart. Coiter contributed to the rise in status of *historia* and the proliferation of anatomical experiments, joining Vesalius, Falloppio, Colombo, and others.[22]

Coiter detailed his shocking vivisection of a young cat, which he put forward as exemplary in his discussion of the motion of the heart. Throughout, he held fast to his supposed observation of the alternating systole and diastole of the auricles and ventricles (he, like Galen and many others, thought of the ventricles as "the heart" proper). Coiter also followed Galen in thinking of "diastole" or expansion as the active phase—in the vivisection of a viper he recorded that the ventricles expanded with such power that it drew the auricles inward and contracted the vena cava.[23] During the diastole of the ventricles of the cat, he saw "no part or fiber of the heart which does not seem to labor," affirming Galen's praise for the strong and hard-working fibers of the heart.[24] He attended closely to the appearances of color and movement: "As the auricles in diastole on account of the filling of the blood and spirits grow red and are extended, so in systole they grow white and settle down and are made flaccid and wrinkly, and by the power of the heart they are drawn somewhat toward the base of

20   Falloppio, quoted in Bylebyl, "Disputation and Description," 239.
21   Coiter, *Observationum anatomicarum chirurgicarumque miscellanea varia*, in *Externarum et internarum...tabulae*, 125. Schullian, "Coiter, Volcher," 342–343.
22   Ragland, "'Making Trials.'"
23   Coiter, *Observationum anatomicarum chirurgicarumque miscellanea varia*, 126.
24   Galen, *On Anatomical Procedures*, trans. Singer, 182.

the heart."[25] He nearly endorsed Realdo Colombo's revisionist account of the alternation of an actively contracting, expulsive heart dilating the arteries, but could not, faced with his observation of the alternating auricles and ventricles, and the actively dilating ventricles. For Coiter, personal experience in dissections and vivisections, described as discrete, historical events, generated and grounded his claims, and tested even celebrated anatomists' theories about the pulse and motion of the heart.

But such experience or experimentation was not decisive for the community of anatomists, who remained split over the motions of the heart and arteries, and in new ways as new claims to discoveries piled up. One leading anatomist, Caspar Bauhin, established and then reversed his opinion on the order of motions, from alternation to simultaneity, based on vivisections.[26]

Thus Johannes Heurnius adopted the anatomists' emphasis on the epistemic power of personal experience and anatomical vivisections, but avoided walking students through all of the complicated controversy knotting texts across the centuries. In fact, he tried to reconcile points from Aristotle and Galen. He taught his students that recent anatomical observation established the true sequence of the motions of the heart and arteries, as noted above. He confirmed Aristotle's notion that there must be a point of rest between contrary motions of systole and diastole, and emphasized that the sense of "touch diligently practiced" could distinguish these motions *and* two different "rests" between them. The rest between dilation and contraction differed from the period of rest between contraction and dilation; all resulted from the same "pulsific faculty."[27]

Heurnius may well have known of Coiter's writings, since his close colleague Paaw knew and mentioned the very same work, which discussed the motions of the heart, in his own lectures and book.[28] Since not even Coiter had used vivisections of frogs to demonstrate visually the synchronicity of the actions of the heart and arteries, it seems likely that Heurnius here followed evidence from Paaw's own dissections and vivisections of animals, most of which did not reach print. Whatever the origin of his claims about the vivisection of frogs, or the truth of his conclusions, Johannes Heurnius combined humanist erudition with the embrace of ongoing improvements in method, including anatomical experiments. In this case, new experiments apparently confirmed

---

25   Coiter, *Observationum anatomicarum chirurgicarumque miscellanea varia*, 124.

26   Bylebyl, "Disputation and Description," 238.

27   Johannes Heurnius, *Institutiones*, 339.

28   Paaw, *Primitiae Anatomicae*, 145. Coiter, *Observationum anatomicarum chirurgicarumque miscellanea varia*, 109.

ancient knowledge. Increasingly, experiments were the foundations and weapons of attacks.

Even in the early 1600s, students questioned professors' demonstrations of the old knowledge. Students who knew some of the new anatomy also at times critiqued their professors' anatomical practices as erroneous and too hide-bound. Isbrand de Diemerbroeck, a student who had matriculated in November 1627, later reported that he saw professors Otto Heurnius and Adrianus Falcoburgius (or Van Valkenburg, 1581–1650) perforate the interventricular septum of the heart when they pushed in their styluses too forcefully. This replicated an error of the ancient anatomists (notably, Galen), he wrote, who thought that some of the blood traveled through pores in the septum from the right to the left ventricles.[29] Vesalius had already expressed skepticism about such pores in the second edition, 1555, of his *Fabrica*, and Realdo Colombo and other anatomists had defended the impenetrability of the septum in their experimental and theoretical arguments for the pulmonary transit of the blood.[30]

In the wake of new anatomical discoveries, professors and students lived out controversies that provoked first-hand observation and experimentation. Through experimentation Gaspare Aselli discovered a new structure, the lacteal vessels. William Harvey argued for a new theory, the circulation of the blood, based on a range of experimental phenomena. Aselli's 1622 discovery (or re-discovery) of the lacteal vessels, which appeared in print in 1627, 1628, and a Leiden edition of 1640, later combined with Harvey's circulation of the blood to raze the foundations of the Galenic system of digestion and the production of the blood.[31] William Harvey's 1628 book, *Anatomical Exercise On the Motion of the Heart and Blood in Animals*, spurred professors and students to debate his experiments, calculations, and argument for the forceful systole and the circulation of the blood.[32] His work provoked ecstasies of interest and tradition-tempered caution.

In 1631, Leiden student Jacobus Svabius (Jacob Swab or Svabe) enthused about the public dissections of his professors, Otto Heurnius and Falcoburgius, in a letter to his mentor, University of Copenhagen professor Ole Worm

---

29 Diemerbroeck, *Opera Omnia Medica et Anatomica*, 287.

30 Shotwell, "Revival of Vivisection," 189.

31 Gabriele Falloppio may well have discovered the lacteals during his anatomy teaching in the 1550s, per Stolberg, "Teaching Anatomy," 65. Aselli, *De lactibus sive Lacteis venis* (Milan, 1627) (Basel, 1628) (Leiden, 1640). Pomata, "*Praxis Historialis*," 118–121.

32 Harvey, *Exercitatio anatomica de motu cordis et sanguinis in animalibus*. Schouten, *Walaeus*. Frank, *Harvey and the Oxford Physiologists*. French, *Harvey's Natural Philosophy*. Van Lieburg, "Early Reception."

(1588–1654). Svabius wrote that he rejoiced and "gloried in my heart" that Heurnius and Falcoburgius held public dissections of human cadavers three times in recent months. After all, "one cannot deny that living inspection of the artificially dissected cadaver is far to be preferred over those handsome and elaborate pictures...though they are not to be deprived of their own praise, since they feed the eyes and mind with the shadowy idea, yet one cannot concede that it is a true idea."[33] Worm asked in reply if the anatomists had yet demonstrated the lacteal vessels purportedly discovered and recently described by Aselli in his 1627 book. Worm had just seen them for the first time that winter, and recommended Svabius see for himself on this "matter of great moment and usefulness."[34]

Svabius' reply moved from Aselli's novel experimental observations to extended remarks on Harvey's 1628 book on the circulation:

> I am well-informed about a certain new and previously unheard-of opinion published by a certain Englishman about the back-and-forth motion of the blood. This matter affected me so much that for the entirety of fully eight days I burned brightly with higher thoughts of it. But yet since I could scarcely satisfy my soul by myself, I opened every bit of the matter to a certain man, industrious and studious for Medicine, *Conring* by name, whom I know familiarly, and who, having been shown the writings of *Harvey*, was then discoursing about the circulation so outstandingly, so subtly, that he seemed nearly to be in the same heresy. Soon, however, he noticed that his mind, itching for the novelty of the matter, was too titillated, too allured, so that this was his position: this contemplation in itself is indeed elegant, and *prima facie* greatly probable, which if *Harvey* had been able to demonstrate by *autopsia* and anatomical procedure, truly he would have carried the whole point. ... Afterward, I also gathered with the Very Famous Men, *Heurnius* and *Falcoburgius*, who both freely said that they were following in *Conring's* opinion, except that they would add that, rather than being bold and rash, we ought to be more cautious and delay in changing ancient things or approving new ones. See here, the judgment of such great Anatomists about so great a matter, which must be checked by experience.[35]

---

33   Jacobus Svabius (Jacob Swab) to Ole Worm, March 1631 in *Olai Wormii et ad eum Doctorum Virorum Epistolae*, Vol. 1, 458. For Worm see Shackelford, "Documenting the Factual and the Artifactual." Grell, "In Search of True Knowledge."

34   Ole Worm to Jacobus Svabius, 1631 in *Olai Wormii...Epistolae*, 459.

35   Jacobus Svabius to Ole Worm, 13 July 1631, in *Olai Wormii...Epistolae*, 460–461. As elsewhere, italics are in the original.

This candid letter from a Leiden medical student, in the context of a conversation about anatomical novelties, shows the epistemological and social activities of that community's response to the serious matter of Harvey's new circulation doctrine. Svabius took time to read and think over Harvey's book, spending eight days swept away by the observations and argument. He then turned naturally to discussion with a trusted fellow student and friend, Hermann Conring, who had shown the right industry and zeal for learning. Harvey's work carried Conring along, too, drawing his mind and discourse into enthusiasm for the new teaching. The fact that Svabius styled Harvey's teaching as a "heresy" should be taken as tongue-in-cheek. After all, he immediately went on to praise the new doctrine as elegant and greatly probable, but lacking the clinching demonstration to the senses of the circulation itself (the blood moving from the heart to the arteries to the veins and back to the heart). Only *autopsia and anatomical procedure*" could directly demonstrate the circulation and carry the point. The Leiden professors expressed a similar position, with the added caution of the professional experts working with the gradually-modified long tradition of Galenic medicine. Even for them, though, "experience" ought to rule on the matter.

Leiden students learned about Harvey's circulation doctrine in university lectures from the early 1630s, too. In 1633, his first year teaching as an "extra-ordinary" professor, and only two years after receiving his Leiden medical doctorate, Johannes Walaeus (1604–1649) gave lectures on medical theory in a "private" institutes of medicine course.[36] Some of these lectures are preserved in student notes, which we will examine here for the first time. In general, Walaeus kept within the "Asclepian" medical philosophy established by Johannes Heurnius, with Hippocratic and Galenic medicine joining Aristotelian natural philosophy on a foundation of the four qualities and elements, temperaments, and faculties.

Walaeus included discussions of chymical phenomena, continuing the Leiden attention to chymistry. But he defended established Galenic-Hippocratic medical principles against rival chymical philosophies. Like Johannes Heurnius, Walaeus taught the plurality of forms, in which the four elements of earth, water, air, and fire compose flesh and fibers of the body, which then make up the other parts. But the substantial forms of the ingredients remain in the mixed bodies, bound under the superior form.[37] In contrast, "Paracelsus lies" when he claims that the four elements are not fundamental, and that he

---

36   Schouten, *Walaeus*. "Institutiones Medicinae ex privato Collegio Joh: Walaei," Sloane MS 658, 1r.

37   Sloane MS 658, 4v.

has extracted the four elements from the air.[38] The Paracelsian principles of Salt, Sulphur, and Mercury must be composed of the elements, since the four elements cannot be drawn out from them, the Sacred Scriptures do not mention them, and one cannot draw out chymical elements from all substances, such as Salt from metals. But Walaeus showed sustained interest in chymical processes. He described how oil can mix with the caput mortuum or residue from sublimation, and even with seven layers of gold foil. The earthy caput mortuum takes on a gold color, imbibing all the gold, and one cannot separate out the gold for fourteen days. This shows how the substantial forms of even the chymical principles can remain subordinated in a true mixture, to be separated out later.[39]

Walaeus took a similarly partial approach to recent innovations in anatomy, including Harvey's circulation doctrine. He accepted the pulmonary transit of the blood, giving credit for its discovery to Realdo Colombo, and agreed that *some* blood is expelled in each contraction of the ventricles of the heart, but only a tiny amount—a half or a third of a grain.[40] He also claimed that yet-unseen vessels or anastomoses connected the veins to the arteries in the parts of the body.

On balance, the senses and reason argued against the circulation of the blood. Walaeus listed two main claims from Harvey in favor of the circulation: First, that there is so much blood expelled in each contraction of the heart that over a very short period of time the liver cannot provide a sufficient supply. Second, that the veins have valves, and these valves impede the flow of the blood from the heart toward the outer parts, as anyone can see if one ties the veins above a valve (toward the heart), and finds that the blood cannot be pushed back through the valves. In response, Walaeus repeated his claim that the heart ejects very little blood in each contraction, that not *all* the veins have valves, and that one can in fact push blood back through the valves, as "the senses witness."[41] He added four further objections to Harvey: that the circulation makes the venous and arterial blood the same, when it perceptibly is not; that nature has then made the veins and arteries different in vain; that Walaeus cannot understand then how the blood in the veins is moved; and that if there is even a little putrefaction in any blood vessel, which was obviously common from corrupt matter causing diseases, the circulation would quickly move it to

---

38   Sloane MS 658, 4r.
39   Sloane MS 658, 5r–5v.
40   Sloane MS 658, 23v–24r.
41   Sloane MS 658, 25v.

the heart, and ruin that source of life, killing people suddenly. "Which is all as absurd as even a blind man can see."[42]

Other Dutch physicians expressed stronger approval for the new circulation doctrine. In 1638, Leiden and Padua graduate Johan van Beverwijck (1594–1647), famed for his Latin and Dutch medical publications, openly endorsed Harvey's theory in his book on kidney stones.[43] Beverwijck very likely finished his book by 1633, and Beverwijck's friend, Isaac Beeckman, also knew of the circulation of the blood doctrine in Dordrecht. Beeckman was Descartes' mentor in corpuscular-mathematical natural philosophy and recorded notes on Harvey's theory in his diary in June 1633, demonstrating that physicians knew of Harvey's book in Dordrecht, too, early in the 1630s.[44] Beeckman even made suggestions in his notes for intravenous infusions, and corrected earlier therapies, such as the use of some purgatives. Yet, as M. J. van Lieburg has pointed out, Van Beverwijck's publications from the later 1630s continued to use the Galenic doctrines of the blood, not Harvey's. Beeckman, unfortunately, kept his writings unpublished during his lifetime.

One early student put his faith in new anatomical teachings into print and his public disputation. In 1634, Franciscus Dele Boë, called Sylvius (François Dele Boë, 1614–1672) presented a public disputation on a variety of medical topics.[45] He dedicated his *Various Medical Positiones* to his father Isaac, but the *Positions* are Sylvius' own work, since he is listed as the "Auth. & Respondens" (Author and Respondent) on the dedication page.[46] If the propositions defended were penned by his professor Vorstius, then Sylvius could only present himself as "Respondens," as is the case for all the other medical disputations before Sylvius that I have viewed. Sylvius' first five propositions deal with the heart, blood, and brain, and they set out themes which Sylvius would elaborate in his later works. The first two propositions defend the claim that "the vital spirit is

---

42   Sloane MS 658, 26r.

43   Van Beverwijck, *De Calculo Renum & Vesicae Liber singularis*, 20–24. Gemert, "Johann van Beverwijck."

44   Van Lieburg, "The Early Reception of Harvey's Theory," 102–105. Van Berkel, *Isaac Beeckman.*

45   In using this form of his name I am following his own signature, as preserved in the following: Archief van notaris Adriaen [Pietersz.] den Oosterlingh, 1663–1691, 1669, Regionaal Archief Leiden, archiefnummer 506, inventarisnummer 1068, aktenummer 202 and aktenummer 283.

46   I have reviewed twenty-seven prior disputations, all of which present the student only as "Respondens." After Sylvius, and especially in the later 1640s and 1650s, "Author and Respondens" is much more common. Franciscus dele Boë Sylvius, *Positiones Variae Medicae* (Leiden, 1634). I have used the translation provided by Gubser, "The *Positiones Variae Medicae* of Franciscus Sylvius."

generated in the heart," and specifically "from the purer parts of the blood."[47] Interestingly, while the second proposition defends the pulmonary transit of the blood, the third accepts the idea that "something" might "sweat through" the ventricular septum. So far, Sylvius has denied the Galenic idea that vital spirits come from natural spirits, while allowing for the possibility of some sort of transit across the septum.

An emphasis on the material and efficient causes of bodily phenomena and disease is well-represented, even in this short treatise. Sylvius reports, for instance, that salt is the material cause of stones [*calculi*] in the body, with heat as the efficient cause. Nausea and epilepsy are both caused by humors or vapors that irritate the stomach and brain. These material explanations are explicitly framed as refutations of superstitious beliefs. Astrology has no bearing on menstrual cycles, temperaments, or the development of epilepsy, and the "silly idea" that a nightmare is caused by witches compressing the body— believed by "old women"—is equally absurd.[48] For Sylvius, even nightmares are caused by the nature of the humors or vapors affecting anatomical structures: "we believe it to be caused by a thick vapor, which obstructs and compresses the organs dedicated to respiration and the posterior part of the brain near the spinal medulla."[49] Here, he continued Leiden's medicalization of superstitions, extending the naturalization of witchcraft from the Leiden medical faculty's earlier consultation over the water test from 1594.

Sylvius' anatomical claims gradually blended innovations into traditional teaching. The nature and activity of acrid [*acer*] humors to produce an irritation [*irritatio*] are foundational to the pathology and anatomy of Sylvius' first medical work. As elsewhere, he moved along established lines in traditional Galenic medicine to produce a more thoroughly material, observational account for diseases others ascribed to the influence of the planets or even witches. This concept of 'irritation' can be found in Galen, in reference to the contraction of the intestines provoked by the irritating 'sting' of the bile.[50] Yet Sylvius' endorsement of the pulmonary transit of the blood also shows that he was willing to join his professor Walaeus and other physicians and anatomists who increasingly questioned Galen's account of the blood and nutrition. His emphasis on material and efficient causation, and on observable substances over distant entities and hidden powers, was in concert not only

---

47   Sylvius, *Positiones*.

48   Sylvius, *Positiones*.

49   Sylvius, *Positiones*, prop. 30, trans. Gubser.

50   Temkin, "The Classical Roots of Glisson's Doctrine of Irritation," and Pagel, "Harvey and Glisson on Irritability with a Note on Van Helmont."

with contemporary Galenism but also Aristotelian thought that increasingly blurred formal and material-structural modes of causation and turned away from the doctrine of signatures, astrology, and less immediately observable causes.[51]

This was by no means the end of the story. By 1640 Sylvius was back in Leiden with a group of experimentally-minded students such as Thomas Bartholin and Roger Drake, teaching anatomy and demonstrating the circulation of the blood in the garden's Ambulacrum.[52] Their experimental replications and extensions of the work of Aselli and Harvey, and integration of chymistry and anatomy, extended Leiden traditions.[53]

2 Early Clinical Training and Anatomies

The professors and Curators of Leiden University formally established clinical instruction for students among the patients in the city's St. Caecilia Hospital in 1636. The sad deaths of patients there often ended in post-mortem dissections, events prized by students and professors alike. Even foreign professors eagerly inquired after the results of these clinical anatomies. But evidence from the period before the founding of regular hospital instruction shows that students witnessed private anatomies of patients and suggests that students accompanied professors when they treated patients prior to 1636.

Historians have long celebrated the institution of hospital teaching at Leiden, and its even stronger revival in the 1650s and 1660s.[54] They have split opinions, though, on whether a request from the medical faculty to begin clinical instruction in 1591 ever materialized in practice. The medical faculty petitioned to begin clinical instruction on the Paduan model, but the Curators postponed the topic until the next meeting and, apparently, never took it up. J. E. Kroon was optimistic, arguing that it would have been unlikely for the Curators to miss an easy chance to improve the reputation and attractiveness of the university.[55] G. A. Lindeboom and Harm Beukers have read the silence in the university archives as denial.[56]

---

51   Maclean, "Foucault's Renaissance Episteme Reassessed," and Pasnau, "Form, Substance, and Mechanism."

52   Schouten, *Walaeus*, 15–17. Ragland, "Mechanism." Drake, *Disputatio medica de circulatione naturalijj.*

53   A more complete account will appear in the subsequent volume.

54   Beukers, "Clinical Teaching."

55   Kroon, *Bijdragen*, 45.

56   Beukers, "Clinical Teaching."

In my view, the evidence from Johannes Heurnius' own education and Paaw's record of dissections in the hospital and elsewhere demonstrates bedside teaching before 1636, and suggests that some form of clinical instruction occurred in the hospital as well. As we saw in the previous chapter, post-mortem dissections in at least 1598 and 1602 happened with students present and occurred *outside* of the anatomical theater.[57] Paaw also performed several post-mortem dissections to find the causes of disease in the hospital in 1593 and 1594.[58] Perhaps the bedside teaching followed the private *consilia* models often practiced in sixteenth-century Italy, in which small groups of students accompanied professors on their private house calls.[59] Johannes Heurnius "saw medical practice" during his studies at Padua, very likely participating in the bedside teaching developed there from the 1540s.[60] He probably carried this mode of instruction into his own teaching in Leiden, giving the students the practical instruction they demanded through a popular style of bedside teaching in private homes. Groups of students could have easily followed Johannes Heurnius, Paaw, Bontius, and others on their visits to patients, and we know that some students witnessed anatomies in private homes, the hospital, or the *forum boarium*. Paaw even appears to have had more favor in the hospital than Otto Heurnius had in 1623, before the establishment of his program of clinical instruction. Otto's request to enter the hospital in 1623 and dissect a cadaver met with a denial.[61]

Whatever the fate of the 1591 request, post-mortem evidence also made it into the regular lectures and faculty books. Johannes Heurnius drew on post-mortem evidence of diseases for his medical lectures and publications. This is not surprising, given his frequent presence at Paaw's post-mortems and his theoretical understanding of the centrality of localizing diseases and treatments in the organs and parts of the body. He described the cause of phthisis, a rotting, wasting of the lungs and chest which often resembled our tuberculosis, in terms of ulcers of the lungs, eroded by salty or acrid matter, which then formed pus and corruption.[62] He confirmed this diagnosis with references to morbid changes of lungs found in cadavers, such as a short reference to the lungs of a printer, which, he wrote, "I saw," whose lungs resembled a "dried apple" due to salty phlegm flowing down.[63] He had a respectable

57   Paaw, *Observationes*, 29, 31.
58   Paaw, *Observationes*, 14, 15, 19.
59   Stolberg, "Bedside Teaching."
60   [Otto Heurnius], "Vita Auctoris."
61   Kroon, *Bijdragen*, 52.
62   Johannes Heurnius, *De morbis pectoris liber*, 100.
63   Heurnius, *De morbis pectoris liber*, 16.

practice as a physician, for instance treating the scholarship students training for proper Reformed ministry at the Staten College, for which he began to be paid one hundred guilders annually in March 1593.[64] The bedside teaching and post-mortem practices of Paaw and Johannes Heurnius developed even further in the clinical-anatomical work of Johannes' son, Otto Heurnius.

3 Founding Regular Bedside Learning at the Hospital

The founding documents of the program of clinical teaching, the Practical College of the University, detail the close association between regular sense-based bedside instruction and clinical anatomies.[65] Professors usually visited patients every other day on the week days, and sometimes more often when patients first entered the hospital and needed urgent care. City physicians continued the care when professors were not present. Students attended on Wednesdays and Saturdays, days without regularly scheduled lectures or church services for the students. In the hospital, students could learn to track the progress of diseases over time according to the visible signs, debate the diagnosis and causes, witness the effects of treatments, and, with God's favor, see the patients cured or stabilized enough to leave. If patients died, regular clinical anatomies revealed the true seats, causes, and progress of the diseases to the senses. Regular bedside instruction combined with post-mortem dissection allowed professors and students to correlate external signs and symptoms observed in living patients with the evidence of the anatomical and humoral changes previously hidden inside their bodies.

To found this program, Otto Heurnius leveraged student interest, the pressure of a recent plague, and worries over competition from an upstart rival program. Regular bedside instruction in hospitals met long standing student interest in practical, bedside teaching, which had also helped to make Italian universities popular destinations for students in the 1500s.[66] In 1635, a violent epidemic attacked Leiden. Students fled or stayed away, forcing the university to cancel lectures for almost a month.[67] Faculty and administrators at Leiden had enjoyed several decades as the only university in the northern Low Countries, with the University of Groningen founded in 1614 and the Amsterdam

---

64   Otterspeer, *Groepsportret*, I, 157.
65   "Collegium Practicum Academiae," per Otto Heurnius, *Historiae*, 5, 11. Beukers, "Clinical Teaching."
66   Stolberg, "Bedside Teaching"; Huisman, *Finger of God*, 128–131.
67   Molhuysen, *Bronnen*, 2, 193.

Athenaeum in 1632 (though the Athenaeum did not confer degrees).[68] Amsterdam and Utrecht were crowding close, and their professors wanted to out-compete Leiden.

A 1636 announcement from Utrecht jolted Leiden professors and administrators into action. In his inaugural oration on 15 April 1636, just a few weeks after the founding of the university, Utrecht professor of medicine Willem van der Straaten announced his plans to create a program of clinical instruction in the local hospital. As Van der Straaten put it, the program would demonstrate in patients' bodies "the veracity of my lectures," and Utrecht would render to the State physicians trained "not so much in theory but in practice."[69] Van der Straaten had studied at Leiden with Paaw and Otto Heurnius, likely inheriting their keen sense of the value of clinical, practical teaching. Ideally, the Utrecht program enhanced learning by forcing the students to debate the causes, prognosis, and treatment for each patient's medical *historia*.[70] Sadly, the program's disorganization brought about its early end. But it did spur the Leiden Curators to allow Otto Heurnius and his colleagues to establish quickly a program of their own—the Curators discussed Otto Heurnius' proposal less than a month later.

Otto Heurnius aimed his proposal for clinical teaching at the Curators' leverage point: fear of declining student enrollment due to the more attractive, practical program at Utrecht.[71] After learning the fundamentals of medical practice from Johannes Heurnius' *practica* curriculum, students could gain repeated, first-hand experience in diagnosis, prognosis, medicinal and surgical treatment, and post-mortem appearances in the local municipal hospital. Like other early university buildings, the hospital had transformed from a religious site, a convent, to a municipal institution, in this case in the 1590s. By 1614, there were two main rooms with 21 beds for men and 23 for women upstairs and two smaller rooms with 11 beds each for convalescing men and women. A separate room or "plague room" contained 13 beds for patients with contagious diseases.[72] On other levels, the city provided room, board, and medical treatment for elderly citizens without means and those deemed insane. Two city doctors and a surgeon would assist the instruction and treat patients regularly. Otto assured the Curators he would not take students into the plague room, with its dangers of deadly contagion, but would "show the causes of death to the

---

68   Van Miert, *Humanism*.
69   Beukers, "Clinical Teaching."
70   Kyper, *Methodus*, 255.
71   Molhuysen, *Bronnen*, 2, 312*.
72   Huisman, *Finger of God*, 126.

students" in the bodies of select patients who had died.[73] He recommended the city surgeon Joannes Camphusius (or Joannes Camphuysen), for the official job, as someone "of good experience besides in surgery, also in anatomy, medicine, and pharmacy." Experience grounded expertise in manual practice, teaching, and witnessing.

All of the plans emphasized the importance of combining clinical observations with the viewing of the injured parts in the bodies of unfortunate patients who died. For the second draft of the plan, the Curators solicited the advice of another professor of medicine, Adolph Vorstius, who led its formulation among the whole medical faculty. They endorsed most of the provisions in the draft, with students and the oldest medical professors visiting the hospital on Wednesdays and Saturdays, along with the two hospital physicians, and on any other days which would not interfere with the official course of lectures. Any extraordinary surgical procedures or rare cases would also draw students whenever possible. At the bedside, students could exercise their skills in the knowledge of diseases, their causes and signs, especially through uroscopy and the pulse, and treatment by indications and remedies. To give students a complete history and record of the medicines used, the hospital doctors should record their treatments. Finally, it was "very profitable and necessary" that surgeons open the bodies of those patients who died of internal diseases, so the students could see with their own eyes the damaged parts and unnatural constitutions.[74]

The official vision for the program in hospital teaching took up the professors' recommendations, a vision they clearly tried to follow in practice: "The Professor, with both the ordinary city doctors ... with the students, together with a good surgeon, will visit the sick persons in the public hospitals, and examine the nature of their internal diseases, as well as all their external accidents, and debate their cures and surgical operations, prescribing medicines according to the order of the hospital, and, also, will open all the dead bodies of the foreign or unbefriended persons there and show the causes of death to the students."[75] The city hospital provided beds set in roomy galleries with large windows, food, and care to patients from among the poor and those with little family support, so that learned professors and wealthy or gentle students exercised social power over them. This power was not total, since the patients that the city physicians recommended for admission had to sign an application

---

73   Molhuysen, *Bronnen*, 2, 312*.

74   Molhuysen, *Bronnen*, 2, 315*.

75   Molhuysen, *Bronnen*, 2, 312*.

and the office of the mayor oversaw the process.[76] And sometimes families of other social levels wanted elite physicians to perform autopsies on their loved ones' bodies, too. Otto Heurnius extended his practice of private anatomies to cadavers well beyond the "foreign and unbefriended," as we will see in the next section. Knowing through direct sensation was too valuable, making autopsies an option for all sorts of bodies.

4   Causes, Histories, and Therapy Displayed in Diseased Bodies

From 1636 to 1641, at least, Otto Heurnius combined newly-vigorous clinical teaching with clinical anatomies—post-mortem dissections in the hospital. Descriptions of twenty-six clinical anatomies include nineteen of them dated from the first period of official hospital teaching, 1636 to 1641, as well as accounts of other post-mortem dissections ranging from 1624 to 1646. Even more detailed than the historical accounts recorded by Paaw, they offer a rich source for understanding Otto Heurnius' practice of clinical anatomy in the context of understanding the causes of diseases and teaching students bed-side practice. Strikingly, as we will see, students could follow their own senses to reason to different emphases and observations. Professors' demonstrations and discussions were not accepted blindly, and students had the power and wit to object. In most of these cases, a surgeon performed the dissection and Otto Heurnius pointed out the morbid appearances and picked out the causes. Many occurred in the hospital itself, in a room adapted for post-mortem dissections and discussion, just off the south entrance.[77] Otto Heurnius explicitly recorded students as present for seven of these clinical anatomies, including one presided over by his colleague in clinical teaching, Ewaldus Screvelius.

In his clinical anatomies, Otto Heurnius elaborated on the embodied erudition of Leiden academic medical pedagogy, combining Galenic precedents with hands-on and sensory experience. In 1634, his planned publications to strengthen the reputation of the university included first of all introductory lectures or "Praelectiones" on practical medicine. Naturally, Otto Heurnius chose to comment and expand on Galen's *On the Affected Places* (*De locis affectis*), the standard work on the pathology and therapy of injured organs and parts of the body from head to foot. This experience-enhanced

76   Lindeboom, *Herman Boerhaave*, 287. Beukers, "Clinical Teaching," 143.
77   Huisman, *Finger of God*, 133–135.

commentary on Galen's essential work of pathology and therapy embraced "the whole of practice."[78]

Despite the scholarly pedigree and practitioners, clinical anatomy was not pleasant. The sights and horrible smells of the internal states of disease-wracked bodies—corruption, stinking pus, wasted organs, hydropsical fluid, morbid blood—did not neatly comport with ideals of bookish learning or gentlemanly sociability. But the admitted disgust only underscores the value students and professors placed on it.

One case illustrates this memorably. In 1640, Ysbet Gillis thought she was pregnant for six months. Then, suddenly, she died. It was some comfort that they found no baby within. Horribly, the swollen belly had developed from the pressure of a wasting liver, an empyema which turned the parenchyma of the liver into pus and flatus: "cut in various places with a razor, and pressed gently with a blunt instrument, the pus burst out onto those students standing nearby."[79] This was hard-won knowledge! Otto Heurnius may not have performed the dissections himself, as Paaw apparently did, but he demonstrated the causes of death in the localized lesions in organs and parts, lesions uncovered by the dissecting actions of expert surgeons. As Paaw did before him, Otto Heurnius presented these skilled and learned surgeons as reliable witnesses.

Only by direct sensation could students and professors really know diseases, and, in the opening of cadavers, perceive directly the material causes of a patient's disease and death. As Otto Heurnius put it in 1639, "with the Chest and Abdomen opened, we detected every cause of the malady."[80] For another patient's body, in 1636, that of the clothmaker Joannes de Neeff, Otto "demonstrated, explaining the causes of death; dissection performed by Mr Joannis Camphusius, ordinary surgeon of the Republic of Leiden"[81] At other times, such as in 1638 with the body of Johannes Hax, they could not locate any clear cause of morbid developments. Hax had sustained a contusion of his ribs, which then began to putrefy. No organ of the abdomen displayed sure signs of preternatual affects; not even the nearby lungs appeared corrupted. A fair amount of pus had collected in the abdomen, but, "When we had accurately investigated the cause of this, we were not able to grasp any cause by ocular confidence, nor comprehend any reason."[82] As always, organs were central. With no morbid changes to organs visible or otherwise perceptible, Otto Heurnius could find

---

78   Molhuysen, *Bronnen*, 2, 191.
79   Otto Heurnius, *Historiae*, in Fernel, *Universa Medicina* (1656), 23.
80   Otto Heurnius, *Historiae*, 19.
81   Otto Heurnius, *Historiae*, 4.
82   Otto Heurnius, *Historiae*, 16.

no seats for impaired faculties and their actions which would generate all that poorly concocted pus. What the senses detected, especially the sense of sight, set the bounds of their inferences to reasons and causes.

Students followed the lead of their professors, though some with prior anatomical training emphasized different phenomena. These pedagogical exercises were not mere demonstrations of existing knowledge that left students passive receptacles. Thomas Bartholin (1616–1680), who came from a family of scholars and physicians in Denmark, described several clinical anatomies in 1638 and 1639. Bartholin's description of the goals of the practice, and its emphasis on things discoverable by the senses, echoed the official pronouncements:

> With the recent sabbath day elapsed, in the public Hospital in individual weeks the proteges of Asclepius and the Practical Professor of Medicine come together, so that they may inquire into the nature of diseases, their causes and remedies, and I was present for the dissection of a human cadaver. We were occupied in the investigation of the hidden cause of death, but truly from the more principal parts, which were preternatural, we found none, for which reason the cause was referred to the spirits or humors.[83]

Otto Heurnius and Bartholin agreed on the standard procedure: check the principal organs (brain, heart, liver) first for morbid lesions, since those governed the chief psychic, vital, and nutritive faculties. Absent perceptible morbid changes to those, check other organs such as the lungs. Without clear evidence of disease, then perhaps the humors or spirits (subtly material vapors) were at fault. Bartholin continued to follow and depart from his professors' teaching. In the public dissection of a criminal in the anatomy theater, Bartholin and the other students "observed nothing peculiar," following the usual tour of the muscles, spleen, liver, and other viscera, but Otto Heurnius "haughtily" taught the wrong anatomy of some of the muscles.[84] Bartholin had the good fortune to be among the "four students picked each week to visit the sick daily" in the hospital. In one cadaver, he noted an unusually large liver and a spleen bigger than any he had ever seen before. The great size of the patient's arteries and veins correlated with his prior suffering from the disease of plethora, caused by an excess of blood.

---

83   Thomas Bartholin to Ole Worm, 3 October 1638, in *Olai Wormii...Epistolae*, 653.
84   Thomas Bartholin to Ole Worm, 4 January 1639, in *Olai Wormii...Epistolae*, 655.

Comparing the accounts of Bartholin and his professor Otto Heurnius on the same cases reveals important differences. Bartholin also sent summaries of his notes on two other hospital dissections, those of Johannes Hax and Thomas Walter. Interestingly, Bartholin largely concurred with his professor Otto Heurnius' account of the spread of corruption and vomica in the case of Hax, but emphasized the morbid spleen and appendix in the cadaver of Walter. While Otto Heurnius had stressed the exsanguinated, denser, dryer, and blacker nature of many of the viscera, Bartholin only described them as "moderate" in appearance.[85]

This clinical teaching at Leiden enacted testing or trial-making in two ways. First, Otto Heurnius tested the students' knowledge by soliciting diagnoses and prognoses at the bedside. As his colleague Albert Kyper described it, "he showed to them the questioning of patients, and asked them in order their opinion about the disease, its causes and Symptoms, the prognosis and care, and in the last place put forth his own opinion."[86] Like most testing, this annoyed the students. They preferred Otto Heurnius simply give them the answer, laying out his own learned opinions on each case. So, he dropped the bedside quizzes, offering only his own explanations. This, no doubt, was easier on the students, and it seems to have fit with prior practices. Having the professors discourse, especially in groups of three or more, on diagnoses and therapies had formed the core teaching of previous practical "colleges" for the University of Padua.[87] If Leiden students changed their minds and wanted to continue presenting their own ideas, though, Otto Heurnius hoped to restore the old method "promptly."

Second, Leiden clinical instruction tested the proffered diagnoses and prognoses by the evidence of a patient's recovery, or, in the unfortunate cases, the anatomical evidence of the patient's disease lesions in the dissected cadaver. Only post-mortem dissections allowed professors and students to detect "every cause of the malady." Without perceptible morbid appearances of organs to license inferences to altered temperaments and impaired faculties, they could not "grasp any cause by ocular confidence, nor comprehend any reason."[88] Naturally, the material causes of diseases met the materials and faculties of medicines in clinical practice.

---

85   Otto Heurnius, *Historiae*, 17. Thomas Bartholin to Ole Worm, 4 January 1639, in *Olai Wormii...Epistolae*, 656.
86   Kyper, *Methodus*, 256.
87   Stolberg, "Bedside Teaching," 641.
88   Otto Heurnius, *Historiae*, 4, 16.

5   Diseases and Remedies from Across the Dutch Empire

Patients, diseases, and remedies came to Leiden from across the geography
and social levels of the emerging Dutch empire. Like Paaw, Otto Heurnius dissected a range of subjects from across the Dutch republic and empire, not just
those of a low or marginal status. In 1617, almost certainly in a private anatomy, he dissected "Aeltje Vergraft, only daughter of Timonis van der Graft, married to Cornelius Sprong, my kinswoman, a noblewoman."[89] In the hospital,
he dissected the body of a young girl of fourteen years, and several artisans,
including clothmakers, woodworkers, and repairers. Otto Heurnius and his
colleagues also tried out novel remedies from the medical traditions of indigenous peoples in Brazil, new chymical treatments, and surgical interventions.

   He treated a foot soldier of the growing Dutch global empire, too. This
case shows not only the resistance of indigenous species but also the clinical practice of Otto Heurnius, as he and his colleagues tried different remedies for the causes and symptoms, including an attempted recreation of an
indigenous treatment. On February 6, 1637, after five weeks of treatment in
the hospital, Otto wrote down the clinical history of a soldier from the Dutch
West Indies Company in Brazil, Thomas van der Guychten. Even the tiniest
inhabitants of Brazil had mounted a counter-attack. The soldier's feet, like
those of many others, became host to tiny parasitic flea-like animals, called
"Ton" after the word of the natives (likely *Tunga penetrans*). These invaders
caused intense burning and itching, and red bumps with white spots in the
middle. Soon, gangrene would set in. In Thomas' case, the tiny fleas penetrated
and corrupted his fingers as well as his toes. Doctors tried remedies including
wraps and ointments with cannabis, absinth, red wine, and honey. The first
ingredient, cannabis, supposedly dulled the pain and itching, and the others
worked against the corruption. Otto Heurnius even assisted in the attempt to
re-create an indigenous remedy for this Brazilian malady, including Peruvian
bark from South America to imitate the color, consistency, and powers of the
indigenous people's "oil of Couroq."[90] Repeated washings and applications of
various ointments—especially those modeled on indigenous remedies—over
the course of a month saw the fevers and paroxysms subside, and the gangrenous spots shrink. With the help of indigenous ingredients and remedies,
applied by the learned physicians (and not the scalpel of the surgeon, who had
failed), this soldier of Dutch empire lived after his brush with minute invaders.

89   Otto Heurnius, *Historiae*, 27.
90   Otto Heurnius, *Historiae*, 8.

In the soldier's case, as in the other histories of successful treatments, the physicians varied their treatments based on their best guesses about what would work—based on similar cases and some theory of drug faculties—and whether they appeared to be working in a particular patient. They needed remedies with faculties of "washing, bathing, restoring flesh, scar-building," and purging of morbid matter. To purge the soldier's body of morbid matter they used known purgatives cassia, rhubarb, agaric, and cinnamon at night and a laxative in the morning. The "golden ointment" of cannabis, honey, tincture of Peruvian bark, and other ingredients worked directly on the wound to fight putrefaction and restore flesh. The patient, Thomas, improved over more than four weeks of hospital care. His fever went away, his bowels opened up, he passed dark-colored morbid matter, and much of his flesh regrew after nearly all of the gangrenous spots healed. As Thomas convalesced, Otto Heurnius varied the remedies. He applied a much gentler purgative three weeks in, when Thomas had no fever and passed only a little dark-colored matter in his urine. Since the purgative used for weeks seemed to work, Otto Heurnius stuck with the recipe but reduced the amounts of rhubarb and other ingredients by a factor of two or three. A resistant spot of gangrene in the toe bone of Thomas' right foot, though, required surgical ablation, and then a new, gentle decoction and ointment to promote further healing.

Interestingly, book learning enabled novel personal experience with new remedies, as Otto Heurnius tried to recreate the indigenous "oil of Couroq" based on the recommendation of the writings of Jean de Lery, a French Protestant colonist who had lived among indigenous peoples in Brazil for a time, and whose book his father had also read.[91] Lery claimed that the "oil of Couroq" ointments worked for the indigenous patients as well as Frenchmen like himself.[92] Book learning and clinical practice went hand-in-hand, even for novel diseases and treatments.

Patients received surgical procedures when Otto Heurnius and the surgeon Joannes Camphusius determined that medicines would be ineffective, but always in conjunction with remedies that would cleanse and restore local intemperances. Petrus Wilhelmus, a muscular, solid young man resisted the plague raging in Leiden in 1635. Twelve hundred people died in *one week* (out of a population of about 50,000), but his "robust nature" repelled the poison of the plague, which settled far from his heart—the seat of the vital faculties—and corrupted his foot.[93] An empiric tried zinc oxide and rose oil, but this

91   Otto Heurnius, *Historiae*, 7. Johannes Heurnius, *Institutiones* (1638), 229.
92   Lery, *Historia Navigationis in Brasiliam quae et America Dicitur*, 137.
93   Van Maanen, "De Leidse bevolkingsaantallen in de 16de en 17de eeuw," 64.

superficial treatment did not work and the rot spread to his foot's cuboidal bones. After the surgeon Camphusius explored the depth of the ulcer, and found the bone corrupted, he and Otto Heurnius determined that all medicines would be ineffective in reaching and cleansing the "porous structure of the bones." Instead, they used general purgatives to purge any loose morbid matter, as well as a cold, wet diet to alter the palpably dry, hot morbid corruption. Then, Camphusius cut out the corrupted bones, "to the wailing and tortured misery of the sick man."[94] Finally, as in the case of the soldier above, Camphusius applied a series of dressings with cannabis, vinegar, red wine, citrus juice, and spirit of vitriol. These cleansed the wound and promoted the growth of new flesh. After three weeks, the cavity regrew new flesh, and the patient recovered his health.

As seen here, Otto Heurnius also used chymical medicines, likely continuing the strong interest in chymistry established at Leiden by his father, Johannes. From at least 1617 to 1635, Otto Heurnius used oil or spirit of vitriol (dilute sulfuric acid) to treat fevers and clean out morbid matter from patients' bodies. Here, he followed the strong recommendation of Paracelsus, who trumpeted vitriol as the best of purgatives for clearing out obstructions.[95] He also applied the iron-based styptic of Paracelsus for a man with a knife-wound in his belly.[96] Most of his remedies relied on plant ingredients, but he clearly adopted some chymical medicines, especially those made by distillation of metal mixtures (oil or spirit of vitriol comes, in our terms, from the distillation of copper or iron sulfate).

When patients died, students and professors could compare the anatomical evidence of the progress of their diseases with their unsuccessful treatment regimens, and with the histories of symptoms and treatments from the successful cases. In every case, contrary to recent claims, Otto Heurnius and his colleagues received permission from the relatives of the deceased, whenever possible.[97] Joannis Pauli's body became a dissection subject only with his wife's permission.[98] Sometimes, the spouse could be shockingly enthusiastic. In 1640, Otto Heurnius and his colleagues obtained permission to dissect the body of sixty-year-old Evert Baerentsen, who had died from an infected aposteme or purulent ulcer of the liver. He had felt pain there, and there was notable swelling for some time. "He died in this state on the 18th of February,

---

94   Otto Heurnius, *Historiae*, 11.
95   Paracelsus, *Paragranum*, in Weeks, *Paracelsus*, 238.
96   Otto Heurnius, *Historiae*, 13.
97   *Pace* Huisman, *Finger of God*, 142.
98   Otto Heurnius, *Historiae*, 26.

but since his wife *had still been noted as alive, we would not open the cadaver without her consent, which on similar occasions was always done from the mandate of the prefects of the hospital.*"[99] When asked, Evert's wife had no compunctions about the autopsy: "Why would I not concede this to you with him dead, whom, while he was living, I often wished to the devil?"[100] As we might expect today, at times family members resisted offering a loved one's body up for dissection, but in other cases years of resentment eased the decision.

6   Tracking Diseases by Clinical Signs and Post-Mortem Evidence

Following Paaw and good Galenic-Hippocratic teaching, Otto Heurnius trained his students to attend carefully to the colors, textures, smells, and tangible changes of bodies living and dead. His practice of combining clinical teaching and anatomies is best seen in full detail, with his humanist learning, attention to colors and textures, reconstruction of the historical progress of the disease, and the witnessing of colleagues and students on display. Otto Heurnius' attention to details and his practical and anatomical learning paint a fine portrait of expert pedagogy, one best seen up close:

> Otto Heurnius, 1636
> In the year 1636, 21st of December, after lunch, the cadaver of *Joannes de Neeff*, of Flanders, was dissected, a clothmaker, a celibate man of 35 years of age. He was of a very soft native constitution, thin, and with a smooth surface of skin. With a sanguineous temperament, inclined toward bile. He lived in Leiden in the neighborhood of the garden of the archers, in the gate area, where in the year 1635 the plague had violently prowled. It caught him in the year 1636 in May with pleuritis [inflammation of the pleural membranes around the lung] in the left side; bloodletting, while the chance still flourished, was neglected, and therefore a rampaging humor changed places, moving from the pleura into the lungs, and made them inflamed, and generated pneumonia, toward which there was a great opportunity in this body due to the tight connections of its parts.
> The cause of such a malady we judged to be a malign pestilent quality which was then nested in those locations and neighbors; whence the humors were violently inflamed and impacted in those parts. Of course, since they had the pestilential thorn, they were seeking the heart for the

---

99   Otto Heurnius, *Historiae*, 23. Italics in original.
100   Otto Heurnius, *Historiae*, 23.

indwelling poison, but were repulsed by the strength of the heart, so they settled into the nearby weaker parts, creating violent pneumonia there with a great coughing of blood by expectoration. At last it crossed over, and the disease was changed into empyema or suppuration of the lungs, then into wretched discharge, for he was spitting out the substance of the lungs turned to pus. With this monstrous wasting disease of the lungs, accompanied by a symptomatic, hectic [chronic and whole-body], and marasmus-like [wasting] fever, and continual wakefulness for the space of two weeks before death, at last in the year 1636, on December 20th, around noon he calmly expired in bed. None of those who were in the same room noticed any struggle in his death.

The mind perpetually stands fixed at that fatal hour. The whole body was dry and sucked out, muscles clearly exhausted, and dried out.

Hard skin through which the viscera could be seen,

Dry bones stuck out under the crooked back

The belly was below the location of the belly, so that you would think it hung from it

The chest, held from the spine as if by wickerwork

[Four line quotation from Ovid, *Metamorphoses* 8.803[101]]

In the left side of the lung we detected that the pleura was unmolested, the lung however was firmly attached to the pleurae, ribs, and pericardium. The membranes there covering the lung were whole, when it was dissected it was shown to be whole and the stain showed itself, for in all those individual wings of the lung, or lobes, there existed abscesses of empyema. The whole parenchyma [the substance of the lungs] was liquefied into a thick pus, white, withered, the greater part of which the wretched sick man had ejected with harsh coughing. For at night and throughout the day he was harassed by this restless vexation. Only the substance of the major vessels, and those of the little connecting membranes, remained dry and bloodless, which was seen in the likeness of a sparse net in texture. To which adhered the thickened and dense purulent matter, mixed with sticky phlegm, just as in we see cling to fishing nets and the swamp grass in lakes. In the right side of the chest the other lobe was plainly swimming freely, not connected by any little nets of the membranes to any part. Outside it was whole and of a natural constitution, but when we felt it to explore whether or not it hid any ulcer, we noticed a hardness in the depth of his upper lobe; then having made a

---

101   Ovid, *Metamorphoses, Volume I: Books 1–8*, trans. Miller, revised by Goold, 460–461.

dissection, we grasped that in the middle region of the parenchyma there was a closed ulcer, and this not insignificant in size, which when dissected poured out much corrupt matter. From this monstrous corrupting of the lung, with the vital spirits and the whole of the blood depraved, thus the temperament of the parts of the whole body was weakened, and their vital strength consumed, and their substance melted. And from this, and from the defect of the natural faculty in cooking and retaining the nutritive juice, with the continual flow [diarrhea] of the belly assisting, thus all the viscera were dried up, so that in the liver, spleen, and kidneys not a drop of blood was detected. All were hard from the dryness, but especially the liver, which was very large, and of an equally dry constitution, without any stones of scirrhus. The substance and color of the pericardium, just as the membranes of the mediastinum, were of the natural constitution, but not covered with any fat. Dissected, a more copious and yellowish matter was seen than is naturally customary.

When the heart was dissected transversely no blood then poured out, except afterward a very little when we investigated and demonstrated the courses of the vessels from their openings, for then from the Aortal Artery and the vena cava a little blood flowed back into the Heart. However the substance of the heart was of a good enough constitution, and its coronary vessels were distended with blood. The omentum was devoid of all fat, so that it was as a bare membrane interwoven with vessels, and it even increased the weakness of the coction of the stomach and intestines. The stomach was small, and its entirety from the bottom through the length, and the many gastric roots from the Portal vein, and the insertion of the gastric aepiploic appendices, were manifestly conspicuous, since they protruded through the omentum, and were also implanted around the intestinal Colon. Indeed the omentum was connected to the Colon at the base of the stomach, whence there is the greatest sympathy of their parts, both on account of this connection and, or especially, on account of the communion of their vessels; whence the appetite and coction of the stomach are destroyed by the stagnating feces in the Colon. This was observed by the very distinguished and very erudite doctor of medicine Sebastian Eckert, Consul of the Republic of Amsterdam, in his notes on the Practice of Dodonaeus, about a certain woman who for a long time was tortured by pain and pica, whether she was dead calm or vexed, and was not able to be placated except after eating raw fish. After death her dissected colon was found distended with dense flatus, by which provocations she was driven to devour raw fish; thus vulgarly it was judged that she had an otter in her belly. *Otto Heurnius*, ordinary Professor of Practical Medicine,

Anatomy, and Surgery, was demonstrating, and explaining the causes of death, with many students of Medicine nearby, and *Dr. Damianus Weissens*, and *Dr. Johannes Moerbergius*, ordinary Physicians of the Republic of Leiden. With *Mr. Joannes Camphusius* administering the dissection, ordinary Surgeon of the Republic of Leiden, particularly appointed to this duty by the Curators of the Academy, and the Governors of the Republic of Leiden.[102]

To mine the riches of this passage, take a step-by-step approach. First, reconstruct the clinical reasoning from the first half of the history. The patient's body naturally tended toward thinness and softness. Contagion from the plague had infected the membrane of his lung on the left side, producing pleurisy. While the inflammation there grew and fluid built up, there was a chance for successful treatment by bloodletting to reduce the inflammation and expel the morbid matter. The corrupt humor then flowed in to the adjacent lungs, producing pneumonia. He coughed up blood and then pus. He suffered from a hectic and wasting fever for two weeks, which dried out his body and drained it, and then he died without a struggle. Naturally, Otto Heurnius' humane sympathy and humanist erudition framed this tragic sight with lines from Ovid's *Metamorphoses*.

Next, compare the evidence and inferences of the post-mortem dissection. Otto Heurnius began by working in order through the anatomical seats of the diseases observed through the patient's symptoms. First, he penetrated to the pleurisy on the side of the left lung, noting the buildup of pus of the empyema. Then, he moved from the site of pleurisy into the lungs, or what remained of the lungs. The substance of the left lung had eroded away and turned to pus, apparently, with sticky pus and phlegm left on the major vessels and their membranes like the sea slime on fishing nets. The right lung, too, had a large hard abscess which opened to pour out more corrupt matter. Most of the other major organs of the chest and abdomen appeared dried out, with no blood in them. The heart seemed healthy, but the obvious connecting vessels between the stomach and colon suggested a strong connection of a similar substance, or "sympathy," for the stagnating corruption from the colon to the stomach.

Throughout, Otto Heurnius concentrated on things revealed to his senses of sight and touch: obvious processes of corruption of the lungs and dried out, wasted viscera. He saw major parts of the lungs apparently turned to pus, and filled with abscesses or ulcers which poured out corrupt fluid when dissected.

---

102   Otto Heurnius, *Historiae*, 1–2.

The major viscera—the liver, kidneys, and spleen, appeared visibly and tangibly dry—he notes that they are hard and without blood. The thickened, dense pus in the lungs was clearly sticky, like the phlegmy gunk often seen clinging to fishing nets.

Throughout his clinical anatomies, Otto Heurnius traced the close interrelations of the generation and movements of morbid matter and the failure of organ actions and faculties. The localization of disease comes through clearly, as the morbid matter moves to different parts and necessarily generates different diseases by impairing or injuring different local actions. Different impairments produce different diseases, from pleurisy in the pleura of the left lung to pneumonia in the neighboring lungs. The morbid matter moved locally, to nearby parts, and according to "sympathy," which again meant anatomical connections, especially vessels for the movement of fluids, and a similarity of temperaments and material structure, as in the case of the colon, stomach, and omentum. Here, Otto Heurnius followed his father's teaching.[103] The patient's anatomical structures mattered greatly for these connections, and for the tendencies toward inflammation, especially since the unusually "tight connections" of his body's parts made blockage, inflammation, and pneumonia more likely. The large, pus-filled ulcer found first as a hardened mass in the lung, then dissected, licensed an inference to the blockage and impairment of the lungs.

In health, according to the best theory, the lungs functioned to give out excess heat from around the heart, the hottest region of the body, and to bring in and refine vital spirits from the air, which the heart would mix with the blood in the left ventricle to make vivifying arterial blood for the whole body. With the lungs putrefying into pus, they could not perform their natural actions and functions, and the body wasted away, deprived of vital arterial blood. He embraced the temperament and faculty theory we saw earlier was a mainstay of Leiden teaching: "thus the temperament of the parts of the whole body was weakened, and their vital strength consumed." Change in qualitative temperament of course weakened the nutritive and other faculties of the body's organs, so that the stomach, intestines, and liver could not turn food into good nutritious venous blood, but instead produced only poorly-concocted matter, in a constant "flow" or diarrhea of the belly.

Like Paaw before him, Otto Heurnius also connected notable features of this case to other, similar ones, for example linking the sticky, purulent matter like that found on fishing nets in the case above to the similar appearances of the

---

103   Johannes Heurnius, *Nova Ratio*, 473.

diseased lungs in the eleventh case. He also connected this case to another one noted by a fellow physician, Sebastian Eckert, in a textual report. This report also marked off the learned physicians' expertise—tutored and confirmed by a post-mortem of the woman suffering from pica—from the vulgar or common story that she had a voracious otter in her belly. And he secured the epistemic status of the appearances of the dissections by noting the witness of students, physicians, and his assisting surgeon, Mr. Camphusius. They had the requisite expertise and official status recognized by the university and the Republic of Leiden. It is worth noting that Otto Heurnius presented himself here and in other recorded cases as not only "demonstrating," in the traditional anatomical practice of showing structures and connections, but also "explaining" the causes of disease and death. Theory met practice at the bedside and the dissecting table.

There are strong continuities in the practice of clinical anatomies from Paaw to Otto Heurnius, especially in their use of their senses. Both, like other anatomists, relied on the senses of sight and touch to detect or grasp "accurately" the state of organs and other parts of the body. Both anatomist-physicians directed their attention to sites of corruption, especially in the form of purulent sores or "vomica" of the lungs, ulcers, scrofulous swelling, or the wasting away of parenchyma into pus. At times, their senses of smell also helped to confirm "very horrible" scents of morbid putrefaction.

Like Paaw, Otto Heurnius attended closely to major organs and the separating membranes of the body, as we see in the case above. He also looked for blockages in major veins, which would indicate that insufficient nutrifying blood could reach the distal organs, or other changes such as coldness or wounds which would harm an organ's normal processes of nutrition and action. Poor coction or nutrition of major organs such as the liver and lungs resulted in the production and buildup of waters (usually yellowish) in the chest and abdomen. They also used touch to assess morbid substances, such as testing how far one could pull sticky phlegm from a diseased heart with the fingers.[104] In this way, they applied the quintessential anatomists' senses of sight and touch to morbid organs and material.[105]

Proper sensory training became a prime feature of Leiden clinical teaching in the anatomy room, too. Whenever he had the chance to dissect a body with his colleagues, Otto Heurnius explicitly taught students to examine all the major organs possible, noting their "structure, tone, and temperament."[106]

---

104   Otto Heurnius, *Historiae*, 24.
105   Klestinec, *Theaters of Anatomy*, 42–54, 73.
106   Otto Heurnius, *Historiae*, 21.

For structure, visual inspection allowed professors and students to judge whether an organ seemed preternaturally large or small, or malformed in some way. Touch and sight together revealed the organs' tone and temperament, sensing morbidly dry, flaccid, swollen, rotting, or discolored body parts (such as livers or ovaries blackened by corrupt vapors, or hearts and kidneys dried out and wasted by insufficient nutritious blood or excess heat and dryness). Sight and touch together indicated an organ's temperament, such as in a visibly shriveled organ dry to the touch, or blackened livers and kidneys from hot diseases.

Otto Heurnius also followed the traces of disease by asking where it hurt, and how—just as he and other Leiden students had been taught for decades in his father's courses (as discussed in chapter five). As Otto Heurnius taught his own students in a 1638 case, it was of great importance in medical practice "to observe and distinguish the various kinds, size, and duration of pains, and from these we know the part affected, the cause of the affect, and the outcome."[107] A jabbing pain indicates an affected membrane, and a spread-out pain a membrane distended with copious matter. An oppressive or heavy pain acts in a fleshy part, and a pulsing pain in the part that suffers, with the arteries woven in it. Different parts had characteristic pains with their common diseases: a heavy pain in the kidney indicated a stone in the flesh or sometimes an abscess, while a pulsing pain meant that the stone cut into the pelvis.

From such site-specific pains, Otto Heurnius taught, together with the "Nature of the injured part," and the constitution of the disease, the physician should derive the foundations of all curative indications, or sure signs for treatment. Pain in a patient's right side, below the heart, strongly suggested an injured liver, especially when combined with the visible signs of a swollen feet and belly.[108] Another patient, coming home drunk one night, had fallen from the top step of a very high staircase, but showed no obvious signs of broken bones. The surgeon drew out eight ounces of blood from the cephalic vein in his head as a preventative against cranial hemorrhage, but the man remained seemingly comatose. When he awoke, he complained that his whole body hurt, and he had a violent pain on the right side of his face, "where the muscle of the lower temporal maxilla is attached."[109] (The anatomical precision of this pain is striking.) Later, when the patient complained of a pain in his forehead, Otto Heurnius or another physician or surgeon touched him there, but the patient felt no pain from that.

---

107   Otto Heurnius, *Historiae*, 16.
108   Otto Heurnius, *Historiae*, 23.
109   Otto Heurnius, *Historiae*, 5.

From the patient's own reported perception of localized pain, and reliable knowledge of the anatomical sites of different types of pains, Otto Heurnius and his students could pinpoint injured parts and identify types of diseases. In this way, they put into daily practice and pedagogical instruction the long Galenic tradition of differential diagnosis of organs and diseases based on the types and locations of pains. Otto Heurnius' father Johannes had mined Galen's writings to develop and practice his own typologies of pains, as we have seen in chapter five.

Leiden hospital pedagogy also used post-mortem dissections to track down the pathways of morbid matter to their bodily origins with a standard method. Otto Heurnius had the surgeon doing the cutting follow a regular pattern of dissecting and examining the major organs of the chest and abdomen, and sometimes the head, not just the morbid organs.[110] In the case of Joannes de Neeff above, the patient's history and symptoms clearly indicated a localized pleurisy and empyema of the lungs generated as a corrupt humor moved from the left pleura to the left lung and then the right. Otto Heurnius and the surgeon Camphusius attended closely to the lesions of the lungs, but also dissected the liver, spleen, kidneys, stomach, heart, omentum, and some vessels of the abdomen. We see similar attention to all the major organs of the chest and abdomen in most of the other dissections, including some cases of systematic dissection well beyond the clear points of injury. In the 1638 case of Johannes Hax who fell and broke ribs on his right side, the gangrene and corruption clearly resided on his right side. Yet Otto Heurnius still carefully dissected both lungs, his heart, and the organs of his abdomen, which showed no organ seriously affected "beyond nature." Thus, they could not grasp any reason for the abundant pus, "by ocular confidence."[111]

Human generation remained a prized topic of investigation, as they had been for Paaw and his colleagues. Given women's bodies, Otto Heurnius and his surgeons always seized the chance to dissect the reproductive organs, looking for the characteristic causes of women's diseases in the uterus and female "testes."[112] Similarly, in two cases of marasmus or wasting disease, they found no clear or exceptional anatomical causes of death, but still dissected all the major organs, including the heart, lungs, pancreas, kidneys, liver, stomach, etc.[113] Making the most of the bodies available, Leiden anatomists dissected sites of interest well beyond the known anatomical seats of a patient's diseases.

---

110   *Pace* Huisman, *Finger of God*, 143, 183.
111   Otto Heurnius, *Historiae*, 16.
112   Otto Heurnius, *Historiae*, numbers 8, 15, 20, 24.
113   Otto Heurnius, *Historiae*, numbers 15 and 20.

Tracking down the causes of disease by following the sensory phenomena of preternatural organs and parts, though, was their primary goal. An exemplary case from the very end of 1639 neatly displays the practice of reasoning back to anatomical disease origins and disease progression from the appearances of the dissected body, *without* the help of a history of symptoms and treatments from a long hospital observation. An older woman, Aeltje Evouts, had her body consumed by atrophy and a concurrent wasting fever and flux of the belly. She "exhaled her spirit placidly," dying a good death in the evening on Christmas Day. As usual, they dissected her body the next day. And, as usual, they worked systematically through the major organs of the chest and abdomen. The liver, the chief organ for the faculty of nutrition, produced nutritive venous blood from the chyle concocted from food and drink in the stomach and intestines. Otto and his colleagues began there, noting the visual and tactile appearance of the liver as "flaccid, outwardly pallid and *inwardly exsanguinated.*"[114] In the left lobe of the liver, near the diaphragm, they found a calloused steatoma the size of a dove's egg (a hard swelling containing a fatty substance, with its own membrane). Working out from the liver, they checked the vessels of the omentum and the parts around the liver. More steatomata appeared in the pylorus, but the passage through it into the intestine still allowed the insertion of a finger. Then they moved farther, to complete the inventory. The heart, spleen, and lungs all appeared pallid, and some exsanguinated. As in almost all the other cases of women's cadavers, they checked the uterus, finding it naturally small given the cessation of menstrual blood. Ultimately, they concluded that the obvious and extensive corruption of the liver had caused the deadly atrophy, with the swelling steatoma compressing the vena cava, blocking the proper flow of nutriment. The most obvious morbid appearance, the large steatoma in the liver, fit with the clinical symptoms to explain the disease and death. Since it was impaired, the liver had made poor blood with poor nutriment, which made it and the heart weak. Weakened by their lack of nutriment, they had only feeble facultative power for their proper actions. The pallid appearance and exsanguination of the heart and liver corroborated their historical inference based on the growth of the steatoma just over the vena cava.

As we have seen from these histories of clinical practice and clinical anatomies, students learned to put their lectures, books, and disputation training into practice at patients' bedsides and crowded around the dissection table in the hospital. Although Otto Heurnius' plan to put the students' own practical recommendations to the test failed after staunch resistance, the success

---

114   Otto Heurnius, *Historiae*, 21. Italics in original.

or failure of the professors' diagnoses and treatments still faced the trial of patients' observed progress. Following the methods from their medical theory and practice courses, which professors such as Otto Heurnius first learned then taught at Leiden, they inspected patients' bodies for observable signs of local impairments: pain, in all its sites and varieties, as reported by the patients, helped to give the first reliable indications of which organs suffered morbid injury; visible signs such as the expectoration of blood and pus, changes in the consistency or color of the urine, diarrhea, or the swollen or wasted appearance of organs body parts all pointed to the seats and qualitative or structural changes of interior disease states (diarrhea and swollen bellies and feet indicated an impaired nutritive faculty of the liver, coughing up blood and pus pointed to pathological matter eroding the substance of the lungs).

Throughout each case, physicians and students tried to make inferences to the qualities and development of morbid affects. Recall how they first described the symptoms of Joannes de Neeff's pleurisy on his left side (signaled by the sharp pain and inflammation there), followed by his coughing up blood and pus, and then his fever and wasting toward death. These urged an inference to a clear history in which pleurisy seated in the pleura on the left side attracted and produced morbid fluid, which caused pus to fill and eat away at the left lung (pneumonia), and then the right, impairing the expiration of heated air (producing a fever) and the inspiration of vital spirit from the air into the arterial blood, reducing the vitality of the blood, and so injuring the nutritive faculty seated in the liver, which could not produce adequately nourishing venous blood, causing wasting and death. In the post-mortem, they found obvious evidence corroborating these inferences.

But not all clinical anatomies confirmed their diagnoses and prognoses. In some bodies, they could find no sensory evidence of diseases or the causes of diseases—they could not grasp causes "by ocular confidence." For all the generous pliability of Galenic theory, these dissections were not blank canvases on which professors painted their preconceived portraits of pathological processes. Inferences to hidden states had to pass the tests clinical anatomies allowed when they made inner organs and parts perceptible to the senses.

7 Making New Knowledge of Phthisis (Consumption)

In the early modern period, phthisis or consumption killed constantly and promiscuously, striking down families and foreigners, rich and poor. Leiden professors' medical diaries and anatomy records brim with terminal cases of patients coughing up phlegm, pus, and blood, burning with fevers, and wasting away into corpses. Patients, families, and healers across early modern Europe experienced the same grim outcomes. Johannes Heurnius reported that the Paduan professor Da Monte drew on his hospital teaching and private practice in the 1540s and 1550s to conclude: "Where one is cured, fully a hundred are dead."[115] By the later 1600s, the English physician Thomas Sydenham warned that those who died of phthisis made up nearly two thirds of those killed by chronic diseases.[116]

Foundational teaching and practice texts also dealt extensively with phthisis. From ancient Hippocratic and Galenic sources to early modern textbooks, healers grappled with this ever-present malady. Like many other sources on pre- and early-modern diseases, these texts consistently argued for a localized understanding of the origins and pathological development of the disease, concentrating on the development of pus, ulcers, and ulceration in the lungs. Hippocratic and Galenic texts, in particular, trained Leiden professors and students to focus their attention on the development of these lesions, tracked through the signs and symptoms of the living patients and ultimately through the visible lesions in dissected lungs. In this section, I present a short history of pathological and therapeutic writings on phthisis, in order to demonstrate the long continuities and gradual innovation displayed in the writings of the early Leiden medical professors.

Around 1600, a traditional emphasis on ulcers or ulceration of the lungs as the defining feature of phthisis came to include a growing recognition of the importance of developing tubercles or swellings in the processes of ulceration. At Leiden, clinical teaching and clinical anatomies generated essential clinical and post-mortem evidence for this recognition. Bedside diagnosis, therapy, and dissection all wove together to produce their knowledge of phthisis from experience with many patients. To show the many layers of continuities and to increase the chances of detecting real changes in the history of "phthisis," I trace the interrelated threads of diagnosis (and some prognosis), pathology, and therapy from the canonical Hippocratic sources through the works of Otto Heurnius.

As is only proper, we first go back to "Hippocrates," especially the ubiquitous *Aphorisms*, which Leiden medical students and professors used as a major source for constructing exams, disputations, lectures, textbooks, and specialized treatises. The Hippocratic *Aphorisms* put forward a terse and influential prognostic warning about phthisis: "After the spitting of blood, spitting

---

115   Johannes Heurnius, *De morbis pectoris liber*, 143.
116   Sydenham, *The Works of Thomas Sydenham*, 332.

of pus."[117] Other texts, especially the *Diseases* books, laid out two origins or types of phthisis: from the buildup of phlegm or from extravasated blood in the lungs.[118] In the first sort, pneumonia or catarrh produced phlegm in the lungs, which stuck there and putrefied, creating pus. This pus ulcerated the lungs, and corrupted them, gradually turned them into pus. As the lung putrefied and developed ulcers, it increasingly failed to nourish itself, and could not serve respiration, so the patient choked and eventually died.[119] In the second sort, violent coughing, screaming, exercise, or some other activity ruptured a blood vessel in the lungs. The extravasated blood stuck there, and then putrefied, beginning a similar morbid development.[120] Hippocratic sources also noted hereditary tendencies: "consumptives beget consumptives."[121] Hippocratic sources also lamented phthisis as the "severest and most troublesome disease, as well as the most fatal."[122]

Descriptions of symptoms from Hippocratic sources traveled through medical texts for centuries. Generally, phthisis revealed itself in the signs of wasting of the body, coughing up phlegm, blood, and pus, and sometimes fever. Their characteristic close descriptions listed fatal signs: curved nails, yellow or greenish stinking pus coughed up, spittle on hot coals produces a "heavy odor" or one like "burnt fat," there is a "heavy" smell from the patient's mouth "like raw fish."[123] For patients without fatal signs, who coughed up white pus, even with bloody streaks, they recommended treatment with mild purgatives such as a bit of hellebore in sweet wine or honey, or a mild emetic such as decoction of lentils.

Hippocratic sources also frequently mentioned nodules or swellings (*phu-mata*) in the lungs of phthisics, which ranged from soft to "hard and uncon-cocted nodules."[124] Although modern sources often translate the Greek words as "tubercles," and the Hippocratic writers may have observed abscesses in the lungs of butchered animals who showed symptoms similar to those of phthisics, they probably had different things in mind than early modern physicians. For the Hippocratic writers, swollen nodules or ulcers in the lung form from eroding bile and phlegm, or heat and exertion, and cause patients

---

117   Hippcrates, *Aphorisms*, 7.15, 197.
118   Cf. Meinecke, "Consumption (Tuberculosis) in Classical Antiquity."
119   Hippocrates, *Diseases* 1.12, 123.
120   Hippocrates, *Diseases* 1.15, 115.
121   Meinecke, "Consumption (Tuberculosis) in Classical Antiquity," 383.
122   Hippocrates, *Epidemics* 3.8, Loeb 253.
123   Hippocrates, *Diseases* 2.48, 50, 58, Loeb 277, 283, 301.
124   Meinecke, "Consumption (Tuberculosis) in Classical Antiquity," 383. Hippocrates, *Diseases* 1.19, Loeb 141–143; *Diseases* 2.57, Loeb 299.

to vomit or cough up blood.[125] Human dissection faced serious taboos in the ancient Greek world, and there are no mentions in these sources of animal dissections, although other authors from at least the 300s performed them.[126] Hippocratic writers seem to have inferred the presence of pulmonary nodules from patients' symptoms: coughing, difficulty breathing, and especially pains in specific locations in their chests. In one passage, the presence of a nodule is correlated with pain "in one place" in a patient's side.[127] Strikingly, they also used succussion or shaking to hear the sloshing or movement of larger amounts of phlegm in the lungs: "succussion is employed here ... the pus makes a splashing sound as it strikes the sides."[128]

Even in the Hippocratic sources, the presence and development of phthisis depended on the changes in the solid parts (organs and membranes) and their interaction with humors. This is consistent with other close studies of diseases from ancient sources, though not with common generalizations about Hippocratic writers ignoring the solid parts of bodies.[129] For the phlegmy sort of phthisis, the stagnant phlegm caused the lungs to ulcerate and putrefy, which impaired their action. The other sort, developing from rotting blood, depended on blood vessels breaking and, later, similar processes of ulceration and putrefaction of the substance of the lungs. The nodules or *phumata* also occurred in the lungs, as well as other parts such as the back, changing solid parts and interfering with their actions.

Phthisis does not appear as communicable or contagious in Hippocratic sources, though by the early 300s BCE Isocrates reported widespread belief in its communicability. Aristotle, writing in the mid-300s, also described phthisis as communicable. Like those suffering from plague, people sick with phthisis exhaled corrupt or poisonous vapors, setting off the development of phthisis in those close by.[130]

Five centuries later, Galen made ulceration of the respiratory organs central to phthisis. He systematized Hippocratic writings on phthisis, added signs from his favorite indicator, the pulse, and greatly expanded therapeutic recommendations. He defined phthisis as an ulceration of the lungs, chest,

---

125   Hippocrates, *Diseases* 1.11, Loeb 121.
126   Von Staden, "The Discovery of the Body."
127   Hippocrates, *Diseases* 2.57, Loeb 299.
128   Hippocrates, *Diseases* 1.15, Loeb 115–166. I thank Domenico Bertoloni Meli for this reference.
129   Wilson, "On the History of Disease-Concepts" traces pleurisy, vs. e.g., Maulitz, "The Pathological Tradition," and Maulitz, "Pathology."
130   Meinecke, "Consumption (Tuberculosis) in Classical Antiquity," 385.

or pharynx accompanied by a cough, fever, and complete emaciation of the body.[131] As always, he defined the disease in terms of injury to a specific bodily action or actions, seated in a specific part or parts. Wasting of the body followed from the impaired action of the lungs due to their ulcers and suppuration. Naturally, the lungs acted to ventilate the heat of the heart, which allowed it to generate vital spirit, and kept the liver well-tempered, so it could perform its function of nourishing blood. Lungs with lesions impaired these vital and nutritive processes.

Galen divided the causes of these ulcers into three types: spitting blood from trauma, cold, excess, or pleurisy (inflammation of the membranes around the lungs); morbid buildup of phlegm in the lungs; and extravasated blood in the lungs from rupture or suppression of blood flow (e.g., of menstruation). He clearly described phthisis as communicable, along with skin diseases and plague: "it is a dangerous thing to associate with people who have it, and especially those who emit such a putrid breath that the homes in which they lie smell bad."[132] His diagnostic signs for phthisis, of both the fatal and the rare curable sort, resembled closely those of the Hippocratic writers, with the addition of a small, weak, faint, and moderately fast pulse.

For treatment, Galen recommended drier climates with calmer winds, against the wetter spring and fall periods associated with phthisis. Like other ancient writers, Galen commended a milk diet, especially the milk of asses and goats, or even human milk. For internal medicines, he recommended especially mountain squill, a plant whose extract thins mucus, diced and put in vinegar for thirty days, as well as pepper, laurel berries, and a compound medicine of myrrh, pomegranate, saffron, castoreum, opium, anise, parsley, and the vapors of boiled ivy. He also handed on the practice of smearing butter on the patient's feet. If the patient spit blood, Galen recommended letting some blood from a vein, as well as vinegar and water taken internally, and the use of hot irons to help dry out and heal internal suppuration from the ulcers.

Medieval physicians tended to follow Galen's advice, especially Avicenna and most Latin authors. Others, such as Isaac Judaeus (c.840–932) in northern Africa, recommended local cures for the drying and wasting of the body, such as cooling breezes and pomegranate juice.[133] He took little notice of claims about lung ulcers, and mentioned nothing about communicability, though other Arabic authors did. "Haly Abbas" (Al-Majusi), writing in Persia in the

---

131   Meinecke, "Consumption (Tuberculosis) in Classical Antiquity," 398–9.
132   Galen, trans. Meinecke, "Consumption (Tuberculosis) in Classical Antiquity," 390. Nutton, "The Seeds of Disease," 5.
133   Bynum, *Spitting Blood*, 28–31.

900s, recommended the use of opium for patients' coughs, as well as goats' milk. Rhazes (al-Razi, 854–925), described patients with phthisis who coughed up blood and phlegm, and other fluids as well, and wasted away with fevers.[134] Rhazes categorized different sorts of phthisis by the locations of the ulcers or abscesses, which he also assigned to patients with pleurisy and pneumonia. If the patient coughed up putrefied bits of lung, death always followed.

Latin physicians encountered similar troubles distinguishing between purulent diseases of the chest. Pneumonia, too, involved ulcer of the lung, so many writers defined phthisis as the more extensive *"ulceration* of the lung."[135] Coughing up pus could mean either empyema (pus and inflammation in and around the lung) or phthisis, but coughing up blood most consistently indicated phthisis.[136] In general, though, they followed ancient precedents in embracing the symptoms of coughing blood and pus (not good or healing pus, but corrupt, bad pus distinguished by its bad odor when burned), fever, and wasting under "phthisis," as well as the ancient causes of local buildup of phlegm and the rupture of blood vessels in the lungs. Faced with the steady decline of so many incurable patients, Latinate medieval physicians stressed their obligation to help, tried various remedies, and praised God "who heals those whom He wishes."[137]

Despite the many ancient and medieval inferences to lung lesions, it is unclear when physicians and surgeons actually first *saw* ulcerated lungs in the bodies of phthisic patients. Arabic and Latin medieval sources, following Galen, consistently defined phthisis in terms of extensive ulcers or ulceration of the lungs, which caused the symptoms of coughing up pus and blood, fever, and wasting. Yet a regular practice of post-mortem dissection does not appear in sources until around 1300.[138] Then, physicians dissected the bodies of saints for marvelous signs of sanctity and the bodies of private patients, often in cases of suspected poisoning.

Antonio Benivieni (1443–1502), a physician in Florence, published short descriptions of 111 cases, over a dozen of which clearly ended in post-mortem dissections. Benivieni's *On Some Hidden and Marvelous Causes of Diseases and Healings* (1507) frequently found the hidden causes by revealing them in dissections. A young man, Juliano, suffered abdominal pains and could not be helped by medicines. He died, and Benivieni "had the body cut open seeking

134   Rhazes, *Continens Rasis*, XCIIv.
135   Demaitre, *Medieval Medicine*, 222.
136   Demaitre, *Medieval Medicine*, 219.
137   Valesco, quoted in Demaitre, *Medieval Medicine*, 226.
138   Park, *Secrets of Women*.

the causes of this grave disease."[139] He found it in the intestines, where a large abscess poured out stinking, black fluid, apparently formed from excess black bile. A man with difficulty breathing died, and in his lungs Benivieni found the "hidden and latent causes" in the black bile and dark blood in his heart, just as Galen suggested in similar cases.[140] A girl of fifteen who coughed up blood seemed to face the certain wasting of phthisis, but found a cure through blood-letting which supposedly alleviated the buildup of her stopped menstrual flow.[141] In Benivieni's time, post-mortem dissections to find the hidden causes of diseases appeared frequently enough that he expressed surprise when one family refused him permission to dissect the body of their relative. Still, none of Benivieni's recorded observations describe actual sensory perceptions of the long-suspected ulcerated lungs.

By the middle of the 1500s, actual post-mortem evidence and concepts of ulcerated lungs appeared tantalizingly close together. Moving to other sources used later at Leiden, we come to Jean Fernel's influential and comprehensive *Universa Medicina* from the mid-1500s. A scholar and successful physician who served the French court, Fernel's work explicitly distinguished between "pathology" and "physiology" (*pathologia* and *physiologia*), and at times grounded his pathology in post-mortem dissections. He followed and condensed the Hippocratic teachings on phthisis. Fernel defined phthisis—using the Latin *tabes* or "wasting"—as "ulceration of the lung by which the whole body is gradually liquefied."[142] The Hippocratic aphorism that spitting blood results in spitting pus, which he quoted, acted as the cornerstone of his pathology, which began with a disturbing cough producing blood, which then turned to pus and eroded the lungs, causing ulceration.[143] But he also mentioned cases from his own practice, noting that "I saw" many patients live happily for a long time after an apparent rupture of a vein in their lungs. He also attested to the "hereditary law" of phthisis after seeing phthisis "attack all the members of the same family in order."[144]

More than the Hippocratic sources, Fernel emphasized the solid parts. He identified the cause of phthisis as two-fold: from the ulcerating, consuming humor in the lungs Hippocrates described, or from "a soft, tender substance of the lungs, one ready for corruption," which many people inherited from their

---

139   Benivieni, *De Abditis Nonnullis ac Mirandis Morborum et Sanationum Causis*, trans. Singer, 83.
140   Benivieni, *De Abditis*, 127.
141   Benivieni, *De Abditis*, 125.
142   Fernel, *Universa Medicina* (1656), 109.
143   Fernel, *Universa Medicina*, 109.
144   Fernel, *Universa Medicina*, 109

parents and carried as a defect "lying hidden" for years. Even without phlegm or other humors in the lungs, these patients' lungs would fail, eventually making their bodies waste away. Solid parts could fail even without morbid humors.

Strikingly, Fernel's attention to the pathology of the solid parts carried over to his practice of post-mortem dissections. Earlier in the same chapter on the diseases of the lungs in which he described phthisis, Fernel described how phlegm or other humors dripping down into the lungs caused a variety of diseases, including "hailstones" (*grandines*). A heavy, slow humor could harden into stones, which are "true *stones*, which we have sometimes noticed filling dissected lungs thickly, some among these were very hard and solid, others just beginning, in the consistency of old cheese, others with the hardness of gypsum."[145] To modern readers, Fernel seems to have observed and described some of the later stages of tubercles, including tubercles filled with cheese-like or caseous matter.[146] He suggested a process of development from some "just beginning" and filled with a cheese-like matter to others hardened to stones. But any connection to phthisis remained unclear.

At Leiden a few decades later, Johannes Heurnius drew on Fernel, Galen, and other sources to craft a new Galenic system of practical medicine, as we have seen in earlier chapters. Johannes Heurnius' discussion of phthisis displays his wide scholarship in ancient, medieval, and early modern sources, and his comprehensive approach. Over nineteen double-column pages, he cited Hippocrates, Galen, Avicenna, Aretaeus, Caelius Aurelianus, Rhazes, Avicenna, John Mesue, Da Monte, and Van Foreest.[147] He defined phthisis much as Fernel had done, as "a cutting away of the whole body, born from ulcer of the lung."[148] Generally, he followed Hippocratic sources on the two sorts of phthisis, the ages of susceptibility (18 to 35 years), the symptoms, and prognosis.

Throughout his works, Johannes Heurnius followed Galen in defining diseases according to impaired actions of the parts, which he reiterated here.[149] Not every wasting counted as phthisis, but only that which followed from ulceration of the lungs. Ulcerated lungs are not able to perform their proper actions of cooling the heart and purifying the vapors going from and to the heart. This impairment inflames the vital spirits in the heart and generates excessive and dirty heat throughout the whole body, causing fever and intemperance of the parts. The parts do not receive the necessary healthy vital spirits and cannot

145   Fernel, *Universa Medicina*, 106.
146   Cf. Stolberg, *Experiencing Illness*, 263, n. 462.
147   Johannes Heurnius, *De morbis pectoris liber*, 137–156.
148   Johannes Heurnius, *De morbis pectoris liber*, 138.
149   Johannes Heurnius, *De morbis pectoris liber*, 138, 140.

receive their own proper nourishment, so the whole body wastes away with a fever. Johannes Heurnius explicitly drew most of this pathology from Galen, as slightly elaborated by later Galenic writers.[150] He also emphasized the hereditary tendency of those with "very tender flesh of the lungs," as well as contagion: "a poisoned air expired in the bedrooms or from the clothes" of the sick.[151]

Johannes Heurnius agreed with the Hippocratic writers that there "ought to be a trial [*periculum*] of the sputum poured on fire," to test whether it is healthy or salty or putrid.[152] To this he added the quick test of immersing the phlegm in hot water—putrid phlegm falls to the bottom, and does not break apart when stirred with a stick. These tests could help students diagnose the "nearly infinite" forms of pus in the early modern world: black, yellow, pure, white, white and green, wide, round, hard, gummy, flowing, lacking odor, fetid, etc.[153]

As in his rational method of curing set out in his courses and textbook, the *New Method*, Johannes Heurnius expanded and systematized therapies for phthisis, joining Galenic with chymical medicines. He echoed Da Monte's caution that where one is cured, a hundred die, but noted that if one followed Galen in cleaning and healing the ulcers, there was hope. Galen, "best of all," set out the way to cure, insofar as it was possible. So Johannes Heurnius used his recipes for washing and drying the ulcers, and recommended a compound of the old and the new, even the New World: "I administer theriac with flowers of Sulphur, and a decoction of guiacum with hawkweed [an astringent and drying herb]...China root," etc.[154] Here Johannes Heurnius' chymical expertise showed in his recommendation of flowers of Sulphur, which formed as mostly pure sulfur in a distillation apparatus. Guiacum and China root recommendations testify to his enthusiasm for "new" medicinal ingredients from the Americas and Asia, specific remedies for fevers of all sorts, which clearly escaped the lists of ancient and medieval pharmacopoeias. He was conflicted on the use of bloodletting, but advised following Galen's qualified recommendations, once again.

Johannes Heurnius followed the trend of including individual histories and empirics' reports to build a comprehensive descriptive account or *historia* of phthisis.[155] For instance, an unnamed empiric recommended a remedy consisting of

---

150   Johannes Heurnius, *De morbis pectoris liber*, 140.

151   Johannes Heurnius, *De morbis pectoris liber*, 139.

152   Johannes Heurnius, *De morbis pectoris liber*, 144.

153   Johannes Heurnius, *De morbis pectoris liber*, 142.

154   Johannes Heurnius, *De morbis pectoris liber*, 145.

155   Pomata, "Sharing Cases." Pomata, *"Praxis Historialis."* Stolberg, "Learning from the Common Folks." Johannes Heurnius, *De morbis pectoris liber,* 147–156.

cooked barley and crabs. Like other ancient and early modern sources, Johannes Heurnius recommended nourishing patients with milk, but added that one should cook the milk with sugar. He included two histories which supported the use of sugar. In the first, a man ate forty pounds of sugar of roses and was cured. The second, from his "greatest friend" Pieter van Foreest, recounted the story of a phthisic nun.[156] Despairing of physicians' cures, the nun tried another remedy, involving three ounces of sugar of roses in the cleaned stomach of a chicken, well-oiled and cooked in water, macerated and then consumed in bed just before sleeping. Since she was emaciated, she also ate two eggs barely cooked, as well as the Sulphur of wine and syrups for her cough. After two months, she was healed. Johannes Heurnius' copious erudition once again demonstrates the breadth and flexibility of late-Renaissance Galenic medicine, as well as its pointed emphasis on localizing the seats of diseases in impaired organs.

Finally, around 1600, physicians across Europe expanded beyond Fernel's reports of the stones in the lungs of some patients with respiratory diseases; they described post-mortem dissections in which they saw and touched the ulcers and abscesses of the lungs of phthisic patients. At Leiden, they did so in the hospital, and "publicly," from at least 1593. Petrus Paaw, Johannes Heurnius' colleague, dissected the bodies of phthisics in Leiden, identifying the characteristic purulent lungs, and even some hardened with stonelike deposits. On November 26, 1593, he "publicly dissected the body of a Young man in the Hospital."[157] As usual, the patient's identity and narrative made no appearance in Paaw's account. Instead, he is listed only as a young man felled by phthisis. His body, though, revealed the details of abscesses in the lungs, some hardened like stones: "Here and in each part of the lung [there were] various purulent abscesses, because in various places phlegm was noticed so hardened in the lung that they seemed to be stones to the touch, and indeed in not a few places it reached a perfect stony hardness."[158] As in other dissections when he touched purulent kidneys (which burst) or lungs, here Paaw used his sense of touch to assess the hardness of morbid matter and determine the strength of membranes.[159]

At least two other dissections revealed lung abscesses to Paaw. One, performed in January of 1597, allowed Paaw to count more than thirty abscesses, one of which "poured out more than four pounds of discharge."[160] In September of the same year, he dissected the body of a woman, at the request of

---

156   Johannes Heurnius, *De morbis pectoris liber*, 155.
157   Paaw, *Observationes*, 15.
158   Paaw, *Observationes*, 15.
159   Paaw, *Observationes*, 9, 28–29.
160   Paaw, *Observationes*, 27.

Dr. Trelcatius. She had died of phthisis, and they found the whole lung purulent: "if you should touch any part, poke it a little bit, white pus would erupt."
For once, local reports came into his narrative, confirming the hereditary dispositions of some phthisics: "they said that this malady was hereditary in the
family, and her brothers had died from it."[161]

Other physicians and surgeons across Europe found the characteristic
lesions of phthisis through post-mortem dissections. In the late 1590s and
early 1600s, Guilhelmus Fabricius Hildanus performed many post-mortem
dissections, in collaboration with local physicians, in order to find the causes
of death in patients' bodies. A polyglot and well-read surgeon, Hildanus combined informal learning from university physicians and ancient texts with
wide surgical experience.[162] He corresponded with learned anatomists such as
Paaw, and many others across Europe, and his practices of collecting, visualization, and publication elaborated on those of physicians in his circle.[163] His
surgical practice, though, inspired a greater emphasis on reporting surgical
cases and body parts in diseased states, including physical specimens for his
museum and many illustrated diseased states, as well as new instruments and
procedures.[164]

Hildanus' observations on phthisis fit the pattern of other learned healers.
A fourteen-year-old girl died in 1600, after suffering from phthisis, which they
characterized by the symptoms of wasting, a continuous cough, and a mild
fever, though no loss of appetite. In her lungs, Hildanus found putrid abscesses,
with pus contained within membranes, one with a pound and a half of pus
inside. Other abscesses, or steatomata, and hard tumors appeared throughout her lungs. She also suffered from a large, gnarled kidney stone, and swollen nodules and steatomata throughout her abdomen, some about the size
of goose eggs.[165] The lungs of a forty-year-old male woodworker, whose body
Hildanus dissected in 1596 while accompanied by two named physicians, also
displayed "tubercles" (*tubercula*) in the intestines, purulent sores in organs
such as the pancreas and kidneys, liver, and lungs, as well as many morbid
"glands" (*glandula*) in the lungs.[166] Working at the same time, both Paaw, the
university professor and physician, and Hildanus, the learned surgeon,

161   Paaw, *Observationes*, 28–29.
162   Bertoloni Meli, "'Ex Museolo Nostro Machaonico.'" Bertoloni Meli, "Gerardus Blasius and
       the Illustrated Amsterdam *Observationes*."
163   Bertoloni Meli, "'Ex Museolo'" and Bertoloni Meli, "Gerardus Blasius and the Illustrated
       Amsterdam *Observationes*."
164   Bertoloni Meli, "'Ex Museolo Nostro Machaonico."
165   Hildanus, *Opera Observationum et Curationum Medico-Chirurgicarum*, 53.
166   Hildanus, *Opera Observationum et Curationum Medico-Chirurgicarum*, 53.

identified similar ranges of abscesses and tubercles in the lungs of phthisic patients' cadavers.

A few decades later, Otto Heurnius, Johannes' son, observed and dissected phthisic bodies in his practice of clinical anatomies in the program of hospital teaching. In 1641, Jacobus Cobier, a woolworker in his forties, developed an acute disease of his chest, which developed morbid matter at the site of pain. He coughed, had difficulty breathing, and, since he was a pauper, was brought to the Leiden hospital. There he lay for three months while the disease became much worse, despite the use of "beneficial" medicines. His phthisis reached "the highest grade," as he developed constant fevers and extreme wasting. He died on November 5th, and Otto dissected the body right away: "I dissected the cadaver the next day...for the benefit of the College of practice," in other words, for Leiden students in their clinical instruction.[167] They found the pleura of the right lung extremely thick, which indicated prolonged inflammation from pleurisy, "so that it was easy to conjecture that here was the beginning and focus of the disease." In other words, Otto correlated Cobier's report of acute pain in one of his lungs with the historical evidence of the progress of pleurisy found in his cadaver. They found the right lung nearly wasted away into pus, so that hardly any of its filaments or vessels remained. "The whole cavity was filled with a very fetid pus, similar to that he had coughed up some seven months before." In the left lung, they found several small abscesses. Clearly, the morbid process had begun in the right lung and progressed through it, then continued on to the left.

In a clear case of phthisis, from 1637, Otto "demonstrated and explained the causes of death" in the body of the unfortunate patient, teaching the students while the surgeon Joannes Camphusius dissected, and two city doctors observed.[168] Hubert Pemble, age 19, a poor Walloon seeking woolwork in the town, had served as a soldier the previous year. Impoverished and sleeping outside on the ground in the winter, he developed frostbite and gangrene on his toes. Surgeons cut back most of his toes on his right foot, and removed all except his big toe on his left. After that, he became sickly, suffering diarrhea, pain in his loins and back, a continual fever, and a very bothersome cough. He coughed up blood and sputum, indicating, Otto taught, that the acrimony of the blood generated by the gangrene had eroded the vessels of his lungs. A couple months later, Pemble developed continual diarrhea from the impairment of his lungs, which prevented his heart from maintaining the proper vital

---

167   Otto Heurnius, *Historiae*, 26.
168   Otto Heurnius, *Historiae*, 10.

heat, disrupting his body' natural faculty of cooking and retaining nourishment. His disease worsened, and he later coughed up a purulent, viscid matter.

Otto followed Galenic precedents. He argued that the wasting of the body, improperly concocted food turned to diarrhea, and coughing up pus indicated the presence and growth of abscesses and ulcers eating away at the lungs. He paid close attention to the pulse, and used Galen's categories for assessing it. It changed from "hard, quick, and frequent" in November to "very hard, worm-like, very quick, and very frequent" in December.[169] This provided clear evidence of the increasingly impaired vital faculty, seated chiefly in the heart.

Pemble wasted away, and developed a "Hippocratic face," his eyes protruding and cheeks sunken, his appearance cadaverous. He was so far gone "when he came under our care," that the violence of the disease overcame the health-bearing efficacy of the medicines. He died January 9th, 1637, in the middle of the night.

Pemble's body, dissected the next day at two o'clock, told a familiar story. His whole body appeared wasted, as by complete dryness. They found nearly the whole substance of the lungs changed into thick pus, with the remainder of it "hardened, tawny, in the likeness of smoked meat of an ashy color." Both lungs showed ulcers and abscesses, some small, some large, with many releasing thick pus. They appeared "marbled with dark and pale droplets."[170] The heart, liver, kidneys, intestines, and stomach seemed fairly natural, though exsanguinated and flaccid. Otto, the surgeon Camphusius, the other doctors, and the "many students of medicine" crowding the table found the characteristic abscesses and spots they expected from the symptoms of expectorated pus, fever, and wasting.

A third case of phthisis, from 1639, showed some of the variation of the lesions in the lungs, while firmly demonstrating "the wasting cause of death seated in the Lung."[171] In the body of David Jarvis, from Scotland, Otto found this cause in the "many tiny tubercles [tubercula] from a crude, viscous matter," that filled up the substance of the lungs. The patient had coughed up blood and pus, and wasted away with a hectic fever. The causes of the disease and its progress seemed obvious in the opened corpse. With the viscous phlegm and pus blocking the lungs' vessels, and the tubercles spreading and making channels and ulcers throughout, the lungs could not perform their proper function of ventilating the vital heat of the heart. The hot, humid temperament of the

---

169   Otto Heurnius, *Historiae*, 10. Galen, *On the Pulse for Beginners*, trans. Singer, 326–328, K
       VIII 456–460.

170   Otto Heurnius, *Historiae*, 10.

171   Otto Heurnius, *Historiae*, 22.

body led to putrefaction, especially when combined with the particular "putrid quality" which "manifold experience" taught was characteristic of phthisics. With the liver overheated and "infected" by this putrid quality, it could not concoct nourishing blood. This intemperance *of the liver* (not of the whole body) came about from the tubercles blocking passages in the lungs, and impaired the liver's faculty of making good nutritive blood. The liver passed on this excessively hot and putrid quality to the venous blood, which then infected other parts of the body, and made them unable to assimilate nourishment from the blood. Otto also directly demonstrated the cause of the clinical effects of phthisics coughing up blood, pointing to the erosion of the lungs and the ulcers while explaining that the ulcers consume the good blood and turn it into the visible pus.

These internal morbid appearances matched the clinical observations of the previous weeks. Students saw the cause of coughing up blood and pus which they had seen during the daily clinical teaching sessions. In the clinical anatomization of these phthisical cadavers, they could see the tubercles, the wasted organs, and the bloody pus in the lungs for themselves. Otto also connected their bedside diagnostic practice of uroscopy with the post-mortem sights of tubercles and pus, noting that they had also seen with their own eyes a thin fluid in the urine and sweat of the patient, which passed off from the body as the sticky pus of the tubercles congealed in the lungs. Bedside symptoms grounded inferences to hidden states and processes. Through clinical anatomies, students could actually see for themselves the later stages of these processes in the bodies of the dead.

8   Later Leiden Pedagogy and a New Theory of Phthisis

As we know too well, the wasting and deaths by consumption or phthisis did not end there. Even by the early 1800s, over one third of the cadavers of patients from the Paris hospitals showed tubercles and putrefaction of the lungs, which physicians working there defined as characteristic of the disease.[172] Even now, a million and a half people around the world die from tuberculosis every year.[173] The story of innovative research on phthisis in Leiden did not end with Otto

---

172   Dubos and Dubos, *The White Plague*, 9. Duffin, *To See with a Better Eye*, 155–156.

173   In 2018, over 1.5 *million* people died from tuberculosis, which remains one of the top ten causes of death worldwide. URL=https://www.who.int/news-room/fact-sheets/detail/tuberculosis#:~:text=A%20total%20of%201.5%20million,with%20tuberculosis(TB)%20worldwide.

Heurnius, either. A few decades later, the gradual addition of new knowledge from the pedagogical practices of clinical teaching and clinical anatomies expanded into an openly experimentalist search for new knowledge. In the 1660s, the Leiden tradition of hospital instruction and clinical anatomies allowed a former student, Franciscus Dele Boë Sylvius, to construct a new theory of phthisis around the gradual development of tubercles in the lungs. Sylvius drew from his Leiden training, experimental projects in chymistry and anatomy, and extensive bedside practice to construct an extensive new system of medicine. Although he still built on the traditional pedagogical practices and used the Galenic notion of disease as an impairment of natural bodily function, Sylvius explicitly set out to re-establish medicine on the more stable foundations of experiments in chymistry, anatomy, and bedside practice.

Historians have long noted Sylvius' eminence as a chymical physician.[174] Here, I will present a short overview of Sylvius' new theory of phthisis or consumption. Educated in the Leiden pedagogical practices of clinical instruction and clinical anatomies, Sylvius then took his medical doctorate at Basel in 1637 and returned to teach anatomy at Leiden in 1638.[175] He also extended his early adoption of the pulmonary transit of the blood to become a noted experimentalist proponent of the circulation of the blood and of chymical physiology and medicine. His new theory of phthisis, founded on clinical anatomies, represents the culmination of Leiden pathological pedagogy and appears as a celebrated innovation deep into the 1700s.

Among early modern physicians, Sylvius has long been credited with pushing physicians' attention to these morbid nodules in the lungs of phthisis patients, for instance by Morgagni in his magisterial 1761 *On the Seats and Causes of Diseases as Investigated by Anatomy*.[176] But the main lines of his work on phthisis remain sketchy and obscure, including his theory of the tubercles as diseased glands, the medical heritage he engaged, the origins of his work in teaching medical students, and especially the importance of his routine clinical post-mortem dissections of hospital patients.[177]

---

174   For Sylvius, see, e.g.: Baumann, *François Dele Boe Sylvius*; Beukers, "Acids Spirits"; Beukers, "Mechanistische Principes"; Beukers, "Het Laboratorium"; Ragland, "Mechanism"; Ragland, "Chymistry and Taste"; Ragland, "Experimental Clinical Medicine"; Smith, *The Body of the Artisan*, ch. 6.

175   Sylvius, *Disputatio de animali motu ejusq; laesionibus* (Basel, 1637).

176   Morgagni, *The Seats and Causes of Diseases Investigated by Anatomy*, trans. Benjamin Alexander, Vol. 1, 656–658. Dubos and Dubos, *The White Plague*, 73. Bynum, *Spitting Blood*, 44.

177   Bynum, *Spitting Blood*, 45, claims he did not relate extrapulmonary tubercles to phthisis. Duffin, *To See with a Better Eye*, 156–157, misses Sylvius' insistence on coughing pus as the inseparable sign, as well as his use of many post-mortem dissections to establish tubercles as central to phthisis and scrofula. Baumann, *Sylvius*, 174–185, gives by far the best

In contrast, previously-unstudied primary sources from student notes from the hospital to Sylvius' own published writings paint a rich, multifaceted picture of this new theory of phthisis, which emerged from Leiden pedagogical practices and Sylvius' new medical system. Sylvius wrote a short treatise on phthisis or consumption and multiple collections of student notes detailed his daily bedside practices and clinical anatomies.[178] Sylvius dissected the bodies of dozens of phthisis patients from the Leiden hospital, where he and students daily observed symptoms, administered remedies, and noted patient progress or declines.[179] His theory centered on developing tubercles he found in dozens of clinical anatomies, and which he correlated with clinical symptoms: "I saw not just once *Glandulous Tubercles in the Lungs*, smaller and larger, in which there was ever varied Pus contained, as shown by dissection. These Tubercles gradually dissipated into Pus, and I consider that the things contained in their thin membranes should be considered *Abscesses*, and from these I recognized that frequently *Phthisis had its origin*."[180] He demonstrated to students the beginnings of tubercles in "little hard particles, which usually developed gradually into abscesses."[181]

Sylvius self-consciously set out to innovate and re-establish medicine on the stronger, more level foundations of experimentation. As he described his project, all of his novel claims depended on "threefold sorts of *Experiments*, called respectively *Anatomical*, *Chymical*, and *Practical*."[182] He began his anatomical and chymical experiments at least by 1639–1640 at Leiden, where his vivisection and chymical experiments with Johannes Walaeus demonstrated the circulation of the blood and investigated the processes of digestion and nutrition.[183] The third kind, practical experiments, involved investigating diseases and trying diagnoses and treatments in medical practice. Like the other kinds of experiments, it "demonstrated things to the Senses," but in patients' bodies living and dead. Upon his return to Leiden as an ordinary professor in 1658, Sylvius reinvigorated clinical instruction and clinical anatomies in the

---

discussion, especially noting Sylvius' division of patients into three groups according to the stages of their disease, based on his extensive clinical observations. But he misses the details of the post-mortems, especially from the students' notes, the importance of the tubercles, and the long reception of Sylvius' work.

178   Franciscus Sylvius, *De phthisi* in *Opera* (1679), 692. Merian, "Casus Medicinales," in Sylvius, *Opera Medica* (1695). Anonymous, "Collegium Nosocomicum," in Sylvius, *Opera Medica* (1681), 709–737. Robert Hepburne, Sloane MS 201.

179   Merian, "Casus" and the "Collegium Nosocomicum" notes give roughly three every two years, making an estimated 21 over Sylvius' fourteen years teaching in Leiden.

180   Sylvius, *Opera* (1679), 692.

181   "Collegium Nosocomicum," 731.

182   Sylvius, "Epistola Apologetica," in *Opera Medica* (1695), 908.

183   Ragland, "Mechanism."

hospital. According to the official course descriptions, in the public hospital Sylvius trained "the students of Medicine in the recognition of diseases by their signs, knowledge by their causes, and curing by their indications. Moreover, whatever about the parts truly affected and the hidden causes of the affects can be captured by the eyes, he lays it all open and makes it clear in the dissection of the dead."[184] After showing the students the success or failure of his remedies in patients' outcomes, failures turned to opportunities for final arbitration through dissection: "in the accurate opening and demonstration of their bodies it was revealed to all whether they had judged rightly or wrongly about that Disease."[185]

Like his predecessors discussed in the previous chapters, Sylvius defined disease in terms of the impairment of the functions of the healthy body. Disease was "a faulty Constitution of a Man impairing some Functions."[186] For Sylvius, too, the number of diseases tracked the number of functions, which followed from the actions of the parts. His major work, the *New Idea of Practical Medicine* clearly aimed to supplant Johannes Heurnius' *New Method of the Practice of Medicine*.[187] In this work, Sylvius primarily organized, diagnosed, and treated diseases according to the various impairments of the functions of men's and women's bodies. Parts of the body often acted in concert to discharge a function, but the physician always had to consider the individual parts, each of which had to be "rightly disposed and constituted" to complete a healthy function. External substances, such as food, drink, and air, had to be in their proper states, too. To know all diseases, the physician needed to account first for the solid parts of the body, then the fluids or other contents, then the state of the sensitive soul, since the "animal functions" of emotion, imagination, memory, and basic appetites could be faulty, too.[188] Most of the time, variations in the chymical humors of the body caused the local impairments of functions which constituted diseases. Chymical medicines, applied with knowledge gained

---

184   Molhuysen, *Bronnen*, 3, 91*.
185   Sylvius, "Epistola Apologetica," 905.
186   Sylvius, *De Methodo Medendi*, ch. 2, in *Opera* (1695), 56. For his predecessors, see chapters 5 and 6. Cf. definitions from his contemporaries, e.g. Plemp, *De fundamentis*, 327: "A disease is a constitution or affect of the living body beyond nature by which primarily a function is injured."
187   Sylvius, *Praxeos Medicae Idea Nova*, 4 Vols. (Leiden and Amsterdam, 1671–1674). The first volume appeared unauthorized, from student notes, in 1663: Franciscus Dele Boë Sylvius, *Medicinae Practicae Academiâ Lugduno-Batavâ Professoris. Disputationum Medicarum Pars Prima Primarias Corporis humani Functiones Naturales ex Anatomicis, Practicis & Chymicis Experimentis deductas complectens* (1663).
188   Sylvius, *De Methodo Medendi*, 57.

from chymical, anatomical, and "practical" experiments, could neutralize the chymical excesses of morbid humors.

Tracing the long history of phthisis through Leiden into the 1600s demonstrates the development of influential anatomical-clinical medicine and teaching, with professors and students committed to the discovery and communication of *new* knowledge, far earlier than much of the reigning historiography allows.[189] The numbers of students trained in this way at Leiden, and the numbers of patients they encountered, living and dead, reached heights unmatched by even the celebrated teaching of Leiden professor Herman Boerhaave, from 1714–1738.[190] During Sylvius' tenure, 1658–1672, over eight hundred students who matriculated in medicine at Leiden learned this sort of medical practice.[191] They encountered up to twelve patients each day in the reserved beds in the hospital, regularly observing eight to ten each day, Monday through Saturday, over the course of several weeks or even several months.[192] One student's extant notes from the hospital teaching from 1659 to 1661 record day-by-day symptoms and medicinal recipes for over fifty patients a year.[193] After the unfortunate deaths of many of these poor patients, students could observe and learn to identify the appearances and causes of diseases in the dissected bodies of fifteen or more patients a year.[194] As student notes indicate, they learned to pass over patients' stories, and even their names, and concentrate their attention instead on perceptible symptoms and reports of sites of pain that indicated the anatomical seat of the disease.[195] In short, they concentrated on the two emphases of the longer *practica* tradition: the diseases and the remedies. Sylvius often tried out new remedies, and students carefully

---

189   Maulitz, "Pathology." Nicolson, "Art of Diagnosis," 805–6. Duffin, *History of Medicine*, 76, 78. This current chapter thus adds significantly to the extension of continuities and varieties of clinical teaching and hospital practice, and the rejection of the "rupture" view, summarized by Lindemann, *Medicine and Society*, 147–148, 162–165, 282. Cf. La Berge and Hannaway, "Paris Medicine."

190   As Harm Beukers and Rina Knoeff have shown definitively, Boerhaave did not deserve his later reputation for clinical teaching. Boerhaave rarely taught in the hospital, and only on some Wednesdays and Saturdays. From 1721 to 1736 the entire hospital teaching program admitted on average only about three patients a year, and zero patients from 1732–1736. Beukers, "Clinical Teaching," 147–148. Knoeff, "Herman Boerhaave at Leiden."

191   Ragland, "Experimental Clinical Medicine," 347.

192   Robert Hepburne, Sloane MS 201, 16r–18r, 19v–21r. Merian, "Casus Medicinales," in Sylvius, *Opera Medica* (1695).

193   Merian, "Casus Medicinales."

194   Ragland, "Experimental Clinical Medicine," 348.

195   Merian, "Casus Medicinales," generally does not list names, writing only of "a hydropsical woman," and other simple descriptors. Robert Heburne usually gave names, but like the other students concentrated on descriptions of diseases and detailed recipes for drugs.

noted their recipes and apparent effects. For the unfortunate patients who did not survive their stay in the hospital, dissection of their cadavers revealed the causes of diseases and death.

By the 1660s, at least, students aimed to innovate, too. They built upon and critiqued their professors' new claims in anatomy, chymistry, and medical theory and practice. Most of all, they jockeyed for precedence and credit for anatomical discoveries.[196] Students such as Nicolaus Steno (Niels Steensen, 1638–1686), Reinier de Graaf (1641–1673), and Jan Swammerdam (1637–1680) identified new structures such as salivary glands, analyzed fluids such as the pancreatic fluid, examined the actions of muscles and nerves, tested new remedies, and investigated pathological lesions in patient cadavers. They often presented their new discoveries and experimental reports in their disputations. Sylvius and other professors encouraged this intention to innovate, and even left bodies in the hospital dissecting room for students to "examine whatever you like" after class.[197]

From dozens of patients' phthisic cadavers, Sylvius reconstructed the development of tubercles and phthisis. The range of sizes and morbid states strongly suggested a developmental pathway for all tubercles, whether phthisic, scrofulous, or otherwise. Tubercles start small, even barely visible, then "increase with age, and gradually pass into Suppuration." Sylvius found a range of tubercular forms in the bodies of phthisis patients from the municipal hospital. There, student notes record Sylvius demonstrating pus-filled abscesses, open ulcers, and dense scatterings of "little hard particles, which usually developed gradually into abscesses."[198]

Sylvius tried to synthesize all of the major causes of phthisis with evidence from clinical anatomies and bedside experience. Like his Galenic teachers, Sylvius defined the proximate cause of phthisis as "an Ulcer staying in the Lungs for a long time, so that from It the emaciation of the Body is excited with a gentle fever."[199] But other antecedent causes also generated the chymical changes in the blood that led to the development of tubercles. Pneumonia or pleurisy could precipitate phthisis, as could contagion, possibly due to acrid chymical vapors exhaled from patients.[200] Sylvius often limited

---

196 E.g., Ragland, "Experimenting." Ragland, "Mechanism." Ragland, "Experimental Clinical Medicine."

197 Nicolaus Steno to Thomas Bartholin, January 9, 1662 in *Thomae Bartholini Epistolarum Medicinalium Centuria III*, 263. Houtzager, "Het experimenteel geneeskundige onderzoek," 61–62.

198 "Collegium Nosocomicum," in Sylvius, *Opera Medica* (1681), 731.

199 Sylvius, *De phthisi*, 690.

200 Sylvius, *De phthisi*, 692–693.

his more certain pathological claims to the perceptible evidence in cadavers. Since he never found blood in the tuberculous capsules turning into pus, Sylvius rejected the ancient Hippocratic belief that extravasated blood generated pus and ulcers. Further, he gave an anatomical "Conjecture and Suspicion" for the apparent hereditary pattern of phthisis: a hereditary disposition of glands made people more or less susceptible to developing the tubercles of scrofula or phthisis.[201] Finally, Sylvius suggested that especially strong grief, just like acrid vapors or food and drink, could cause the lymph to become acrid and sticky, which made it build up in the glands. Like his predecessors, he knew that phthisis was rarely cured, and he also used Sulphur-based remedies to cleanse ulcers and improve patients' breathing. He added the regular use of opioid remedies, such as laudanum, to ease breathing and pain.

Post-mortem observation of these morbid tubercles allowed Sylvius to connect scrofula, characterized by swollen nodules and pain, especially in the neck and head, with phthisis, a wasting and respiratory disease.[202] In the hospital patients' bodies, he "saw them presented and distributed throughout all the Viscera and Flesh of our Body." He found such glandulous tubercles "*manifest in a strumous or scrofulous constitution*" in the sides of the neck and the mesentery. Throughout the body, and prominently in the lungs, these tubercles developed along the same morbid path: glands normally invisible in healthy patients swelled, built up morbid matter such as phlegm or pus within their membranes, and then became distinct purulent vesicles which could rupture into open ulcers. In the lungs, these abscessed tubercles, especially open ones, were the "proximate cause" of phthisis, since they generated the "pus continually excreted by coughing" which was the "inseparable sign" of phthisis.[203]

Differential diagnosis correlating patients' symptoms and evidence from clinical anatomies allowed Sylvius to distinguish phthisis from similar diseases. He divided pus from phlegm based on their origins, chymical make-up, and properties. Pus came from enkindled blood in vessels or organs which stagnated and lost its chymical spirits and volatile particles, leaving the acidic and saline parts to become sharper and generate an effervescence with the oily parts. Pus appeared thicker, and often stank of corruption. Phlegm, in contrast, derived from saliva, which changed gradually in its passage through the stomach and intestines.[204] This chymical change also generated heat, and blood

---

201   Sylvius, *De phthisi*, 690.
202   *Pace* Bynum, *Spitting Blood*, 45.
203   Sylvius, *De phthisi*, 690, 691, 689.
204   Sylvius, *De Methodo Medendi*, in *Opera Medica* (1695), 97.

corrupted into pus.[205] Taking pus as the "inseparable sign" allowed Sylvius to distinguish phthisis from pneumonia, which he defined as the inflammation of the lungs due to stagnant blood in their blood vessels and lacked this sort of pus.[206] This pus, of course, came from the tubercles and ulcers he observed in clinical anatomies, tubercles whose development formed the core of his new theory.

Other physicians made pathological discoveries from post-mortem dissections, too. At the same time Sylvius made his clinical anatomies, the Leiden professor of anatomy, Johannes van Horne (1621–1670), also dissected phthisic patients. One case strongly corroborated Sylvius' observations on tubercles: "On the 7th of June in 1663, Johannes van Horne dissected a male cadaver killed by phthisis in the Academic Hospital of Leiden." Very many "glands" were conspicuous in the mesentery, "some the size of peas, others the size of beans." There were very many abscesses in the left lung, "like grains," while the "whole Lung was occupied with scattered Tubercles with pus." In the right lung, there was an abscess in the cavity, and very many small ones throughout the whole lung."[207] In England, the chymical physician and active Royal Society member Thomas Willis (1621–1675) published his accounts of phthisis in the mid-1670s.[208] He continued some ancient precedents, such as diagnosing "phthisis of the back" from excessive venery, and suggested that the disease of the lungs arose from problems of chymical excess of the blood.[209] Willis did not insist on ulcers as necessary for the disease, but defined phthisis as "a withering away of the whole body arising from an ill formation of the Lungs."[210] His post-mortem dissections of private patients did not always uncover ulcers, but displayed "little swellings, or stones, or sandy matter throughout the whole."[211] Sometimes, he found "one or two ulcers, with a callus around" them, likely from the buildup of serum in the lungs, which filled little bladders until they burst.[212] Patients with only a few, bounded ulcers suffered only from coughing up some spittle and yellow matter every morning, and could live this way for some time.

Physicians and surgeons across Europe sought the causes and tracks of diseases in dissected cadavers; they especially hunted phthisis. The erudite

---

205   Sylvius, *Idea Nova*, in *Opera Medica* (1695), 282.
206   Sylvius, *Idea Nova*, 208.
207   Bonet, *Sepulchretum sive Anatomia Practica, ex Cadaveribus Morbo Denatis*, Vol. 1, 567.
208   Frank, *Harvey and the Oxford Physiologists*. Willis, *Pharmaceutice rationalis*.
209   Hippocrates, *Diseases* 2.51, Loeb 285. Willis, *Pharmaceutice rationalis*, 27.
210   Willis, *Pharmaceutice rationalis*, 30.
211   Willis, *Pharmaceutice rationalis*, 29.
212   Willis, *Pharmaceutice rationalis*, 31.

Genevan physician Théophile Bonet (1620–1689), compiled a vast "*Graveyard*" of reports of thousands of post-mortem dissections, mostly from 469 different authors, but some from his own practice.[213] Drawing from accounts from over two dozen physicians and surgeons, Bonet compiled and discussed over 168 reports of post-mortem dissections of "phthisis" patients, recounted with commentary over eighty-nine pages. He concluded that phthisis, or a wasting of the body, very often proceeded from ulcer of the lung, but not always. Other dissections showed wasting from morbid states of other parts of the body, such as the bowels. Interestingly, fifteen descriptions of post-mortems from Leiden dot his pages, with nine histories from Otto Heurnius, two from Paaw, one from Johannes Heurnius, one from Van Horne, and two from Sylvius.[214] He also commended Willis for his chymical explanations, as well as Sylvius for his theory of the glandular nature of the tubercles, which could explain the apparent hereditary patterns of phthisis.

A century later, Giovanni Battista Morgagni famously expanded and re-ordered the vast scholarly graveyard of Bonet and his other predecessors with his own post-mortem pathological dissections. His *On the Seats and Causes of Diseases Investigated by Anatomy* (1761) is the fruit of the long early modern practices of post-mortem pathological investigations, as well as Morgagni's practice and teaching as professor of anatomy at Padua from 1715–1771. Morgagni had avoided dissecting the contagious bodies of those killed by phthisis, completing only one, but often found ulcers and tubercles in other bodies. He explicitly followed Sylvius in thinking that hereditary variations in glands explained the apparent hereditary patterns of phthisis.[215] Yet some patients' bodies clearly showed a great deal of pus in the lungs, others' very little, and some not at all— Morgagni concluded that Sylvius was probably right that the final group of patients lost any pus from the drying and healing of their ulcers.[216] Morgagni linked these varied appearances of tubercles and ulcers in size and contents by a familiar story: phlegm coming down or a swelling in the lungs stagnated, and let out corrupt and acrid matter, which spread through the lungs, eating out ulcers and spreading, like the branches and nodules of a fungus, throughout the lungs.

213   Bonet, *Sepulchretum*, 545–634. Irons, "Théophile Bonet, 1620–1689." Rinaldi, "Organising Pathological Knowledge."

214   Bonet, *Sepulchretum*, 559, 561, 565, 575, 576, 582, 586, 590, 560, 563, 591, 577, 579.

215   Morgagni, *The Seats and Causes of Diseases Investigated by Anatomy*, trans. Alexander, Vol. 1, 657.

216   Morgagni, *The Seats and Causes of Diseases Investigated by Anatomy*, trans. Alexander, Vol. 1, 658–9.

Last of all, we should mention R. T. H. Laennec (1781–1826), a leader in the new pathological anatomy around 1800 and a figure often presented as making a decisive turn. As the story goes, Laennec used new methods of post-mortem dissection to unite his concept of phthisis around tubercles, correlating patients' symptoms with a fine-grained history of tubercular development.[217] For Laennec, tubercles revealed in dozens of post-mortem dissections took center stage, and only tuberculous pulmonary phthisis counted as phthisis. Here, Laennec explicitly corrected the 1810 account of his friend, G. L. Bayle (1774–1814), which used material from his dissections of nine hundred hospital patients to provisionally articulate six species of phthisis, including tuberculous, granulous, melanous, ulcerous, calculous, and cancerous forms.[218] In contrast Laennec described one phthisis with various symptoms and four main types of tubercles: miliary (like grains of millet), crude, granular, and encysted. These types echo the observations of many earlier pathological anatomists we have met, who wrote frequently about little hard particles, sandy matter, droplets the size of peas and beans, tubercles with cheese-like contents, hard stones, and steatomata with membranes. Of course, Laennec had created a new diagnostic tool, the stethoscope, and built a vast interpretive practice around the music of diseases, from the gurgling of early phthisis to the "metallic tinkling" of healed tubercular fistulas.[219] Earlier physicians, notably Sylvius, had also correlated symptoms, even "inseparable signs" and post-mortem lesions.

There are striking similarities between the foundations and causes of the theories of phthisis of Sylvius and Laennec, separated by a century and a half. Laennec unified his theory more tightly around the development of tubercles, but for both the stages of tubercles revealed in dozens of post-mortem dissections, and correlated with symptoms, constituted the core identity of phthisis. Laennec also joined Sylvius in rejecting extravasated blood as an antecedent cause, based on its absence prior to the formation of tubercles in cadavers.[220] Both distinguished phthisis from pneumonia by the presence of developing tubercles, and both identified strong grief as an important antecedent cause. Laennec had been struck by the deep religious grief of women in a religious community, most of whom phthisis struck down over ten years.[221] After all, he was hard-pressed to explain non-hereditary waves in other terms. In contrast to Sylvius and most other writers on phthisis, Laennec boldly rejected the idea that phthisis was contagious! Although he would die of the disease a few years

---

217   Duffin, *To See with a Better Eye*, 156–158. Bynum, *Spitting Blood*, 56–62.
218   Rey, "Diagnostic différentiel et espèces nosologiques."
219   Laennec, *Treatise*, 308, 313–317.
220   Laennec, *Treatise*, 301.
221   Laennec, *Treatise*, 303.

later, at the time he composed his treatise he was still confident in his own experience. He had cut his finger while sawing tuberculous vertebrae, and a tubercle developed which he cauterized. No other symptoms followed, so he doubted contagion.[222]

Laennec's definition of the "new" science of pathological anatomy in the *Dictionary of Medical Sciences* summed up his approach: "Pathological anatomy is a science which has the goal of the knowledge of the visible alterations which the state of disease produced in the organs of the human body. The opening of cadavers is the means of acquiring this knowledge; but, in order for it to become of direct use and an immediate application to practical medicine, it must be joined to the observation of symptoms or the alterations of functions which coincide with each species of alteration of the organs."[223] This could have been written at Leiden two centuries earlier·

The similarity of the methods and theories of Sylvius and Laennec comes as a great surprise for our master narrative in the history of medicine. Many historians still maintain that post-mortem dissections and clinical teaching were not set up to produce new knowledge and that the productive correlation of symptoms and post-mortem appearances had to wait for the Paris hospital medicine around 1800.[224] But the strong similarities between the theories of Sylvius and Laennec should turn our gaze toward the longer histories of pedagogy and pathology. Even the altered "functions" of bodies and organs still played an important role. Recall that since at least 1636 the official course listings at Leiden advertised the regular correlation of symptoms and the lesions and causes of diseases found in clinical anatomies. "The Professor, with both the ordinary city doctors ... with the students, together with a good surgeon, will visit the sick persons in the public hospitals, and examine the nature of their internal diseases, as well as all their external accidents, and debate their cures and surgical operations, prescribing medicines according to the order of the hospital, and, also, will open all the dead bodies of the foreign or unbefriended persons there and show the causes of death to the students."[225] A century and a half before the supposed emergence of "modern" hospital medicine and pathology, we find a striking tradition at Leiden.[226] Official university practices founded on ancient Galenic medicine could foster the production of gradual and even precocious new knowledge.

---

222   Laennec, *Treatise*, 304–305.

223   Laennec, "Anatomie Pathologique," *Dictionnaire des Sciences Médicales*, ed. Nicolas Adelon (1812–1822), Vol. 2, 46–47.

224   E.g., Maulitz, "Pathology." Bynum, *History of Medicine*, 15, 55. But see Lindemann, *Medicine and Society*, 147–148, 282. Stolberg, "Post-mortems."

225   Molhuysen, *Bronnen*, 3, 312*.

226   E.g., Bynum, *History of Medicine*, 55–57.

9   Conclusions

The early, Galenic-Hippocratic program of clinical teaching and post-mortem dissections at Leiden bore fruit in student sensory engagement (the foundation of knowledge), practical experience in diagnosis and treatment, and even the gradual addition of knowledge to existing traditions of pathology. Professors and students conjectured diagnoses based on a wide range of signs or evidence perceptible to the senses, signs emphasized in Galenic practical medicine. Otto Heurnius felt patients' pulses and used Galen's categories—"hard," "wormlike," etc.—to assess the changes to the vital organs' temperaments and so the vital faculty seated in the heart. Students learned to follow Hippocratic and Galenic methods by attending closely to the visible changes in patients' faces, mouths, hands, and feet, and infer the hidden changes in their organs' faculties and temperaments from the locations of pain and other signs of injured bodily actions. As ever, patients' excreta, from the colors and consistency of coughed up pus and blood to the visible details of their urine and feces, gave clues for inferences to hidden changes of organs' temperament-based faculties. This was Galenic medicine embodied in a range of pedagogical practices in one place.

Although they embraced traditional language, ideas, and methods, this was a medical and pedagogical culture that embraced personal experience with new cures, knowledge from empirics, new global medicines, and even chymistry. Otto Heurnius' father Johannes, like his eminent friend Pieter van Foreest, took care to pass on recommendations from his own practice, try new remedies, and pass on case histories and empirics' recipes for specifics. Eating forty pounds of sugar to cure phthisis did not obviously fit with ancient or medieval practices, although medieval physicians had gradually shifted from honey-based sweet medicines to sugar-based compounds from Arabic sources. Johannes Heurnius' chymical practice also broke the limits of earlier Galenic therapies, signaled especially by his recommendation of flowers of Sulphur for phthisics. Based on his own experience with patients, Johannes Heurnius combined Galenic theriac, global guiacum and China root, and chymical Sulphur into his remedy against the deadly and daily disease of phthisis.

Otto Heurnius also showed experience-based openness to new remedies and diseases, highlighted by his attempt to make a substitute for the indigenous "oil of Couroq" to treat the corruption in a Dutch soldier's feet caused by the counterattack of tiny Brazilian parasites. In their openness to communicating and testing new, non-canonical remedies and diseases, Leiden physicians displayed a commitment to personal experience as the ground of therapy which Renaissance physicians elsewhere shared.[227] As Dioscorides and Galen had admonished, and early modern physicians faced with a far wider world of medicinals and diseases knew well, personal experience played a vital and ineliminable role in knowing how to cure.

Similarly, experience with patients' bodies living and dead in regular clinical anatomies generated gradual innovation in pathology. Early modern physicians increasingly found a range of morbid tubercles and ulcers in the lungs, from many small droplets or specks like seeds, to large abscesses and purulent ulcers. Like others across Europe, they found the "seat" and "cause" of phthisis in these morbid developments in the lungs. In Leiden medical teaching the establishment of an extensive and intentional program of clinical anatomies supplied two sources of experience necessary for pathological innovation: frequent hospital bedside observation and treatment over time, combined with regular post-mortem dissections and close attention to the morbid appearances in patients' bodies. Galenic pedagogy produced cumulative and novel pathological findings. Just a few decades later, in the middle of the 1600s, a former student and now professor of medicine at Leiden, Franciscus Sylvius, extended this tradition of clinical observation and clinical anatomies with his new chymical system of medicine. Sylvius' formation in the Leiden practices of clinical teaching and clinical anatomies, along with his early anatomical investigations in the wakes of Aselli and Harvey, gave him a productive set of practices for generating new knowledge. Even tempered by their professors' caution for revolutionary new doctrines such as the circulation of the blood, which they could not sense directly, other students showed similar interest in novelties.

Before Sylvius and other physicians aiming to re-found medicine, medieval and early modern physicians followed Galen's example and identified ulcers of the lungs, chest, and pharynx as the cause of phthisis. By the late Renaissance they localized their definitions more precisely, limiting the proximate cause to ulcers of the lungs. Johannes Heurnius, like Fernel before him, defined phthisis as wasting of the body caused by ulcer of the lung. He also remarked on the apparently hereditary and clearly contagious nature of the disease. Before Johannes Heurnius, Jean Fernel had identified "stones" in the lungs of dissected patients' bodies, and some with the consistency of "old cheese," but did not explicitly link these with phthisis. Petrus Paaw dissected bodies of phthisis patients, and revealed to sight and touch the purulent abscesses in their lungs, some with a "stony hardness."

---

227   Stolberg, "Empiricism," 507–512.

Otto Heurnius, performing his regular clinical instruction and anatomies in the hospital a few decades later, went even further. Like his father Johannes, Otto located the cause of the symptoms of phthisis—the wasting, fever, and coughing up pus and blood—in ulcers of the lungs. He described a range of morbid abscesses and "tubercles." He found lungs filled with "many tiny tubercles," lungs "marbled with dark and pale drops," and lungs bearing huge abscesses or consumed by pus. Like Galen, Fernel, and his father Johannes, Otto described the process by which ulcers impaired the action and function of the lungs: they blocked the healthy ventilation of the heart and caused the buildup of heat, which spoiled the temperament of bodily organs and especially the proper concoction of nourishing blood in the liver. He did not, though, explicitly string together the range of morbid appearances in the lungs, or describe clearly a regular developmental path for the tubercles, as the later Leiden professor, Franciscus Sylvius, did in the 1660s. (Although the growth of abscesses from smaller to larger forms is strongly *implicit* in his account of them eating and eroding the substance of the lungs.) Nor did Otto insist on coughing up pus as the inseparable sign of phthisis or link the primary causes of scrofula and phthisis as the development of the *same* sort of tubercles in different parts of the body. Again, by the 1660s, Sylvius would connect the dots of all of these morbid appearances and clinical phenomena to found a new theory of phthisis centered on the gradual development and morbid states of tubercles.

Even in the late 1500s and early 1600s, Leiden professors such as Petrus Paaw and Otto Heurnius insisted on finding the causes of disease and death in the dissected bodies of patients, the correlation of symptoms with hidden and revealed anatomical disease states, and, by 1636 under Otto, the combination of regular post-mortem dissection with clinical instruction in the hospital serving many dozens of poor patients during a student's education there. Students built on this program through the seventeenth century. By the 1660s, former Leiden student Thomas Bartholin acquired a reputation as an eminent anatomist and physician. He collected post-mortem observations from his own practice and reports from other physicians. The planned title for his unrealized printed collection fit well with the Leiden tradition: *Practical anatomy from those dead by disease for investigating the affected seat*.[228] Bartholin also printed post-mortem reports from his Leiden professors in other works, for instance Paaw's diary of observations.[229]

Around the same time in Geneva, the erudite physician Théophile Bonet (1620–1689) compiled a vast *Graveyard* (1679) of thousands of post-mortem

---

228   Rinaldi, "Organizing Pathological Knowledge," 43.
229   Paaw, *Observationes*, printed with Bartholin, *Historiarum Anatomicarum Rariorum* (1657).

reports from nearly five hundred authors, and his own practice, for similar ends. For example, he recorded at least one hundred and sixty-eight reports of post-mortem dissections of phthisis patients, with commentary. As mentioned, fifteen descriptions of post-mortems from Leiden dot his.[230] Bonet's *Graveyard, or practical Anatomy from Cadavers dead by Disease, Proposing Histories and Observations of nearly all affects of the human Body, and revealing their hidden Causes* also fits with earlier Galenic practices and language.[231]

Remarkably, even by the 1630s and 1640s the Leiden practice of clinical anatomy began to approach famed physician and anatomist William Harvey's later ideal of anatomy-based pathology. In his 1649 reply to the eminent Parisian anatomist Jean Riolan, Harvey insisted on the necessity of dissecting diseased cadavers, rather than merely healthy bodies, for understanding the "seats of all diseases." As Harvey stressed, and other anatomists agreed, "there is no knowledge [*scientia*] which does not arise from acquaintance-knowledge [*cognitio*], nor any sure and fully known knowing [*notitia*] which does not draw its origin from sense."[232] Harvey had planned and hoped for a sense-based science of pathology, which would not only investigate the places of diseases from the cadavers of the healthy, but from many diseased bodies. "So that I might undertake to relate, from many dissections of the bodies of the sick, complete with the most serious and most marvelous affects, in what manner and how the interior parts are changed in situation, size, constitution, figure, substance, and the other sensory accidents, from their natural form and appearance (as all Anatomists commonly describe), and how in various and marvelous ways they are affected."[233]

Influential Dutch physicians carried on the Leiden program. Nicolaes (or Nicolaas) Tulp (1593–1674), immortalized in Rembrandt's painting of his anatomical practice, also pursued pathological anatomy. Tulp studied under Paaw at Leiden University from 1611 to 1614, taking his MD in 1614. In his 1641 *Medical Observations*, Tulp praised the use of *observationes*, as demonstrated by anatomy, "the true eye of medicine."[234] In this preface, he urged his son, Petrus, to avoid futile trifles and silly disputations, and turn his mind to anatomical

---

230 Bonet, *Sepulchretum*, 559, 561, 565, 575, 576, 582, 586, 590, 560, 563, 591, 577, 579.

231 Bonet, *Sepulchretum*, title page. I have attempted to keep his capitalization.

232 Harvey, *Exercitatio Anatomica I, Exercitationes Duae Anatomicae de Circulatione Sanguinis* (1649), 2.

233 Harvey, *Exercitatio*, 3.

234 Tulp, *Observationum medicarum libri tres*, *2v.

dissections: "descend to the interior parts, and inquire not just into the nature of the viscera, but especially into the locations, and causes, of hidden diseases." By these, Tulp wrote, "you will know rightly" and pass on the light of real knowledge to others.[235] Tulp's *Observations* enjoyed popularity in Latin and Dutch editions for over a century. Tulp described over a hundred and fifty notable cases of disease, with case histories, references to ancient medical sources, and sometimes post-mortem dissections. Strikingly, his 1641 work contains a number of detailed illustrations of diseased organs and patients, from polypous hearts to arterial calculi, expectorated parts of lungs, tapeworms, "spina bifida," a term he coined, and of course kidney and bladder stones. Tulp tended to have illustrations of the rare or "monstrous" things, including conjoined twins and an orangutan.[236] In addition to his busy private practice, Tulp became the anatomical praelector for the Amsterdam Guild of Surgeons in 1628, and also had access to patients from the Amsterdam hospital. Sint Pieters Gasthuis could house hundreds of patients, especially during the years of warfare, and Tulp mentioned treating then dissecting some bodies "in the public hospital."[237] Like other Dutch physicians, Tulp performed some surgical and anatomical procedures himself, and collaborated with city surgeons and physicians.[238]

By the 1660s, Leiden professors and students expanded and intensified their clinical anatomies, making systematic investigations of diseases such as phthisis to produce new *theories* of their causes, progress, and treatment. The main theory centered on the gradual development of tubercles in the lungs. These tubercles, and their varied appearances, already appear in Leiden clinical anatomies under the reigning Galenic-Hippocratic tradition. Already in the 1630s, and perhaps earlier, post-mortem dissections appear regularly as the capstones of medical teaching and practice. This sophisticated practice, already cultivated at Leiden across four decades, and later expanded further with experiments and much more frequent clinical teaching, drew students to the university and fostered gradual and dramatic innovations. In this tradition, Petrus Balen's death and dissection, described in the introduction of this book, appear not surprising, but all too familiar.

---

235   Tulp, *Observationum medicarum libri tres*, *4.

236   Bertoloni Meli, "Gerardus Blasius," 229–239.

237   Tulp, *Observationum medicarum libri tres*, 47, 154. Wesdorp, "The Physician Dr. Nicolaes Tulp," 142.

238   De Moulin, *History of Surgery*, 219.

Even before the rise of experimentalism and widespread experimental practices, Leiden medical practitioners drew on ancient models and developed university pedagogical institutions to produce gradual progress in their knowledge of healthy and diseased organs and parts in their patients' living and lifeless bodies. The fact that this progress and localization appear in the main courses on medical practice at Leiden, and the popular courses and textbooks from the late sixteenth century, which later served as the main teaching texts for a popular medical school for at least five decades, gives further reasons to question Foucault's influential claim that the "great break" in all the history of Western medicine "dates precisely from the moment clinical experience became the anatomo-clinical gaze."[239] In this view, physicians concentrated only on surface symptoms before the later 1700s, and did not practice a "gaze" which moved vertically into the anatomical depths of patients' bodies, either in imagination or clinical dissections. The basic story of Foucault is still accepted in recent authoritative sources, despite important qualifications by many historians.[240] As Wilson, Wear, Stolberg, and others have shown, especially very recently, pathological theory and post-mortem dissection emphasized localized, anatomically-based disease states well before Bichat around 1800.[241] In the early modern period, post-mortem dissections in private and public settings became increasingly common by the middle of the 1600s, and hospitals were key sites in which, as David Harley has argued, physicians excised the perspectives of the patient as they dissected their bodies for pathological knowledge.[242] In the next volume, we will see 1660s Leiden students and professors practicing anatomical-clinical medicine in an explicitly experimentalist, persistently innovative, and strikingly productive pedagogical culture.[243] But these later experimentalists built on the earlier pedagogical practices of teaching, learning, and curing cultivated from 1575 to the 1640s. The evidence from this earlier period, gathered across lectures, textbooks, student disputations, medical diaries, and eyewitness accounts, paints a vivid portrait of the interconnected vital organs of Leiden pedagogy. Laennec's sketch of the "new" science of pathological anatomy strongly resembles the pedagogical practices from two centuries earlier.

---

239   Foucault, *The Birth of the Clinic*, 179.

240   Maulitz, "Pathology," 371. In contrast, see, e.g.: La Berge and Hannaway, eds., *Constructing*. De Renzi et al., eds., *Pathology in Practice*. Lindemann, *Medicine*, 148, 159–162, 282.

241   Wilson, "On the History of Disease-Concepts." Wear, *Knowledge & Practice*, 117–124, 146–148. Stolberg, "Post-mortems."

242   Harley, "Political Post-Mortems."

243   For early discussions, see Ragland, "Mechanism, the Senses, and Reason"; Ragland, "Chymistry and Taste"; Ragland, "Experimental Clinical Medicine."

Training in the lecture hall, garden, theater, hospital, and private rooms all shared philosophical principles of intelligibility—especially material temperaments and faculties—and the unifying goal of preserving healthy bodies and restoring diseased bodies to health. From plants to chymicals to bedside observation and post-mortem pus, knowledge of the "sick parts" and their cures came from their senses as guided by theory—in their terms, from experience and reason.

A Microcosm of Medical Learning and Practices

Some fifteen hundred students matriculated in medicine at Leiden from 1575–1640.[1] What did these medical students learn and how did they learn it? What practices helped make them into practicing physicians? They heard lectures on Hippocratic aphorisms and Galenic notions of physiology, disease, and pulse diagnosis. They witnessed public anatomies in the theater, clinical anatomies in the hospital dissecting room, and private anatomies in private rooms. Outside the lecture hall and dissecting rooms, they learned about medicinal "simples" in the garden, and also heard chymical lectures in the medical practice course. Medical professors engaged in humanist research in ancient sources *and* in their direct sensation and manipulation of plants, medicines, chymical processes, living patients, and especially patients' cadavers. Their research drew on and blended into their teaching, with new lectures on medical theory and practice appearing as textbooks, new anatomical claims popping up in lectures, and humanist quotations from Ovid adorning descriptions of post-mortem dissections of phthisic cadavers in the hospital.

I would like to highlight five main conclusions. First, this was Galenic medicine, with Galen's example, sources, method, and terminology as the foundation. Second, professors and students at Leiden and other medical schools grounded their claims to knowledge in the senses and in the principles of natural philosophy, especially the primary qualities. Third, from the garden to the bedside and the dissecting table, knowledge depended on embodied engagement with material things. Fourth, building *with* ancient models and methods rather than against them, professors and students generated real innovations in pathology, healthy anatomy, and therapy. Fifth, the scholarly and civic expertise and authority of these physicians rested on the combination of their discursive erudition and experience with material objects.

First and foremost, students encountered a medical curriculum founded on largely Galenic ideas and methods, and integrated by the language, histories, texts, and practices of attention cultivated by that tradition. Galen's works, made alive by vigorous humanist scholarship, structured many of their categories, goals, terms, and anecdotes. At times, his words blended into their writing smoothly, without citations or authorial markers. Contrary to widely repeated

---

1 Prögler, *English Students at Leiden University*, plate 14.

© EVAN R. RAGLAND, 2022 | DOI:10.1163/9789004515727_010

narratives, this tradition put knowledge of the changes and functions of organs and body parts at the center of theory and practice. After all, physicians defined disease in terms of the impaired functions of organs and simple parts. In diagnosis, they aimed to identify the impaired part or parts from the signs and symptoms of impaired functions. Students learned to combine reports of patients' pains with the evidence of their impaired functions such as respiration and nutrition, and the analysis of pulse and excrement variations, to pinpoint the impaired part and the nature of the impairment.

As Galen had taught across his works, basic matter theory formed the foundation of physiology, diagnosis, and pathology. The basic hot, cold, wet, and dry qualities mixed to form the different temperaments or complexions of organs and parts. The "imbalance" that characterized many diseases was emphatically not the imbalance of amounts of humoral fluids in general in a patient's body.[2] Rather, the "imbalance" or bad mixtures of diseases referred almost always to specific imbalances of the hot, cold, wet, and dry primary qualities that made up the different temperaments of different organs and simple parts. This was true from Galen through the academic medicine of the medieval period and into early modern academic medicine in Italy, the Low Countries, and elsewhere.[3]

The standard story about Galenic medicine is that anatomy "did not have direct practical use in treating diseases."[4] When we look into the details of Galenic medicine, whether in Galen's own works or in its early modern revivals and extensions, we see that the standard story is false. From the practice of bloodletting along vascular lines to the knowledge of diseased and healthy parts and their treatment, the details of organs and simple parts mattered deeply. After all, as Paaw put it in an echo of many earlier anatomists, the "profit" of the "business" of anatomy came from training students to be practical physicians, who knew from anatomy "the affects and diseases of the individual parts of the whole body," and how to cure the sick parts.[5] Despite the brief warnings

---

2   Joel Kaye's conclusion is worth repeating, that Galen *never* "drew a simple equation between health and the balance (or the proper blending) of the four humors themselves." Kaye, *History of Balance*, 168.

3   Cf. Ottoson, *Scholastic*, 130–132. Siraisi, *Avicenna in the Renaissance*, 296–315. Pace, e.g., Maclean, *Logic, Signs, and Nature*, 241 and Lindemann, *Medicine*, 17–18.

4   Cook, *Matters of Exchange*, 37. For similar remarks, see, e.g., Bynum, *History of Medicine*, 15, 55. Cunningham, *Anatomist Anatomis'd*, 197. French, *Dissection and Vivisection*, 2 and throughout.

5   Paaw, *Primitiae*, unpag. preface.

of some past eminent historians, we have often substituted vague claims about humors for the impaired organs and parts at the heart of Galenic medicine.[6]

At Leiden, the leading teaching professor Johannes Heurnius drew on his humanist learning, his medical practice, and chymical processes to build the central teaching lectures and textbooks of this period. He sought to construct a precise rational method that could unite the head-to-toe survey of diseases and remedies of the teaching of medical practice tradition with the philosophical causes of the medical theory tradition. As his lectures and textbooks moved through the body and the healthy and morbid temperaments and structures of its organs and parts, Johannes Heurnius followed Galen's *Art of Medicine*, *Method of Medicine*, and *Affected Places*. But he also systematized Galen's sprawling works though sixteen categories of causes, precise weights and measures for medicinal ingredients, an expanded pharmacopoeia that embraced drugs beyond the ancient Mediterranean, chymical processes and medicines, tips from his own practice, and some post-mortem dissections. Of course, he always emphasized the importance of beginning with "the part occupied by the disease, the disease, and its cause."[7] Like other professors at Leiden and across Europe, he cultivated and extended the educational formation he had received at Padua, especially. Lines of pedagogy shaped practices and ideas across this period, producing shared activities and culture for thousands of physicians.

New anatomists eclipsed Galen's anatomical knowledge even as they drew on his work. The importance of anatomy for medical knowledge and practice, especially pathology and therapy, grew into three different types of anatomies: private, public, and clinical. In private rooms, the anatomy theater, and the hospital, professors, surgeons, and students gave perceptible embodiment to the anatomical knowledge cultivated and refined from Galen on. Although the three types of anatomies admitted different spectators into different places, they all aimed to complete the Galenic emphasis on diseases as impaired functions and injured parts by finding the causes of diseases and death in the cadavers of patients.

Pedagogical traditions and innovations grew on this Galenic foundation, with Galenic scaffolding. Professors grew the anatomy teaching tradition quickly. As early as 1582, professors performed anatomical dissections aimed at understanding the body's parts, organs, and their healthy actions. From at least

---

6   Temkin, *Galenism*, 17–18, 138, n. 10. Riese, *Conception*, 41–45. For recent work, see, e.g., Stolberg, "Post-mortems."

7   Heurnius, *Institutiones*, 534.

1587, the courses on practical medicine provided a rational method for targeting those morbid affects of the organs and specific parts with precisely-measured medicines to ameliorate morbid temperaments of the parts and to purge local developments of morbid matter. Medical theory in the standard medical theory or *Institutes* course, taught from 1592 through the 1640s, provided the theoretical foundations for knowing and treating such diseases in their local "seats" in bodily organs. Paaw performed post-mortem dissections to find the causes of disease and death at least by 1591, and students attended such private anatomies by 1598, if not earlier. From 1593, public anatomies displayed healthy and diseased bodies in the university's anatomy theater. In private and clinical anatomies, dissections of diseased bodies revealed the local changes to solid and humoral parts that constituted diseases and their causes. By at least 1636, and probably earlier, students visited patients in the hospital. Throughout this period, students eagerly attended regular post-mortem dissections in private rooms, the hospital, and the anatomy theater to learn the phenomena and facts of bodies and diseases first-hand.

Second, practices, values, histories, and maxims of medicine taught to students all emphasized the foundations of a supposedly unified Galenic-Hippocratic tradition in the senses and the best natural philosophy. Professors presented a unified medical tradition and system of knowledge, at times glossing over real difficulties such as in the theory of temperaments. These were undergraduate surveys and topical courses, after all. And to be persuaded, one had to accept the epistemological force of arguments for the primacy of hot, cold, dry, and wet qualities constituting and changing stuff in the world. Of course, this view drew power from everyday experience, rational argumentation, and the apparent poverty of crude atomist accounts, as well as the seemingly unified front of Aristotle, Galen, and "Hippocrates." It also drew power from the practitioners' deep trust in the senses to perceive the true causes of things. Indeed, the orientation of Leiden professors went well beyond the "resolutely practical and descriptive," and they confidently taught the causes of diseases with a framework and curative indications, indications that pointed to causes, culled from a Galenic theoretical system of diseases and drugs.[8]

Third, practices varied from the garden to the lecture hall, and from the hospital to the anatomy chambers, but they all depended on embodied learning about material objects. Students had to learn to read, write, dispute, see, smell, identify, taste, diagnose, prognose, treat, and comport rightly in group settings. And all while avoiding a violent or drunken end (or both), and dodging

---

8   *Pace* Cook, *Matters of Exchange*, 111.

eruptions of morbid matter during bedside instruction and post-mortem dis-sections. Ancient ideals of reason and experience, as well as more specific models and maxims, emphasized knowing first-hand through the senses in anatomy, chymistry, and botany, and motivated even the innovative practices of clinical anatomies in the hospital. Students learned to perceive and under-stand material things.

Professors and students consistently focused on material properties, changes, and explanations. When they thought about how the best books and disputation practices trained a student's "wit" or *ingenium*, they followed Galen in thinking about these pedagogical practices as shaping students' brains into a finer substance for swifter reasoning. They consistently grounded the faculties of body parts and medicinal substances in the observation of their regular material changes and effects, and in their basic mixtures of hot, cold, wet, and dry qualities. After all, these qualities were the fundamental active powers of the material world. Physicians often avoided explaining faculties of bodies in terms of the soul, leaving that way of speaking to philosophers. Rather, the faculties of organs or medicinal ingredients arose from their basic mixture, in relation to some other object. The gallbladder visibly retains and expels bile, so it has faculties for retention and expulsion; aloe cleanses eyes, so it has a faculty for cleansing. The rational schemes of primary qualitative mixtures, their degrees, and higher-order faculties based on these mixtures did not usually work out in practice (though Johannes Heurnius and others cer-tainly tried). But the material powers of things, discovered by direct sensation and the study of their effects, constituted the core of faculty theory. In this, of course, they followed Galen's example in his works on faculties and medicines, notably *Simple Drugs*.

In gardens and on herborizing field trips, professors and students trained to know plants and their faculties by direct sensory engagement and textual tradition. Petrus Paaw and Johannes Heurnius had to study hard with samples from the garden of Hoghelande. Students filled their workbooks on the univer-sity garden's plants with names and uses. They attempted to fit plants' faculties into the rational ground of their primary mixtures of qualities, but most often they followed traditions of the teaching of medical practice and listed ingredi-ents by their faculties and doses "proven by long use."

When they turned to patients' bodies, materials and material explanation also distinguished the Galenic search for the three most important things to know: the disease, the cause(s) of the disease, and the remedies. Following Galen, influential professors such as Da Monte at Padua and Johannes Heurnius at Leiden emphasized what they called material causes. These included qual-itative alterations to parts that caused local intemperances, and so made a part's faculties malfunction. (Da Monte called qualitative changes "incorporeal material causes.") They scrutinized many kinds of material causes: the putrefaction of solids and humors, changes to the qualities of organs or humors, ruptures, breaks, obstructions of vessels, the concretion of matter around arthritic joints, and the formation of ulcers, abscesses, and tubercles. In short, professors and students came to know and treat many kinds of material changes. In the bodies of living patients, they tracked down diseases to their anatomical seats by examining patients' faces, feet, arms, hands, and excrements. They attended to the causal influences of food, drink, air, and contagion, among other causes natural, non-natural, and divine. In their anatomies, professors and surgeons looked for the visible and tangible effects of qualitative changes in "burnt" or desiccated organs. They also noted the causes of diseases and death in morbid material accretions such as abscesses or blockages in ducts, organ putrefaction, preternatural humors they could sense and measure, and even small amounts of matter where it should not be, such as the yolk-like liquid in the hearts of two women felled by sudden death. When they adopted Aristotelian categories of causes, like Galen they materialized them. Efficient causes were often proximate material and qualitative causes, formal causes reduced to the shape and structure of body parts, and final causes dropped out—diseases impaired final causes. Of course, as Galen and Aristotle agreed, knowing the use or function of a part was essential for understanding the healthy body. Anatomy mattered for knowing healthy and diseased parts. Professors also materialized and debunked claims about witchcraft and rejected the doctrine of signatures as superstition.

Surprisingly, these students of Galenic medicine learned chymical operations and recipes as well, and earlier than 1587. Close readings of the textbooks and lecture notes of Leiden professors and students reveal a learned and practical medicine that embraced chymistry far earlier than reigning narratives allow.[9] Traditional ideals of knowing materials through the senses and finding treatments that work also motivated the welcoming embrace of chymical processes, and some chymical theory, and the use of chymical remedies. Johannes Heurnius' youthful enthusiasm for Paracelsian chymistry and transmutation lived on in his teaching, but in a domesticated form more appropriate to the standards of the official examinations and degrees. He still praised and taught

---

9 *Pace* Powers, *Inventing Chemistry*, 47, 6–8, 62, 91, 169. Powers maintains that there was no chymical instruction before 1642, and that before Boerhaave's pedagogical reforms in the early 1700s Leiden chymical teaching was marginal, low status, and aimed primarily at the production of remedies rather than knowledge. For some later revisions to this story, see, e.g., Ragland, "Chymistry" and Ragland, "Experimental Clinical Medicine."

chymistry as necessary and useful for medicine and life, and folded chymists into his lineage of the true medicine by claiming that Democritus taught Hippocrates the art of chymistry. Other professors, such as Johannes Walaeus, continued to teach some chymistry into the 1630s, even as they kept to their Galenic-Hippocratic foundations and principles.

Professors modeled how to know medicines from personal experience in their lectures and especially in their clinical teaching. Johannes Heurnius testified to the effectiveness of chymical remedies from his own practice, for example in his recommendation of oil of vitriol for all sorts of complaints, or of the flowers of Sulphur to treat phthisis. Similarly, his son Otto Heurnius practiced and taught from his own direct experience trying old and new drugs on patients. He used ingredients from ancient pharmacopoeias, as well as novel substances from the New World and Asia, and chymical productions made by laboratory processes. In the university garden, too, Otto Heurnius cultivated knowledge about useful substances, teaching students to identify plants by their visible features and to correlate types and appearances with medicinal faculties known through textual traditions and informal trials in patients' bodies. In the hospital, we can see physicians showing students the practice of making incremental tweaks to remedies based on a patient's observed progress. In the case of our foot soldier of the growing Dutch empire, Otto Heurnius attempted to recreate the indigenous remedy, the "oil of Couroq," and kept administering the same purgative mixture that had worked for weeks, but reduced the amounts to lessen the facultative powers of the ingredients. Surgeons such as Joannes Camphusius worked regularly with professors such as Otto Heurnius to excise corrupt parts, dress wounds, and dissect bodies to establish the legal causes of death. With expert surgeons and physicians at their sides, Leiden students learned the proper balance between medicinal treatments and surgical interventions.

Anatomy, like natural history and clinical instruction, aimed mainly at developing techniques of sense-based observation, memory, and reporting. Following long pedagogical traditions from ancient models and newly extended practices, students learned to track the phenomena and describe them closely. Rational systems of organs, faculties, actions, and their diseases ordered their attention and descriptions, but did not eclipse the phenomena.

In the practices of clinical teaching and clinical anatomies in the hospital, professors such as Otto Heurnius could correlate patients' symptoms with the visible and tactile morbid changes of their organs and parts revealed in dissections. Of course, this was something Paaw had done as well in private and public dissections. Paaw, like Dodonaeus, performed post-mortem dissections as an extension of his own educational formation in Italy. Paaw and

Otto Heurnius also played legal roles in the city as experts on the causes of death, especially in cases of suspected murder by poisoning or witchcraft. But Otto Heurnius had more frequent contact with more patients, and their cadavers, through the regular instruction in the hospital set up in 1636. From patients in their hospital beds to chymicals, plants, and dissected bodies, students learned to sense and know a world of medical objects.

Fourth, building *upon* and *with* ancient models and texts, rather than against them, these institutionalized pedagogical practices cultivated genuine innovations in pathology, therapy, and anatomy. Even here, professors contined to build with Galenic materials, enriched by chymistry and new anatomical and clinical practices and knowledge. Our history of phthisis or consumption demonstrates the productivity of pedagogy for gradual innovations in pathology and therapy. Physicians from at least the Hippocratic writers on had used signs to make inferences to the hidden phlegm, pus, swellings, erosion, and ulcers they thought caused phthisis. Galen reasoned from the expectorated pus and blood, difficulty breathing, fever, and impaired nutrition to ulceration of the lung as the proximate cause. By the 1590s, Paaw at Leiden joined other physicians and surgeons in cutting into bodies to reveal and sense directly these inferred ulcers. He also found hardened stones and pus-filled abscesses in the lungs of phthisic patients. From the mid-1630s, Otto Heurnius had more bodies to examine, and reported a more detailed range of morbid appearances. In the teaching hospital, he observed and treated the symptoms of several phthisic patients; clinical anatomies of the bodies of the unfortunates uncovered a spectrum of morbid states, from lungs "marbled with dark and pale droplets," to "many tiny tubercles" formed from a "crude, viscous matter," to larger and smaller abscesses and open ulcers.[10] To treat these morbid lesions, physicians drew on ancient traditions, such as the nutrifying power of milk, but added chymical medicines, empiric sugar cures, and other darts to throw at their deadly foe.

Professors and students also accumulated anatomical innovations beyond pathological anatomy. Paaw staked his claim to new bones in the inner ear and new insights into treatment. Controversies over the action of the pulse—did the heart and arteries pulse simultaneously, or alternately?—pushed Leiden professors to experiment on live frogs. Although their work often confirmed Galen's explanations, students inspected, and even swooned over, more radical innovations. Students felt the attraction of radical anatomical doctrines developed through close descriptions of particulars and sophisticated experiments,

---

10   Otto Heurnius, *Historiae*, 10, 22.

especially those of Aselli on the lacteals and Harvey on the circulation of the blood. Increasingly, from at least 1631, they debated these claims and even publicly defended them. Franciscus Sylvius' 1634 disputation defended the pulmonary transit of the blood, in line with his professor Johannes Walaeus' lectures from 1633. A few years later, around 1640, students aggressively defended the circulation and extended Harvey's lines of experimental investigation.[11]

By looking ahead to clinical anatomies in the 1660s, we saw how the institutionalized pedagogical practices of clinical teaching and clinical anatomies at Leiden fostered significant innovations in the pathology of Sylvius. Trained as a student and later returned to teach his new experimentalist, chymical medicine, Sylvius correlated extensive clinical observations with dozens of clinical anatomies to construct a new theory of phthisis around the development of tubercles in the lungs. He used the standard definition of disease as impaired bodily function. He also extended the earlier attention to tubercles and ulcers throughout the body, and presented the similar developmental pathways of tubercles in scrofula and phthisis as a way to associate the two diseases. Like his predecessors, he described the passing on of phthisis by contagion and hereditary dispositions. He also used the lung-cleansing Sulphur remedies of his forebears, and added other chymical remedies to neutralize acids and alkalis, and laudanum to dull pain. Later eminent physicians such as Morgagni celebrated Sylvius' new pathology and etiology of phthisis based on post-mortem dissections. Even Laennec's fine-grained studies of consumptive tubercles and symptoms from the early 1800s show striking similarities to those generated from Leiden pedagogical traditions nearly two centuries earlier. His definition of pathological anatomy also bears a remarkable (genealogical?) resemblance to the course descriptions and methodological statements of Leiden hospital teaching.

Fifth, and finally, the scholarly and civic expertise of physicians depended on their deep intellectual and bodily engagement with things *hand in hand with* their bookish study of texts. Discursive study and skill earned students degrees and licences. It also provided physicians with a shared set of concepts and models for knowing particulars. As with humanists across Europe, these physicians and students sought to know particulars and incorporate them into their systems and histories of knowledge.[12] A predilection for facts, attested by witnesses with the right expertise, flourished. As in natural history, this likely grew from humanist values and practices of discursive expertise. These values and practices came about not from leaving texts and the ancients behind, but

---

11   Schouten, *Walaeus*, 15–17. Ragland, "Mechanism." Drake, *Disputatio.*

12   Ogilvie, *Science of Describing*, 116. See also the sources in the following note.

from adding to this copious humanist erudition the experience of particulars demanded by ancient texts, from the needs of practice, and from the world overflowing with new things to know. This elevation of *historia*, well known from historians' studies of natural history, anatomical texts, humanist scholarship, and other subjects, also mutually reinforced legal forms of witnessing.[13] In natural history, experts earned credibility across a variety of social backgrounds, from the acutely erudite Clusius to learned apothecaries such as Dirck Cluyt and Christiaan Porret, to noble women, students, and contacts in foreign lands.[14] Dirck's son Outgert Cluyt joined apothecary training to Leiden University medical education. His perilous journeys across the Mediterranean in search of new medicines introduced him to the learned Jewish doctors and dangerous pirates of the region. Johannes Heurnius took careful note of the wonders he saw as a student in Italy or in Paris with Petrus Ramus, and attested to the particular truths of chymistry in his own courses. Teaching at Leiden, Johannes Heurnius and Petrus Paaw practiced their hands-on plant identification skills with the garden and collection of the Leiden naturalist Johan van Hoghelande. Heurnius also pushed students toward fine precision of weights and measures when they mined ancient and early modern texts on drugs for useful remedies.

Anatomical practices and forms of writing corroborated this trend of communities of experts establishing facts about the natural world. Surgeons acted as witnesses of the facts of public, private, and clinical anatomies. Paaw, Johannes Heurnius, and Otto Heurnius all described what they had seen and felt (and sometimes smelled). After all, the explicit central goal of anatomy was to train students to be practical physicians by revealing to their senses the phenomena of healthy and diseased bodies and parts. Especially in post-mortem dissections, professors took care to name the expert witnesses—notably physicians *and* surgeons—whose expertise and status grounded their reports of the phenomena uncovered in dissected cadavers. There were often high legal and social stakes for the conclusions of their dissections, including for professors themselves. Paaw confidently identified evidence of murder by poison in several bodies, and also cleared his colleague Johannes Heurnius of accusations of poisoning a patient. Paaw also critiqued rival anatomists based on what he himself had seen, and argued for his priority in identifying small bones of the ear. Similarly, the anatomist Volcher Coiter narrated what he had seen in his anatomical experiments and dissections, greatly expanding the more limited historical narrative styles of anatomists such as Berengario, Vesalius, Colombo,

---

13   Pomata, "Praxis Historialis." Pomata, "A Word of the Empirics." Pomata, "Observation
      Rising." Findlen, *Possessing Nature.* Ogilvie, *Science of Describing.*
14   Cf. Egmond, *World.*

and Valverde.[15] In university medicine, pharmacology, natural history, clinical practice, and anatomy, then, facts took their establishment from communities of witnesses who achieved credibility based on their trained expertise. These expert witnesses shared, but at times debated and denied, claims to facts. Discursive skill and erudition, together with perceived and trained practical abilities, made early modern physicians, and made them credible experts.

Clearly, communities of practitioners at Leiden and other universities trained students in the practices of being a physician. Practices are now often at the heart of histories of science and medicine, but practices are not merely activities, or whatever people happened to do.[16] They are complex, sustained, goal-oriented, and communally-cultivated. Pedagogical cultures train students in practices in this sense, and in so doing make them into physicians and other distinct community members. Further, histories of practices are not neatly separable from histories of ideas, disciplinary ideals, or rational methodologies. Rather, as I have tried to show in this book, the wide range of practices that constituted the making of early modern physicians always combined discourse and sensation, ideas and objects. Our histories have to embrace this range, too. This approach may look somewhat "internalist," but detailing communities of practitioners and their practices necessarily demands that we attend closely to how things look from the inside, though with our eyes open to much broader connections and contexts.

The rich sources and practices of early modern universities are ripe for the picking. The histories of early modern science and medicine rightly display the scholarly bounty acquired from other plots, such as the famed scientific societies, courts, households, frontiers, commercial exchanges, indigenous communities, and many more groups and sites of knowing and doing. But shared pedagogy made shared practices and cultures, and changes to pedagogy produced broad and deep effects. If we want to understand how many thousands of people came to share the sophisticated and productive practices of knowing and doing surveyed above—and many more in mathematics, natural philosophy, and medicine across Europe and the wider world—surely universities call for more attention.[17]

---

15   Ragland, "'Making Trials.'"

16   For a recent historiographic discussion, see Hicks and Stapleford, "Virtues of Scientific Practice."

17   For some examples of the significance of pedagogy for modern science, see Kaiser, *Pedagogy and the Practice of Science.* For excellent studies of sixteenth- and early seventeenth-century pedagogy and science, see, for example: Findlen, *Possessing Nature.* Feingold, *Mathematicians' Apprenticeship.* Dear, *Discipline and Experience.* Klestinec, *Theaters of Anatomy.* Moran, *Andreas Libavius.*

Of course, it would be absurdly provincial to claim Leiden academic culture, or even the broader academic or medical cultures, created all or most of the new sciences or ways of knowing in the early modern period. But across European academic medicine we see a striking pattern. Increasingly, professors, students, and physicians combined the scholarly revival of ancient methods and ideals with a growing elevation and dependence on their own sensory experience or experiments, alongside the elevation of disciplines to greater philosophical status.

This book joins a chorus of studies on sixteenth-century humanist anatomy, natural history, and medicine focused mostly on other places to argue strongly for the priority of academic culture. This culture had demonstrable roots in the learned cultures at Italian, German, and other universities, which built models and methods from ancient sources. Pedagogical formation, humanist research in ancient sources, embodied engagement with things, and the goal of finding knowledge and practices that worked to treat the sick combined to make physicians who they were, and so made much of academic medical culture what it was. If there are important effects from the values and tastes of the political and commercial elites, they are not at all obvious in the sources from these communities. These academic cultures, which emphasized personal experience, exact description, clear communication of facts, and even making trials or experiments, clearly pre-date the rise of the remarkable Dutch global trade empire.[18]

The culture and developments in academic medicine were, perhaps unsurprisingly, first and foremost academic. That pedagogy was an important mode of cultivating medical and scientific practices and practitioners should not surprise us; that is what pedagogical formation does. Similar training formed the medical men who made up large or predominant parts of seventeenth-century scientific societies, including the English Royal Society, the French Académie des Sciences, and especially the German Academia Naturae Curiosorum.[19]

We now know much better how Leiden University medical education made students into physicians. Pedagogy made students practitioners in a variety of practices. Even our short course of study in the rich flood of sources from that time and place has rendered up serious revisions for standard narratives about Galenic medicine and the much longer histories of pathology and clinical practice. Contrary to widespread claims, organs and other body parts were vital to Galenic medical theory, pathology, and therapy. Students and professors

---

18   *Pace* Cook, *Matters of Exchange.* See the introduction for more discussion.
19   Cook, "New Philosophy and Medicine in Seventeenth-Century England," 403–404; Stroup, *A Company of Scientists*, 172; and Barnett, "Medical Authority and Princely Patronage."

eagerly engaged in pathological dissections, in private, public, and clinical settings, and built new knowledge of the sick parts and their treatments. Standard courses welcomed chymical practices and medicines as necessary for health and life. Professors developed ancient knowledge and methods into systems that secured their reputations and made gradual innovations possible. Material causes and objects of study from plants to chymical substances, and from living bodies to morbid cadavers, took center stage as the sources of knowledge and practical experience for practicing physicians. Bookish, discursive expertise inspired, guided, and framed sensory experience with things. This was a complex culture that displayed the productive interplay of tradition and innovation. There were many more sites of educational formation and practice, and more times of both change and conservation. Surely there is much more to learn about other places and times that similarly made early modern academic medicine out of books and disputations, medicines and ingredients, bodies living and dead.

Bibliography

Archival Sources

Archief van notaris Adriaen [Pietersz.] den Oosterlingh, 1663–1691, 1669, Regionaal Archief Leiden, archiefnummer 506, inventarisnummer 1068, aktenummer 202 and aktenummer 283.

Robert Hepburne, Sloane MS 201, British Library.

Sloane MS 658, British Library.

Sloane MS 3528, British Library.

Carolus Clusius to Justus Lipsius, Oct. 8 1594, CLU C316. Leiden University.

Carolus Clusius to Joachim Camerarius II, Nov. 22, 1592. CLU C290. Leiden University.

Petrus Paaw to Carolus Clusius, August 1593, Leiden University Library, VUL 101:214.

Printed Primary Sources

Adamus, Melchior. *Vitae Germanorum Medicorum*. Heidelberg: Impensis heredum Jonae Rosae, Excudit Johannes Georgius Geyder, Acad. Typogr., 1620.

Adelon, Nicolas. *Dictionnaire des Sciences Médicales*. Paris: C. L. F. Panckoucke, 1812–1822.

Agricola, Georgius (Georg). *Libri quinque de Mensuris & Ponderibus*. Paris: Excludebat Christianus Wechelus, 1533.

Album studiosorum Academiae Lugduno-Batavae MDLXXV–MDCCCLXXV. Edited by G. de Reu. The Hague: Apud Martinum Nijhoff, 1875.

Antonius, Donatus. *Nonnulla Opuscula Nunc Primum in Unum Collecta*. Venice, 1561.

Aristotle. *Metaphysics, Volume I: Books 1–9*. Translated by Hugh Tredennick. Loeb Classical Library 271. Cambridge, MA: Harvard University Press, 1933.

Aristotle. *Nichomachean Ethics*. Translated by H. Rackham. Loeb Classical Library 73. Cambridge, MA: Harvard University Press, 1926.

Aristotle. *On the Soul. Parva Naturalia. On Breath*. Translated by W. S. Hett. Loeb Classical Library 288. Cambridge, MA: Harvard University Press, 1957.

Aristotle. *Physics*. Translated by R. P. Hardie and R. K. Gaye. In *The Complete Works of Aristotle*, edited by Jonathan Barnes. 2 vols. Princeton: Princeton University Press, 1984.

Aselli, Gaspare *De Lactibus Sive Lacteis Venis Quarto Vasorum Mesaraicorurn Genere Novo Invento Gasparis Asellii Cremonensis Anatomici Ticinensis Dissertatio*. Milan, 1627.

Atti della nazione germanica artista nello Studio di Padova, edited by Antonio Favaro. 2 vols. Venice: A Spese della Societa, 1911–1912.

Avicenna (Ibn Sina). *Liber Canonis, de medicinis cordialibus, et cantica.* Translated by Andrea Alpago. Venice: Giunta, 1544.

Avicenna (Ibn Sina). *Liber Canonis Avicenne revisus.* Venice, 1507.

Bartholin, Thomas. *Thomae Bartholini Epistolarum Medicinalium, Century IV.* The Hague, 1740.

Benivieni, Antonio. *De Abditis Nonnullis Ac Mirandis Morborum et Sanationum Causis.* Translated by Charles Singer. Springfield: Charles C. Thomas, 1954.

Berengario da Carpi, Giacamo. *Commentaria cum amplissimis additionibus super anatomiam Mundini una cum textu ejusdem in pristinum et verum nitorem redacto.* Bologna: Hieronymum de Benedectis, 1521.

Blancken, Gerard. *Catalogus Antiquarum, et Novarum Rerum, ex Longe Dissitis Terrarum Oris, Quarum Visendarum Copia Lugduni in Batavis, in Anatomia Publica.* Leiden: Danielis van der Boxe, 1671.

Boerhaave, Herman. "Discourse on Chemistry Purging Itself of Its Own Errors." In *Boerhaave's Orations.* Translated with introductions and notes by E. Kegel-Brinkgreve and A. M. Luyendijk-Elshout, 180–213. Leiden: E. J. Brill / Leiden University Press, 1983.

Bonet, Theophilus. *Sepulchretum Sive Anatomia Practica, Ex Cadaveribus Morbo Denatis, Vol. 1.* Geneva: Leonardus Chouet, 1679.

Bronchorst (Bronckhorst), Everardus. *Diarium sive Adversaria Omnium quae Gesta Sunt in Academia Leydensi (1591–1627),* edited by J. C. van Slee. The Hague: Martinus Nijhoff, 1898.

Brouchuisius, Danielis (Daniel van Broekhuizen), ed. *Secreta Alchimiae magnalia D. Thomae Aquinatis, De Corporibus supercoelestibus, & quòd in rebus inferioribus inueniantur, quoque modo extrahantur: De Lapide minerali, animali, plantali. Item Thesaurus Alchimiae secretissimus, quem dedit fratri suo Reinaldo. Accessit et Ioannis de Rupescissa Liber lucis, ac Raymundi Lullij opus pulcherrimum, quod inscribitur Clauicula & Apertorium: in quo omnia quae in opere Alchimiae requiruntur, venustè declarantur, & sine quo, vt ipse testatur Lullius, alij sui Libri intellegi nequeunt. Opusculua studiosis artis secretissimae, vt summè necessaria, ita lectu iucundissima. Opera Danielis Brovcvisii artium & medicinae Doctoris nunc primùm in lucem edita. cum Praefatione D. Ioannis Huernij* [sic]. Cologne: Nicolaus Bohm-bargen, 1579.

Cockeram, Henry. *English Dictionarie.* London, 1623.

Coiter, Volcher. *Externarum et internarum principalium humani corporis partium tabulae.* Nuremberg: Theodoricus Gerlatzenus, 1573.

Coiter, Volcher. *Lectiones Gabrielis Fallopii de Partibus Similaribus Humani Corporis... His Accessere Diversorum Animalium Sceletorum Explicationes Iconibus Artificiosis.* Nuremberg: In Officinia Theodorici Gerlachii, 1575.

Coiter, Volcher. *Observationum anatomicarum chirurgicarumque miscellanea varia, in Externarum et internarum principalium humani corporis partium tabulae.* Nuremberg: Theodoricus Gerlatzenus, 1573.

Cordus, Euricius. *Botanologicon.* Cologne, 1534.

Cotgrave, Randle. *Randle Cotgrave, A Dictionarie of the French and English Tongues.* London: Adam Islip, 1611.

Da Forli, Jacopo. *Expositio super tres libros Tegni Galeni.* Pavia, 1487.

Da Monte, Giambattista. *In Nonum Librum Rhasis ad Mansorem Regem Arabum, Expositio.* Venice: Apud Baltassarem Constantinum ad Signum Divi Georgii, 1554.

Da Monte, Giambattista. *Lectiones...In secundam Fen primi Canonis Avicennae.* Venice: Vincentius Valgrisius, 1557.

Da Monte, Giambattista. *Opuscula uaria praeclara.* Basel: Per Petrum Pernem, 1558.

De Graaf, Reinier. *Disputatio Medica de Natura et Usu Succi Pancreatici.* Leiden, 1664.

De Raey, Johannes. *Clavis philosophiae naturalis, seu introductio ad naturae contemplationem Aristotelico-Cartesiana.* Leiden: Johannis & Danielis Elsevier, 1651.

[De Raey, Johannes]. *Disputatio Philosophica de Mundi Systemate & Elementis. Prima.* Respondent Carolous Loten. Leiden, 1661.

[De Raey, Johannes]. *Disputationum physicarum ad Problemata Aristotelis, Prima de praecognitis in genere.* Respondent Casparus ter Haars. Leiden: Francisci Hackii, 1651.

Descartes, René. *Discourse on Method.* In *The Philosophical Writings of Descartes.* Translated by John Cottingham, Robert Stoothoff, and Dugald Murdoch. 2 vols. Cambridge: Cambridge University Press, 1985. [CSM]

Dioscorides, Pedanius. *De materia medica.* Translated by Lily Y. Beck. Altertumswissenschaftliche Texte und Studien 38. Hildesheim: Olms, 2005.

Dodonaeus (Dodoens), Rembertus (Rembert). *Medicinalium Observationum exempla rara* Cologne: Apud Maternum Cholinum, 1581.

Dodonaeus (Dodoens), Rembertus (Rembert). *Stirpium Historiae Pemptades Sex.* Antwerp: Christophorus Plantinus, 1583.

Drake, Roger. *Disputatio Medica de Circulatione Naturali. Seu, Cordis & Sanguinis Motu Circulari. Pro Cl. Harveio, Thesis II.* Leiden: Wilhelmi Christiani, 1640.

Eden, Richard. *A treatyse of the newe* India. London: In Lombard strete, by [S. Mierdman for] Edward Sutton, [1553].

Falloppio (Falloppia), Gabriele. *Observationes Anatomicae.* Venice: Apud Marcum Antonium Vlmum, 1561.

Fernel, Jean. *Universa Medicina Primùm quidem studio & diligentiâ Guiljelmi Plantii, Cennomanni elimata, Nunc autem notis, observationibus, & remediis secretis Ioann. & Othonis HeurnI, Ultraject. et Aliorum Praestantissimorum Medicorum scholiis illustrata. Cui accedunt Casus & observationes rariores, Quas Cl. D.D. Otho Heurnius in Academia Leydensi Primarius Medicinae practicae, Anatomiae & Chirurgiae Professor, in diario practico annotavit.* Utrecht: Gisbertus à Zijll & Theodorus ab Ackersdijck, 1656.

Fernel, Jean. *Pathologiae Libri VII* in *Medicina.* Paris: Apud Andream Wechelum, 1554.

Fernel, Jean. *Physiologia*. In *The Physiologia of Jean Fernel (1567)*. Translated and Annotated by John M. Forrester. Philadelphia: American Philosophical Society, 2003.

Ferrier, Auger. *Vera medendi methodus, duobus libris comprehensa*. Leiden: Ex Officina Ludovici, 1574.

Florentius, Henricus (respondent). *Disputatio Medica de Exulceratione Renum*. Leiden, 1611.

Fuchs, Leonhart. *De Historia Stirpium Commentarii Insignes*. Basel, 1542.

Fuchs, Leonhart. *De Medendis Singularum Humani Corporis Partium A Summo Capite ad Imos Usque Pedes Passionibus ac Febribus*. Basel, 1539.

Fuchs, Leonhart. *Institutionum medicinae, ad Hippocratis, Galeni, aliorúmque veterum scripta rectè intelligenda mirè vtiles Libri quinque*. Leiden: Apud Sebastianum Barptolomaei Honorati, 1555.

Fuchs, Leonhart. *Institutionum medicinae Libri quinque*. Basel: Typis Conradi Vvaldkirchij, 1605.

Galen. *Claudii Galeni Pergameni Ars Medica*. Translated by Martinus Akakia. Venice: Ex Officina Erasmiana, apud Vincentium Vaugrius, prope horologium Divi Marci, 1544.

Galen. *De Affectorum Locorum Notitia, libri sex, Guilielmo Copo Basiliensi interprete*. Paris: officina Simonis Colinaei, 1520.

Galen. *De simplicium medicamentorum facultatibus libri XI*. Translated by Theodoricus Gaudanus. Leiden, Gulielmus Rouillius, 1561.

Galen. *De Symptomatum Differentiis* in Galen, *Claudii Galeni Pergameni de Morborum et Symptomatum Differentiis et Causis libri sex Gulielmo Copo Basileiensi interprete*. Paris: Ex officina Christiani Wecheli, 1546.

Galen. *Extraordinem Classium Libri*. Venice: Apud Ivntas, 1556.

Galen. *Method of Medicine*. Translated by Ian Johnston and G. H. R. Horsley. Loeb Classical Library 516. Cambridge, MA: Harvard University Press, 2011.

Galen. *Mixtures*. In *Galen: Selected Works*. Translated with an Introduction and Notes by P. N. Singer, 202–295. Oxford and New York: Oxford University Press, 1997.

Galen. *On Anatomical Procedures: Translation of the Surviving Books with Introduction and Notes*, translated by Charles Singer. New York: Oxford University Press, 1956.

Galen. *Galen on Anatomical Procedures: The Later Books*. Translated by W. L. H. Duckworth. Cambridge: Cambridge University Press, 1962.

Galen, *On Prognostics*, ch. 11, in *Source Book of Medical History*, edited and translated by Logan Clendening, 50–51. New York: Dover, 1960.

Galen. *On the Pulse for Beginners*. In *Galen: Selected Works*. Translated with an Introduction and Notes by P. N. Singer, 325–344. Oxford and New York: Oxford University Press, 1997.

Galen. *On the Causes of Diseases*. In *Galen: On Diseases and Symptoms*. Translated by Ian Johnston, 157–179. Cambridge: Cambridge University Press, 2011.

Galen. *On the Differentia of Diseases*. In *Galen: On Diseases and Symptoms*. Translated by Ian Johnston, 131–156. Cambridge: Cambridge University Press, 2011.

Galen. *Omnia, quae extant*. Translated by Johannes Baptista Rasarius. Venice: Vincentius Valgrisius, 1562.

Galen. *On the Natural Faculties*. Translated by A. J. Brock. Loeb Classical Library 71. Cambridge, MA: Harvard University Press, 1916.

Galen. *On the Usefulness of the Parts of the Body*. Translated by Margaret T. May. 2 vols. Ithaca: Cornell University Press, 1968.

Galen. *The Art of Medicine*. In *Galen: Selected Works*. Translated with an Introduction and Notes by P. N. Singer, 345–396. Oxford and New York: Oxford University Press, 1997.

Galen. *The Construction of the Embryo*. In *Galen: Selected Works*. Translated with an Introduction and Notes by P. N. Singer, 177–201. Oxford and New York: Oxford University Press, 1997.

Galen. *The Soul's Dependence on the Body*. Translated by P. N. Singer. In *Galen: Selected Works*. Translated with an Introduction and Notes by P. N. Singer, 151–176. Oxford and New York: Oxford University Press, 1997.

Pseudo-Galen, *On Theriac to Piso*. Translated by Robert Leigh. In *On Theriac to Piso, Attributed to Galen: A Critical Edition with Translation and Commentary*. Leiden: Brill, 2016.

Gesner, Conrad. *Euonymus, Sive de Remediis Secretis...Pars Secunda*. Leiden: Apid Bartholom. Vincentium, 1572.

Goclenius, Rudolph. *Lexicon Philosophicum*. Frankfurt, 1613.

Gryllus (Gryll), Laurentius (Lorenz). *De Sapore Dulci et Amaro*. Prague, 1566.

Harvey, William. *Exercitatio Anatomica I, Exercitationes Duae Anatomicae de Circulatione Sanguinis*. Rotterdam: Arnold Leers, 1649.

Harvey, William. *Exercitationes de Generatione Animalium. Amsterdam*: Apud Ludovicum Elzevirium, 1651.

[Heereboord, Adrianus]. *Disputatio Philosophica de Metaphysicae Constitutione*. Respondent Franciscus Nysius. Leiden, 1659.

Herodotus. *The Persian Wars*. Translated by A. D. Godley. Loeb Classical Library 117. Cambridge, MA: Harvard University Press, 2004.

Heseler, Baldasar. *Andreas Vesalius' First Public Anatomy at Bologna, 1540*. Translated by Ruben Eriksson. Uppsala: Almqvist & Wiksell, 1959.

Heurnius (van Heurne), Johannes. *De Historie, Natuere ende Beduidenisse der erschrickelicke Comeet*. 1577.

Heurnius (van Heurne), Johannes. *De Morbis Pectoris Liber*. Leiden: Ex Officina Plantiniana, Raphelingii, 1602.

Heurnius (van Heurne), Johannes. *De morbis qui in singulis partibus humani capitis insidere consueverunt*. Leiden: Franciscus Raphelingius, 1594.

Heurnius (van Heurne), Johannes. *Hippocratis Coi Aphorismi Graecè, & Latinè.* Leiden: Ex Officina Plantiniana, 1609.

Heurnius (van Heurne), Johannes. *Institutiones Medicinae, Exceptae è dictantis eius ore. Accessit modus studendi eorum qui Medicinae operam suam dicarunt.* Leiden: Ex Officina Plantiniana, Apud Franciscum Raphelengium, 1592.

Heurnius (van Heurne), Johannes. *Institutiones Medicinae. Editio altera, priore emendatior, operâ auctoris filii Othonis Heurnii.* Leiden: Ex officina Plantiniana, Raphelingii, 1609.

Heurnius (van Heurne), Johannes. *Institutiones medicinae.* Leiden: Ex Officina Ioannis Maire, 1638.

Heurnius (van Heurne), Johannes. *Opera Omnia: tam ad Theoriam, quam at Praxin Medicam Spectantia.* 2 Vols. Leiden: Sumptibus Ioannis Antonii Hvgvetan, & Marci Antonii Ravavd, 1658.

Heurnius (van Heurne), Johannes. *Praxis Medicinae Nova Ratio.* Leiden: Ex Officina Plantiniana, Apud Franciscum Raphelingium, 1587.

Heurnius (van Heurne), Johannes. *Praxis Medicinae Nova Ratio.* Leiden: Ex Officina Plantiniana, Raphelingij, 1609.

Heurnius (van Heurne), Johannes. *Praxis Medicinae Nova Ratio.* Rotterdam: Ex Officinâ Arnoldi Leers, 1650.

Heurnius (van Heurne), Otto. *Historiae et Observationes quaedam Rariores ex Praxi et Diario* in Jean Fernel, *Universa Medicina Primùm quidem studio & diligentiâ Guiljelmi Plantii, Cennomanni elimata, Nunc autem notis, observationibus, & remediis secretis Ioann. & Othonis HeurnI, Ultraject. et Aliorum Praestantissimorum Medicorum scholiis illustrata. Cui accedunt Casus & observationes rariores, Quas Cl. D.D. Otho Heurnius in Academia Leydensi Primarius Medicinae practicae, Anatomiae & Chirurgiae Professor, in diario practico annotavit.* Utrecht: Gisbertus à Zijll & Theodorus ab Ackersdijck, 1656.

[Heurnius, Otto] "Vita Auctoris." In *Ioannis Heurnii Vltraiectini...Opera Omnia.* Leiden: Ex Officina Plantiniana Raphelingii, 1609.

Hexham, Henry. *Het Groot Woorden-Boeck: Gestalt in 't Nederduytsch, End in 't Engelsch.* Rotterdam: Arnout Leers, 1648.

Hildanus, Guilhelmus Fabricius. *Opera Observationum et Curationum Medico-Chirurgicarum.* Frankfurt: Sumptibus Ioan Ludov Dufour, 1682.

Hippocrates. *Affections. Diseases 1. Diseases 2.* Translated by Paul Potter. Loeb Classical Library 472. Cambridge, MA: Harvard University Press, 1988.

Hippocrates. *Ancient Medicine. Airs, Waters, Places. Epidemics 1 and 3. The Oath. The Precepts. Nutriment.* Translated by W. H. S. Jones. Loeb Classical Library 147. Cambridge, MA: Harvard University Press, 1923.

Hippocrates. *Epidemics 2, 4–7.* Edited and translated by Wesley D. Smith. Loeb Classical Library 477. Cambridge, MA: Harvard University Press, 1994.

Hippocrates, Heracleitus. *Nature of Man. Regimen in Health. Humours. Aphorisms. Regimen 1–3. Dreams. Heracleitus: On the Universe.* Translated by W. H. S. Jones. Loeb Classical Library 150. Cambridge, MA: Harvard University Press, 1931.

Hippocrates. *On Ancient Medicine.* Translated by Mark J. Schiefsky. In *Hippocrates 'On Ancient Medicine': Translated with Introduction and Commentary.* Leiden: Brill, 2005.

Jacchaeus (Jack), Gilbertus. *Institutiones medicae.* Leiden: Ioannes Maire, 1624.

Kyper, Albert. *Institutiones Medicae.* Amsterdam, Apud Joannem Janssonium, 1654.

Kyper, Albert. *Medicinam Rite Discendi et Exercendi Methodus.* Leiden: Apud Heironymum de Vogel, 1643.

Kyper, Albert. *Transsumpta Medica, Ea ex Physicis repetentia, Quibus Continentur Medicinae Fundamenta* in *Institutiones Medicae.* Amsterdam, Apud Joannem Janssonium, 1654.

Laennec, R. T. H. *A Treatise on the Diseases of the Chest.* Translated by John Forbes. London: Henry Renshaw, 1834.

Lange, Johannes. *Epistolarum Medicinalium Volumen Tripartitum.* Frankfurt: Apud heredes Andreae Wecheli, 1589.

Laurentius, Andreas. *Historia Anatomica, Humani Corporis Partes Singulas Uberrime Enodans.* Frankfurt, 1602.

Lery, Jean. *Historia Navigationis in Brasiliam quae et America Dicitur.* Second Edition. Geneva, 1594.

Locke, John. *An Essay concerning Humane Understanding.* London, 1690.

Pseudo-Llull, Raymund. *De Secretis Naturae, Seu de Quinta Essentia Liber Unus.* Cologne: Apud Ioannem Birckmannum, 1567.

Mattioli, Pietro Andrea. *Commentarii in Sex Libros Pedacii Dioscoridis Anazarbei de Medica Materia.* Venice: Ex Officina Valgrisiana, 1565.

Menage, M. *Menagiana.* Amsterdam: Pierre de Coup, 1716.

Merian, Joachim "Casus Medicinales," in Franciscus Dele Boë Sylvius, *Opera Medica.* Utrecht and Amsterdam: Apud Guillelmum van de Water and Apud Antonium Schelte, 1695.

Meursius, Joannis. *Athenae Batavae.* Leiden: Apud Andream Cloucquium, et Elsevirios, 1625.

Morgagni, Giovanni Battista. *The Seats and Causes of Diseases Investigated by Anatomy.* Translated by Benjamin Alexander. 2 vols. Mount Kisco, NY: Futura Publishing Company, Inc., 1980.

Orlers, J. J. *Beschrijvinge der Stadt Leyden.* Leiden: Door Andries Janz. Cloeting tot Delft. Ende Abraham Commelijn tot Leyden, 1641.

Ps.-Orpheus. *Musaei Opusculum de Herone et Leandro, Orphei Argonautica, Eiusdem Hymni, Orpheus de Lapidibus.* Venice, 1517.

Ovid. *Metamorphoses, Volume I: Books 1–8*. Translated by Frank Justus Miller. Revised by G. P. Goold. Loeb Classical Library 42. Cambridge, MA: Harvard University Press, 1916.

Paaw, Petrus. *Hortus Publicus Academiae Lugduno-Batavae*. Leiden: Christophorus Raphelingius, 1601.

Paaw, Petrus. *Observationes Anatomicae*, printed with Thomas Bartholin, *Historiarum Anatomicarum Rariorum*, Centuriae III & IV. Copenhagen: Ex Typographia Adriani Vlacq, 1657.

Paaw, Petrus. *Primitiae Anatomicae de Humani Corporis Ossibus*. Leiden: Ex Officina Iusi à Colster, 1615.

Paracelsus, and Andrew Weeks. *Paracelsus (Theophrastus Bombastus von Hohenheim, 1493–1541): Essential Theoretical Writings*. Leiden; Boston: Brill, 2008.

Petreivs, Nicolavs (respondent). *Disputatio inauguralis de cholera hvmida*. Leiden, 1614.

Plato. *Charmides* in *Charmides. Alcibiades I and II. Hipparchus. The Lovers. Theages. Minos. Epinomis*. Translated by W. R. M. Lamb. Loeb Classical Library 201. Cambridge, MA: Harvard University Press, 1927.

Plato. *Euthyphro. Apology. Crito. Phaedo. Phaedrus*. Translated by Harold North Fowler. Loeb Classical Library 36. Cambridge, MA: Harvard University Press, 1914.

Plato. *Timaeus, Critias, Cleitophon, Menexenus, Epistles*. Translated by R. G. Bury. Cambridge, Mass.: Loeb Classical Library 234. Cambridge, MA: Harvard University Press, 1929.

Plemp, Vopiscus Fortunatus. *De fundamentis medicinae libri sex*. Leuven: Typis ac Sumptibus Iacobi Zegersii, 1638.

Pliny. *Historia Mundi Naturalis*. Frankfurt, 1582.

Rhazes (Muhammad ibn Zakariya al-Razi). *Continens Rasis* (1509).

Sallust. *The War with Catiline*, in *The War with Catiline. The War with Jugurtha*. Translated by J. C. Rolfe. Loeb Classical Library 116. Cambridge, MA: Harvard University Press, 2013.

Sandifort, Eduard. *Mvsevm Anatomicvm Academiae Lvgdvno-Batavae*. 4 vols. Leiden: J. Luchtmans, 1793–1835.

Santorio, Santorio. *Commentaria in primam fen primi libri canonis Avicennae*. Venice, 1626.

Schvttivs, Diodorus (respondent). *Theses Medicae de Natura Febris*. Leiden, 1616.

Severinus, Petrus. *Idea Medicinae Philosophicae*. Basle: Ex Officina Sixti Henricopetri, 1571.

Stevin, Simon. *De Beghinselen der Weeghconst*. Leiden: Inde Druckerye van Chirstoffel Plantijn, By Françoys van Raphelinghen, 1586

Stevin, Simon. *The Principal Works of Simon Stevin Vol. 1: General Introduction. Mechanics*, edited by E. J. Dijksterhuis. Translated by C. Dikshoorn. 2 vols. Amsterdam: C. V. Swets & Zeitlinger, 1955.

[Stuart, David]. *Disputatio Eclectica de Unione Animae & Corporis. Pars Prima.* Respondent Guiljelmus à Nieuwenhuysen. Leiden, 1664.

Sydenham, Thomas. *The Works of Thomas Sydenham, M.D.* Edited by William Alexander Greenhill and R. G. Latham. London, 1848.

Sylvius, Franciscus Dele Boë. *Disputatio de Animali Motu Ejusq; Laesionibus.* Basel, 1637.

Sylvius, Franciscus Dele Boë. *Medicinae Practicae Academiâ Lugduno-Batavâ Professoris. Disputationum Medicarum Pars Prima Primarias Corporis humani Functiones Naturales ex Anatomicis, Practicis & Chymicis Experimentis deductas complectens.* Amsterdam: Apud Johannem van den Bergh, 1663.

Sylvius, Franciscus Dele Boë. *Opera Medica.* Amsterdam: Apud Danielem Elsevirium et Abrahamum Wolfgang, 1679.

Sylvius, Franciscus Dele Boë. *Opera Medica...Accessit huic Editioni hactenus ineditum Collegium Nosocomicum ab Authore habitum.* Geneva: Apud Samvelem de Tovrnes, 1681.

Sylvius, Franciscus Dele Boë. *Opera Medica...Editio Nova, Cui accedunt Casus Medicinales.* Utrecht and Amsterdam: Apud Guillelmum van de Water and Apud Antonium Schelte, 1695.

Sylvius, Franciscus Dele Boë. *Positiones Variae Medicae.* Leiden, 1634.

Sylvius, Franciscus Dele Boë. *Praxeos Medicae Idea Nova*, 4 Vols. (Leiden and Amsterdam, 1671–1674)

Tulp, Nicolaas. *Observationum medicarum libri tres.* Amsterdam: Apud Ludovicum Elzevirium, 1641.

Thomas Willis. *Pharmaceutice Rationalis, or, an Exercitation of the Operations of Medicines in Humane Bodies.* London: T. Dring, C. Harper, and J. Leigh, 1678.

Van Beverwijck, Johan. *De Calculo Renum & Vesicae Liber singularis.* Leiden: Ex Officina Elseviriorum, 1638.

Van Beverwijck, Johan. *Schat Der Ongesontheyt.* Dordrecht: Jasper Gorssz., 1644.

Van Diemerbroeck, Ijsbrand (or Ysbrand). *Anatome Corporis Humani, Plurimis Novis Inventis Instructa, Variisque Observationibus, & Paradoxis, Cùm Medicis, Tum Physiologicis Adornata.* Leiden, 1679.

Varolio, Costanzo. *Anatomiae.* Frankfurt, 1591.

Vesalius, Andreas. *De Humani Corporis Fabrica Libri Septem.* Basel, 1543.

Vesalius, Andreas. *De Humani Corporis Fabrica Libri Septem.* Basel, 1555.

Vesalius, Andreas. *Epistola, rationem modumque propinandi radices Chynae decocti.* Basel, 1546.

Vesalius, Andreas. *"The China Root Epistle": A New Translation and Critical Edition.* Edited and translated by Daniel H. Garrison. Cambridge: Cambridge University Press, 2015.

Vinshemius, Menelaus. *Disputatio Inauguralis de Hydrope.* Leiden, 1612.

Vlaxcq, Theodorus (respondent). *Theses medicae de ictero.* Leiden, 1616.

Worm, Ole, et al. *Olai Wormii et ad Eum Doctorum Virorum Epistolae.* Copenhagen, 1751.

Secondary Sources

Ahsmann, Margareet. *Collegia en Colleges: Juridisch onderwijs aan de Leidse Universiteit 1575–1630 in het bijzonder het disputeren.* Groningen: Wolters-Noordhoff/Egbert Forsten, 1990.

Anstey, Peter. *The Philosophy of Robert Boyle.* London: Routledge, 2000.

Arrizabalaga, Jon, John Henderson, and R. K French. *The Great Pox: The French Disease in Renaissance Europe.* New Haven and London: Yale University Press, 1997.

Ballester, Luis Garcia. "Soul and Body: Disease of the Soul and Disease of the Body in Galen's Medical Thought." In *Le opere psicologiche di Galeno; atti del terzo colloquio galenico internazionale, Pavia, 10–12 settembre 1986*, edited Paola Manuli and Mario Vegretti, 117–152. Napoli: Bibliopolis, 1988.

Banchetti-Robino, Marina Paola. *The Chemical Philosophy of Robert Boyle: Mechanism, Chymical Atoms, and Emergence.* New York: Oxford University Press, 2020.

Banga, J. *Geschiedenis van de Geneeskunde En van Hare Beoefenaren in Nederland.* Leeuwarden: W. Eekhoff, 1868.

Barge, J. A. J. *De Oudste Inventaris Der Oudste Academische Anatomie in Nederland.* Leiden: H. E. Stenfert Kroese, 1934.

Barnett, Frances Mason. "Medical Authority and Princely Patronage: The Academia Naturae Curiosorum, 1652–1693." PhD. diss. University of North Carolina, 1995.

Barrera, Antonio. "Local Herbs, Global Medicines: Commerce, Knowledge, and Commodities in Spanish America." In *Merchants and Marvels: Commerce, Science, and Art in Early Modern Europe*, edited by Pamela H. Smith and Paula Findlen, 163–181. New York and London: Routledge, 2002.

Baumann, E. D. *François Dele Boe Sylvius.* Leiden: E. J. Brill, 1949.

Bayer, Greg. "Coming to Know Principles in Posterior Analytics II 19." *Apeiron* 30, no. 2 (June 1, 1997): 109–42.

Bellis, Delphine. "Empiricism without Metaphysics: Regius' Cartesian Natural Philosophy." In *Cartesian Empiricisms*, edited by Mihnea Dobre and Tammy Nyden, 151–83. Dordrecht: Springer, 2013.

Bennett, J. A. "The Mechanics' Philosophy and the Mechanical Philosophy." *History of Science* 24 (1986): 1–28.

Berryman, Sylvia. "Galen and the Mechanical Philosophy." *Apeiron* 35, no. 3 (September 1, 2002): 235–54.

Bertoloni Meli, Domenico. "'Ex Museolo Nostro Machaonico': Collecting, Publishing, and Visualization in Fabricius Hildanus." *Journal of the History of Medicine and Allied Sciences* 72, no. 1 (2017): 98–116.

Bertoloni Meli, Domenico. "Gerardus Blasius and the Illustrated Amsterdam Observationes from Nicolaas Tulp to Frederik Ruysch." In *Professors, Physicians and Prac-*

tices in the History of Medicine, edited by Gideon Manning and Cynthia Klestinec. 227–269. Dordrecht: Springer, 2017.

Bertoloni Meli, Domenico. *Mechanism: A Visual, Lexical, and Conceptual History*. Pittsburgh: University of Pittsburgh Press, 2019.

Bertoloni Meli, Domenico. *Mechanism, Experiment, Disease: Marcello Malpighi and Seventeenth-Century Anatomy*. Baltimore: Johns Hopkins University Press, 2011.

Bertoloni Meli, Domenico. "The Color of Blood: Between Sense Experience and Epistemic Significance." In *Histories of Scientific Observation*, edited by Lorraine Daston and Elizabeth Lunbeck, 117–134. Chicago: University of Chicago Press, 2011.

Bertoloni Meli, Domenico. *Thinking with Objects: The Transformation of Mechanics in the Seventeenth Century*. Baltimore: Johns Hopkins University Press, 2006.

Bertoloni Meli, Domenico. *Visualizing Disease: The Art and History of Pathological Illustrations*. Chicago: University of Chicago Press, 2017.

Beukers, Harm. "Acid Spirits and Alkaline Salts: The Iatrochemistry of Franciscus Dele Boë, Sylvius." *Sartoniana* 12 (1999): 39–58.

Beukers, Harm. "Clinical Teaching in Leiden from Its Beginning Until the End of the Eighteenth Century." *Clio Medica* 21, no. 1/4 (1988): 139–152.

Beukers, Harm. "Het Laboratorium van Sylvius." *Tijdschrift Voor de Geschiedenis Der Geneeskunde, Natuurwetenschappen, Wiskunde en Teckniek*, 3 (1980): 28–36.

Beukers, Harm. "Mechanistische Principes Bij Franciscus Dele Boë." *Tijdschrift Voor de Geschiedenis Der Geneeskunde, Natuurwetenschappen, Wiskunde en Teckniek*, 5 (1982): 6–15.

Beukers, Harm. "Studying Medicine In Leiden In The 1630s." In '*A man very well studyed': New Contexts for Thomas Browne*, edited by Richard Todd and Kathryn Murphy. Leiden: Brill, 2008.

Blair, Ann. *The Theater of Nature: Jean Bodin and Renaissance Science*. Princeton. N.J.: Princeton University Press, 1997.

Blank, Andreas. *Biomedical Ontology and the Metaphysics of Composite Substances: 1540–1670*. Munich: Philosophia Verlag, 2010.

Blank, Andreas. "Sennert and Leibniz on Animate Atoms." In *Machines of Nature and Corporeal Substances in Leibniz*, edited by Justin E. H. Smith and Ohad Nachtomy. Dordrecht: Springer, 2011.

Boss, Jeffrey. "The 'Methodus Medendi' as an Index of Change in the Philosophy of Medical Science in the Sixteenth and Seventeenth Centuries." *History and Philosophy of the Life Sciences* 1 (1979): 13–42.

Bouley, Bradford A. *Pious Postmortems: Anatomy, Sanctity, and the Catholic Church in Early Modern Europe*. Philadelphia: University of Pennsylvania Press, 2017.

Brennessel, Barbara, Michael D. C. Drout, and Robyn Gravel. "A Reassessment of the Efficacy of Anglo-Saxon Medicine." *Anglo-Saxon England* 34 (2005): 183–95.

Brüning, Volker Fritz. *Bibliographie der alchemistischen Literatur*. 2 vols. München: KG Saur, 2004.

Bylebyl, Jerome J. "Commentary." In *A Celebration of Medical History*, edited by Lloyd G. Stevenson, 200–211. Baltimore: Johns Hopkins University Press, 1982.

Bylebyl, Jerome J. "Disputation and Description in the Renaissance Pulse Controversy." *Medical Renaissance of the Sixteenth Century*, edited by A. Wear, R. K. French, and I. M. Lonie. Cambridge: Cambridge University Press, 1985.

Bylebyl, Jerome J. "Medicine, Philosophy, and Humanism in Renaissance Italy." In *Science and the Arts in the Renaissance*, edited by John W. Shirley and F. David Hoeniger, 27–49. Washington, D.C.: Folger Books, 1985.

Bylebyl, Jerome J. "Teaching *Methodus Medendi* in the Renaissance." In *Galen's Method of Healing*, edited by Fridolf Kudlein and Richard Durling, 157–189. Leiden: Brill, 1991.

Bylebyl, Jerome. "The Manifest and the Hidden in the Renaissance Clinic." In *Medicine and the Five Senses*, edited by W. F. Bynum and Roy Porter. Cambridge: Cambridge University Press, 1993.

Bylebyl, Jerome. "The School of Padua: Humanistic Medicine in the Sixteenth Century." In *Health, Medicine and Mortality in the Sixteenth Century*, edited by Charles Webster, 335–370. Cambridge: Cambridge University Press, 1979.

Bynum, Helen. *Spitting Blood: The History of Tuberculosis*. Oxford: Oxford University Press, 2012.

Bynum, W. F. *The History of Medicine: A Very Short Introduction*. Oxford: Oxford University Press, 2008.

Cadden, Joan. *Meanings of Sex Difference in the Middle Ages: Medicine, Natural Philosophy and Culture*. Cambridge: Cambridge University Press, 1993.

Camerota, Michele, and Mario Helbing. "Galileo and Pisan Aristotelianism: Galileo's 'De Motu Antiquiora' and the Quaestiones de Motu Elementorum of the Pisan Professors." *Early Science and Medicine* 5, no. 4 (2000): 319–65.

Chang, Ku-ming (Kevin). "Alchemy as Studies of Life and Matter: Reconsidering the Place of Vitalism in Early Modern Chemistry." *Isis* 102, no. 2 (June 2011): 322–29.

Cheung, Tobias. "Omnis Fibra Ex Fibra: Fibre Œconomies in Bonnet's and Diderot's Models of Organic Order." *Early Science and Medicine* 15, no. 1/2 (2010): 66–104.

Clericuzio, Antonio. "Teaching Chemistry and Chemical Textbooks in France. From Beguin to Lemery." *Science and Education* 15 (2006): 335–355.

Clendening, Logan, ed. *Source Book of Medical History*. New York: Dover, 1960.

Cohen, H. Floris. *How Modern Science Came into the World: Four Civilizations, One Seventeenth-Century Breakthrough*. Amsterdam: Amsterdam University Press, 2010.

Cook, Harold J. *Matters of Exchange: Commerce, Medicine, and Science in the Dutch Golden Age*. New Haven: Yale University Press, 2007.

Cook, Harold J. "Medicine." In *The Cambridge History of Science. Early Modern Science*, edited by Katharine Park and Lorraine Daston, 3:407–34. The Cambridge History of Science. Cambridge: Cambridge University Press, 2006.

Cook, Harold J. "The New Philosophy and Medicine in Seventeenth-Century England." In *Reappraisals of the Scientific Revolution*, edited by David C. Lindberg and Robert S. Westman, 397–436. Cambridge: Cambridge University Press, 1990.

Cook, Harold J. "The New Philosophy in the Low Countries." In *The Scientific Revolution in National Context*, edited by Roy Porter and Mikuláš Teich, 115–149. Cambridge: Cambridge University Press, 1992.

Cooper, Alix. *Inventing the Indigenous: Local Knowledge and Natural History in Early Modern Europe*. Cambridge: Cambridge University Press, 2007.

Copenhaver, Brian P. "Natural Magic, Hermetism, and Occultism in Early Modern Science." In *Reappraisals of the Scientific Revolution*, edited by David Lindberg and Robert Westman, 261–301. Cambridge: Cambridge University Press, 1990.

Corcilius, Klaus. "Faculties in Ancient Philosophy." In *The Faculties: A History*, edited by Dominik Perler, 19–58. Oxford and New York: Oxford University Press, 2015.

Crombie, A. C. *Robert Grosseteste and the Origins of Experimental Science 1100–1700*. Oxford: Clarendon Press, 1953.

Crowther, Kathleen M. *Adam and Eve in the Protestant Reformation*. Cambridge: Cambridge University Press, 2013.

Cunningham, Andrew. *The Anatomist Anatomis'd: An Experimental Discipline in Enlightenment Europe*. Farnham: Ashgate, 2010.

Cunningham, Andrew. "The Bartholins, the Platters and Laurentius Gryllus: the *peregrinatio medica* in the Sixteenth and Seventeenth Centuries." In *Centres of Medical Excellence?*, edited by O. P. Grell, A. Cunningham, and J. Arrizabalaga, 3–16. Surrey and Burlington: Ashgate, 2010.

Cunningham, Andrew. "Fabricius and the 'Aristotle Project' in Anatomical Teaching and Research at Padua." In *The Medical Renaissance of the Sixteenth Century*, edited by A. Wear, R. K. French, and I. M. Lonie, 195–222. Cambridge: Cambridge University Press, 1985.

Daston, Lorraine. "Baconian Facts, Academic Civility, and the Prehistory of Objectivity." *Annals of Scholarship* 8 (1991): 337–364.

Dear, Peter. *Discipline and Experience: The Mathematical Way in the Scientific Revolution*. University of Chicago Press, 1995.

Debru, Armelle. In *The Cambridge Companion to Galen*, edited by R. J. Hankinson, 263–282. Cambridge Companions to Philosophy. Cambridge: Cambridge University Press, 2008.

Debus, Allen G. "Chemistry and the Universities in the Seventeenth Century." *Estudos Avançados* 4 (1990): 173–196.

Deer Richardson, Linda. "The Generation of Disease: Occult Causes and Diseases of the Total Substance." In *The Medical Renaissance of the Sixteenth Century*, edited by A. Wear, R. K. French, and I. M. Lonie, 175–194. Cambridge: Cambridge University Press, 1985.

De Jonge, H. J. "The Study of the New Testament."n *Leiden University in the Seventeenth Century: An Exchange of Learning*, edited by Th. H. Lunsingh Scheurleer and G. H. M. Posthumus Meyjes, 65–109. Leiden: University of Leiden Press / E. J. Brill, 1975.

Demaitre, Luke. *Medieval Medicine: The Art of Healing from Head to Toe*. Santa Barbara: Praeger, 2013.

De Moulin, Daniel. *A History of Surgery with Emphasis on the Netherlands*. Dordrecht: Martinus Nijhoff Publishers, 1988.

De Renzi, Silvia, Marco Bresadola, and Maria Conforti, eds. *Pathology in Practice: Diseases and Dissections in Early Modern Europe*. London and New York: Routledge, 2018.

De Renzi, Silvia, Marco Bresadola, and Maria Conforti. "Pathological Dissections in Early Modern Europe: Practice and Knowledge." In *Pathology in Practice: Diseases and Dissections in Early Modern Europe*, edited by De Renzi, Bresadola, and Conforti, 3–19. London and New York: Routledge, 2018.

De Renzi, Silvia. "Seats and Series: Dissecting Diseases in the Seventeenth Century." In *Pathology in Practice: Diseases and Dissections in Early Modern Europe*, edited by Silvia De Renzi, Marco Bresadola, and Maria Conforti, 84–98. London and New York: Routledge, 2018.

DeVun, Leah. *Prophecy, Alchemy, and the End of Time: John of Rupescissa in the Late Middle Ages*. New York: Columbia University Press, 2009.

De Wreede, Liesbeth. "Willebrord Snellius (1580–1626): a Humanist Reshaping the Mathematical Sciences." PhD. diss. Utrecht University, 2007

Dijksterhuis, E. J. *Simon Stevin: Science in the Netherlands Around 1600*. Edited by R. Hooykaas and M. G. J. Minnaert. The Hague: Martinus Nijhoff, 1970.

DiMeo, Michelle and Sara Pennell, eds. *Reading and Writing Recipe Books, 1550–1800*. Manchester: Manchester University Press, 2013.

Distelzweig, Peter M. "Fabricius's Galeno-Aristotelian Teleomechanics of Muscle." In *The Life Sciences in Early Modern Philosophy*, edited by Ohad Nachtomy and Justin E. H. Smith, 65–84. Oxford and New York: Oxford University Press, 2014.

Distelzweig, Peter M. "The Use of *Usus* and the Function of *Functio* Teleology and Its Limits in Descartes's Physiology." *Journal of the History of Philosophy* 53, no. 3 (2015): 377–99.

Donato, Maria Pia. *Sudden Death: Medicine and Religion in Eighteenth-Century Rome*. Translated by Valentina Mazzei. Surrey: Ashgate, 2014.

Donini, Pierluigi. "Psychology." In *The Cambridge Companion to Galen*, edited by R. J. Hankinson, 184–209. Cambridge Companions to Philosophy. Cambridge: Cambridge University Press, 2008.

Dubos, René and Jean Dubos. *The White Plague: Tuberculosis, Man, and Society*. New Brunswick: Rutgers University Press, 1996.

Dupré, Sven. "Inside the 'Camera Obscura': Kepler's Experiment and Theory of Optical Imagery." *Early Science and Medicine*, 13 (2008): 219–244.

Durling, Richard. "A Chronological Census of Renaissance Editions and Translations of Galen." *Journal of the Warburg and Courtauld Institutes* 24, no. 3, 4 (1961): 230–305.

Duffin, Jacalyn. *History of Medicine: A Scandalously Short Introduction*. Second Edition. Toronto: University of Toronto Press, 2010.

Duffin, Jacalyn. *To See with a Better Eye: A Life of R. T. H. Laennec*. Princeton: Princeton University Press, 1998.

Eamon, William. *Science and the Secrets of Nature: Books of Secrets in Medieval and Early Modern Culture*. Princeton, NJ: Princeton University Press, 1994.

Edelstein, Emma J., and Ludwig Edelstein. *Asclepius: Collection and Interpretation of the Testimonies*. Johns Hopkins University Press, 1998.

Egmond, Florike. "Experimenting with Living Nature: Documented Practices of Sixteenth-Century Naturalists and Naturalia Collectors." *Journal of Early Modern Studies* 6 (2017): 21–45.

Egmond, Florike. *Het Visboek: De Wereld Volgens Adriaen Coenen*. Zutphen: Walburg Pers, 2005.

Egmond, Florike. *The World of Carolus Clusius: Natural History in the Making, 1550–1610*. London: Pickering and Chatto, 2010.

Estes, J. Worth. "The European Reception of the First Drugs from the New World." *Pharmacy in History* (1995): 3–23.

Feingold, Mordechai. *The Mathematicians' Apprenticeship: Science, Universities, and Society in England, 1560–1640*. New York: Cambridge University Press, 1984.

Findlen, Paula. "Controlling the Experiment: Rhetoric, Court Patronage, and the Experimental Method of Francesco Redi." *History of Science* 31 (1993): 35–64.

Findlen, Paula. "Empty Signs? Reading the Book of Nature in Renaissance Europe." *Studies in the History and Philosophy of Science* 21 (1990): 511–518.

Findlen, Paula. *Possessing Nature: Museums, Collecting, and Scientific Culture in Early Modern Italy*. Berkeley: University of California Press, 1994.

Findlen, Paula. "The Formation of a Scientific Community: Natural History in Sixteenth-Century Italy." In *Natural Particulars: Nature and the Disciplines in Renaissance Europe*, edited by Anthony Grafton and Nancy Siraisi, 369–400. Cambridge, MA.: MIT Press, 1999.

Fissell, Mary E. "The Disappearance of the Patient's Narrative and the Invention of Hospital Medicine." In *British Medicine in an Age of Reform*, edited by R. K. French and A. Wear, 92–109. London: Routledge, 1991.

Frank, Robert G. "Medicine." In *The History of the University of Oxford: Volume IV Seventeenth-Century Oxford*, edited by Nicholas Tyacke, 505–558. Oxford: Oxford University Press, 1997.

Frank, Robert G. *William Harvey and the Oxford Physiologists: Scientific Ideas and Social Interaction*. Berkeley: University of California Press, 1980.

Frede, Michael. "On Galen's Epistemology." In *Galen: Galen: Problems and Prospects*, edited by Vivian Nutton, 65–86. London: The Wellcome Institute for the History of Medicine, 1981.

French, Roger. "Berengario da Carpi and the Use of Commentary in Anatomical Teaching. In *The Medical Renaissance of the Sixteenth Century*, edited by Andrew Wear, Roger K. French, and I. M. Lonie, 42–74. Cambridge: Cambridge University Press, 1985.

French, R.K. *Canonical Medicine: Gentile Da Foligno and Scholasticism*. Leiden: Brill, 2001.

French, Roger. *Dissection and Vivisection in the European Renaissance*. Burlington, VT: Ashgate, 1999.

French, Roger Kenneth. *Medicine before Science: The Business of Medicine from the Middle Ages to the Enlightenment*. Cambridge: Cambridge University Press, 2010.

French, Roger. *William Harvey's Natural Philosophy*. Cambridge: Cambridge University Press, 1994.

Frietsch, Ute. "Alchemy and the Early Modern University: An Introduction." *Ambix* 68, no. 2–3 (August 2021): 119–34.

Foucault, Michel. *The Birth of the Clinic: An Archaeology of Medical Perception*. Translated by A. M. Sheridan Smith. New York: Vintage Books, 1975.

Garber, Dan. "Descartes and Experiment in the Discourse and Essays." In *Essays on the Philosophy and Science of René Descartes*, edited by Stephen Voss, 288–310. New York: Oxford University Press, 1993.

Gascoigne, John. "A reappraisal of the role of the universities in the Scientific Revolution." In *Reappraisals of the Scientific Revolution*, edited by David C. Lindberg and Robert S. Westman, 207–260. Cambridge: Cambridge University Press, 1990.

Gibbs, Frederick W. *Poison, Medicine, and Disease in Late Medieval and Early Modern Europe*. Abingdon and New York: Routledge, 2019.

Goldgar, Anne. *Impolite Learning: Conduct and Community in the Republic of Letters, 1680–1750*. New Haven, CT and London: Yale University Press, 1995.

Goldgar, Anne. *Tulipmania: Money, Honor, and Knowledge in the Dutch Golden Age*. Chicago: University of Chicago Press, 2008.

Gómez, Pablo F. *The Experiential Caribbean: Creating Knowledge and Healing in the Early Modern Atlantic*. Chapel Hill: University of North Carolina Press, 2017.

Goodey, C. F. *A History of Intelligence and "Intellectual Disability": The Shaping of Psychology in Early Modern Europe*. Burlington, VA: Ashgate, 2011.

Goulding, Robert. "Thomas Harriot's Optics, between Experiment and Imagination: The Case of Mr Bulkeley's Glass." *Archive for History of Exact Sciences* 68, no. 2 (2014): 137–78.

Gourevitch, Danielle. "The Paths of Knowledge: Medicine in the Roman World." In *Western Medical Thought*, edited by Mirko D. Grmek, translated by Antony Shugaar, 104–138. Cambridge, MA: Harvard University Press, 1998.

Grafton, Anthony. "A Sketch Map of a Lost Continent." In *Worlds Made by Words: Scholarship and Community in the Modern West*. Cambridge, MA and London, England: Harvard University Press, 2009, 9–34.

Grafton, Anthony. *Bring Out Your Dead: The Past as Revelation*. Cambridge, MA: Harvard University Press, 2004.

Grafton, Anthony. "Civic Humanism and Scientific Scholarship at Leiden." In *The University and the City: From Medieval Origins to the Present*, edited by Thomas Bender, 59–78. New York: Oxford University Press, 1988.

Grafton, Anthony. *Joseph Scaliger: A Study in the History of Classical Scholarship*. 2 vols. Oxford: Clarendon Press, 1983 and 1993.

Grafton, Anthony. "Libraries and Lecture Halls." In *The Cambridge History of Science, Vol. 3: Early Modern Science*, edited by Katharine Park and Lorraine Daston, 238–250. Cambridge: Cambridge Univ. Press, 2006.

Grafton, Anthony. "The New Science and the Traditions of Humanism." In *Bring Out Your Dead: The Past as Revelation*, by Anthony Grafton, 97–117. Cambridge, MA: Harvard University Press, 2004.

Grell, Ole Peter, Andrew Cunningham, and Jon Arrizabalaga, eds. *Centres of Medical Excellence?: Medical Travel and Education in Europe*. Burlington: Ashgate, 2010.

Grell, Ole Peter. "In Search of True Knowledge: Ole Worm (1588–1654) and the New Philosophy." In *Making Knowledge in Early Modern Europe: Practices, Objects, and Texts, 1400–1800*, edited by Pamela H. Smith and Benjamin Schmidt, 214–232. Chicago: The University of Chicago Press, 2007.

Grendler, Paul F. *The Universities of the Italian Renaissance*. Baltimore: Johns Hopkins Press, 2002.

Gubser, Alfred. "The Positiones Variae Medicae of Franciscus Sylvius." *History of Medicine* 40, no. 1 (1966): 72–80.

Guerrini, Anita. *The Courtier's Anatomists: Animals and Humans in Louis XIV's Paris*. Chicago and London: University of Chicago Press, 2015.

Hackett, Jeremiah. "Roger Bacon on *Scientia Experimentalis*." In *Roger Bacon and the Sciences: Commemorative Essays*, edited by Jeremiah Hackett, 277–315. Leiden: Brill, 1997.

Hankinson, James (R. J.). "Actions and Passions: Affection, Emotion, and Moral Self-Management in Galen's Philosophical Psychology." In *Passions and Perceptions: Studies in Hellenistic Philosophy of Mind*, edited by Jacques Brunschwig and Martha C. Nussbaum, 184–222. Cambridge: Cambridge University Press, 1993.

Hankinson, R. J. "Causes and Empiricism: A Problem in the Interpretation of Later Greek Medical Method." *Phronesis* 32 (1987): 329–348.

Hankinson, R. J. "Epistemology." In *The Cambridge Companion to Galen*, edited by R. J. Hankinson, 157–83. Cambridge Companions to Philosophy. Cambridge: Cambridge University Press, 2008.

Hankinson, Robert J. "Galen and the Ontology of Powers." *British Journal for the History of Philosophy* 22 (2014): 951–973.

Hankinson, Robert J. "Partitioning the Soul: Galen on the Anatomy of the Psychic Functions and Mental Illness." In *Partitioning the Soul: Debates from Plato to Leibniz*, edited by Klaus Corcilius and Dominik Perler, 85–106. Berlin and Boston, Walter de Gruyter, 2014.

Hankinson, R. J. "Philosophy of Nature." In *The Cambridge Companion to Galen*, edited by R. J. Hankinson, 210–41. Cambridge Companions to Philosophy. Cambridge: Cambridge University Press, 2008.

Hankinson, R. J. "Substance, Element, Quality, Mixture: Galen's Physics and His Hippocratic Inheritance." *Aitia* 7.2 (2017). http://journals.openedition.org/aitia/1863; DOI: https://doi.org/10.4000/aitia.1863

Hannaway, Owen. *The Chemists and the Word: The Didactic Origins of Chemistry*. Baltimore: Johns Hopkins University Press, 1975.

Harley, David. "Political Post-Mortems and Morbid Anatomy in Seventeenth-Century England." *Social History of Medicine* 7, no. 1 (1994): 1–28.

Harrison Peter. *The Fall of Man and the Foundations of Modern Science*. Cambridge: Cambridge University Press, 2007.

Harskamp, Jaap. *Dissertatio medica inauguralis: Leyden Medical Dissertations in the British Library, 1593–1746: A Catalogue of the Sloane-Inspired Collection*. London: Wellcome Institute for the History of Medicine, 1997

Haskins, Charles Homer. *The Rise of Universities*. New York: Henry Holt and Company, 1923.

Hendriksen, Marieke M. A. *Elegant Anatomy: The Eighteenth-Century Leiden Anatomical Collections*. Leiden: Brill, 2015.

Henry, John. "Occult Qualities and the Experimental Philosophy: Active Principles in Pre-Newtonian Matter Theory." *History of Science* 24, no. 4 (December 1, 1986): 335–81.

Henry, John. *The Scientific Revolution and the Origins of Modern Science*. New York: Palgrave, 2002.

Hicks, Daniel J., and Thomas A. Stapleford. "The Virtues of Scientific Practice: MacIntyre, Virtue Ethics, and the Historiography of Science." *Isis* 107, no. 3 (September 20, 2016): 449–72.

Hirai, Hiro. *Medical Humanism and Natural Philosophy: Renaissance Debates on Matter, Life and the Soul*. Leiden: Brill, 2011.

Houtzager, H. L. "Enkele medici rond de prins van Oranje en het postmortale onderzoek van de prins." *Jaarboek Vereniging 'Oranje-Nassau Museum'* (1984): 84–100.

Houtzager, H. L. "Het experimenteel geneeskundige onderzoek in ons land ten tijde van Reinier de Graaf." In *Reinier de Graaf*, edited by H. L. Houtzager, 53–82. Rotterdam: Erasmus Publishing, 1991.

Houtzager, H. L. "Het Leids Anatomisch Onderzoek ten Tijde van Pieter Paaw en Diens Uitgave van de *Epitome* van Vesalius." *Scientiarum Historia* 21 (1995): 43–48.

Houtzager, H. L. ed. *Reinier de Graaf, 1641–1673: In Sijn Leven Nauwkeurig Ontleder En Gelukkig Genesheer Tot Delft.* Rotterdam: Erasmus Publishing, 1991.

Huguet-Termes, Teresa. "New World Materia Medica in Spanish Renaissance Medicine: From Scholarly Reception to Practical Impact." *Medical History* (2001): 359–376.

Hulshoff Pol, Elfriede. "The Library." In *Leiden University in the Seventeenth Century: An Exchange of Learning*, edited by Th. H. Lunsingh Scheurleer and G. H. M. Posthumus Meyjes, 394–459. Leiden: University of Leiden Press / E. J. Brill, 1975.

Huisman, Frank. *Stadsbelang en Standsbesef: Gezondheidszorg en Medisch Beroep in Groningen 1500–1730.* Rotterdam: Erasmus Publishing, 1992.

Huisman, Tim. *The Finger of God: Anatomical Practice in 17th Century Leiden.* Leiden: Primavera Pers, 2009.

Hunter, Michael, ed. *Robert Boyle Reconsidered.* Cambridge: Cambridge University Press, 1994.

Irons, Ernest E. "Théophile Bonet, 1620–1689: His Influence on the Science and Practice of Medicine." *Bulletin of the History of Medicine* 12 (1942): 623–65.

Israel, Jonathan. *The Dutch Republic: Its Rise, Greatness, and Fall, 1477–1806.* New York: Oxford University Press, 1995.

Jacquart, Danielle. "Anatomy, Physiology, and Medical Theory." In *The Cambridge History of Science: Volume 2: Medieval Science*, edited by David C. Lindberg and Michael H. Shank, 2:590–610. The Cambridge History of Science. Cambridge: Cambridge University Press, 2013.

Janson, Theodorus, ed. *Isaaci Casauboni Epistolae.* Rotterdam: Casparis Fritsch and Michaelis Böhm, 1709.

Jewson, N. D. "The Disappearance of the Sick-Man from Medical Cosmology, 1770–1870." *Sociology* 10, no. 2 (1976): 225–44.

Johansen, Thomas Kjeller. *The Powers of Aristotle's Soul.* Oxford: Oxford University Press, 2012.

Johnston, Ian. *Galen: On Diseases and Symptoms.* Cambridge: Cambridge University Press, 2011.

Jorink, Eric. *Reading the Book of Nature in the Dutch Golden Age, 1575–1715.* Translated by Peter Mason. Leiden: Brill, 2011.

Jouanna, Jacques. "Hippocrates as Galen's Teacher." In *Hippocrates and Medical Education*, edited by Manfred Horstmanshoff and Cornelis van Tilburg, 1–21. Leiden: Brill, 2010.

Jouanna, Jacques. *Hippocrates.* Translated by M. B. Debevoise. Baltimore; London: The John Hopkins University Press, 1999.

Kahn, Didier. "The First Private and Public Courses of Chymistry in Paris (and Italy) from Jean Beguin to William Davisson." *Ambix* 68, no. 2–3 (August 2021): 247–72.

Kaiser, David. "Introduction." In *Pedagogy and the Practice of Science: Historical and Contemporary Perspectives*, edited by David Kaiser, 1–10. Cambridge, MA: The MIT Press, 2005

Kaiser, David, ed. *Pedagogy and the Practice of Science: Historical and Contemporary Perspectives*. Cambridge, MA: The MIT Press, 2005.

Kaye, Joel. *A History of Balance, 1250–1375: The Emergence of a New Model of Equilibrium and Its Impact on Thought*. Cambridge: Cambridge University Press, 2014.

Keel, Othmar. *L'avenement de la medicine clinique moderne en Europe, 1750–1815*. Montreal: Presses de l'Université de Montreal, 2001.

King, Helen. "Female Fluids in the Hippocratic Corpus: How Solid Was the Humoral Body?" In *The Body in Balance*, edited by Peregrine Horden and Elisabeth Hsu, 1st ed., 25–52. New York: Berghahn Books, 2013.

King, Helen. *The One-Sex Body on Trial: The Classical and Early Modern Evidence*. London and New York: Routledge, 2016.

Klein, Joel A. "Alchemical Histories, Chymical Education, and Chymical Medicine in Sixteenth- and Seventeenth-Century Wittenberg." In *Alchimie und Wissenschaft des 16. Jahrhunderts: Fallstudien aus Wittenberg und vergleichbare Befunde. Tagungen des Landesmuseums fur Vorgeschichte Halle*, 15 (2016): 195–204.

Klein, Joel A. "Daniel Sennert and the Chymico-Atomical Reform of Medicine." In *Medicine, Natural Philosophy and Religion in Post-Reformation Scandinavia*, edited by Ole Peter Grell and Andrew Cunningham, 20–37. London and New York: Routledge, 2016.

Klerk, Saskia. "Galen Reconsidered. Studying Drug Properties and the Foundations of Medicine in the Dutch Republic, ca. 1550–1700." PhD. diss. Utrecht University, 2015.

Klerk, Saskia. "The Trouble with Opium. Taste, Reason and Experience in Late Galenic Pharmacology with Special Regard to the University of Leiden, 1575–1625." *Early Science and Medicine* 19 (2014): 287–316.

Klestinec, Cynthia. *Theaters of Anatomy: Students, Teachers, and Traditions of Dissection in Renaissance Venice*. Baltimore: Johns Hopkins, 2011.

Knoeff, Rina. *Herman Boerhaave (1668–1738): Calvinist Chemist and Physician*. Amsterdam: Koninklijke Nederlandse Akademie van Wetenschappen, 2002.

Knoeff, Rina. "Herman Boerhaave at Leiden: Communis Europae Praeceptor." In *Centres of Medical Excellence? Medical Travel and Education in Europe, 1500–1789*, edited by Ole Peter Grell, Andrew Cunningham, and Jon Arrizabalaga, 269–86. Farnham and Burlington: Ashgate, 2010.

Krafft, Fritz. "The Magic Word Chymiatria – and the Attractiveness of Medical Education at Marburg, 1608–1620: A Somewhat Different Reflection on Attendance." In *History of Universities* XXVI/1 (Oxford: Oxford University Press, 2012.): 1–116.

Kroon, Just Emile. *Bijgraden Tot de Geschiedenis van Het Geneeskundig Onderwijs Aan de Leidsche Universiteit 1575–1625*. Leiden: S. C. van Doesburgh, 1911.

Kuhn, Thomas S. "Mathematical vs. Experimental Traditions in the Development of Physical Science." *Journal of Interdisciplinary History* 7 (1976): 1–31.

Kusukawa, Sachiko. *Picturing the Book of Nature: Image, Text, and Argument in Sixteenth-Century Human Anatomy and Medical Botany*. Chicago: University of Chicago Press, 2012.

La Berge, Ann and Caroline Hannaway, eds. *Constructing Paris Medicine*. Amsterdam: Rodopi, 1998.

La Berge, Ann and Caroline Hannaway. "Paris Medicine: Perspectives Past and Present." In *Constructing Paris Medicine*, edited by Ann La Berge and Caroline Hannaway. Amsterdam: Rodopi, 1998.

Laqueur, Thomas. *Making Sex - Body and Gender from the Greeks to Freud*. Cambridge, MA: Harvard UP, 1992.

Levitin, Dmitri. *Ancient Wisdom in the Age of the New Science: Histories of Philosophy in England, c. 1640–1700*. Cambridge: Cambridge University Press, 2015.

Levitin, Dmitri. "Early Modern Experimental Philosophy: A Non-Anglocentric Overview." In *Experiment, Speculation, and Religion in Early Modern Philosophy*, edited by Peter Anstey and Alberto Vanzo, 229–291. New York: Routledge, 2019.

Levitin, Dmitri. "The Experimentalist as Humanist: Robert Boyle on the History of Philosophy." *Annals of Science* 71, no. 2 (2014): 149–182.

Lehoux, Daryn. "Observers, Objects, and the Embedded Eye: Or, Seeing and Knowing in Ptolemy and Galen." *Isis* 98, no. 3 (2007): 447–67.

Leigh, Robert. *On Theriac to Piso, Attributed to Galen: A Critical Edition with Translation and Commentary*. Leiden: Brill, 2016.

Leijenhorst, Cees, and Christoph Lüthy. "The Erosion of Aristotelianism. Confessional Physics in Early Modern Germany and the Dutch Republic." In *The Dynamics of Aristotelian Natural Philosophy from Antiquity to the Seventeenth Century*, edited by Cees Leijenhorst, Christoph Lüthy, and Johannes M.M.H. Thijssen, 375–411. Leiden: Brill, 2002.

Leong, Elaine. *Recipes and Everyday Knowledge: Medicine, Science, and the Household in Early Modern England*. University of Chicago Press, 2018.

Leong, Elaine and Alisha Rankin. "Testing Drugs and Trying Cures." *Special Issue: Bulletin of the History of Medicine* 91, no. 2 (2017): 157–182.

Leong, Elaine and Alisha Rankin, eds., "Testing Drugs and Trying Cures." Special issue, *Bulletin of the History of Medicine* 91 (2017): 157–429.

Lind, L.R. *Studies in Pre-Vesalian Anatomy: Biography, Translations, Documents*. Philadelphia, Pa.: The American Philosophical Society, 1975.

Lindeboom, G. A. *Dutch Medical Biography: A Biographical Dictionary of Dutch Physicians and Surgeons, 1475–1975*. Amsterdam: Rodopi, 1984.

Lindeboom, G. A. *Herman Boerhaave: The Man and His Work*. London: Methuen & Co Ltd, 1968.

Lindemann, Mary. *Medicine and Society in Early Modern Europe*. Second Edition. Cambridge: Cambridge University Press, 2010.

Lloyd, G. E. R. "Experiment in Early Greek Philosophy and Medicine." In *Methods and Problems in Greek Science: Selected Papers*. Cambridge: Cambridge Univ. Press, 1991.

Long, Esmond R. *A History of Pathology*. New York, Dover Publications, 1965.

Long, Pamela O. *Artisan/Practitioners and the Rise of the New Sciences, 1400–1600*. Corvallis, OR: Oregon State University Press, 2014.

Long, Pamela O. *Openness, Secrecy, Authorship: Technical Arts and the Culture of Knowledge from Antiquity to the Renaissance*. Baltimore: Johns Hopkins University Press, 2004.

Lonie, Iain M. "The 'Paris Hippocrates': Teaching and Research at Paris in the Second Half of the Sixteenth Century." In *The Medical Renaissance of the Sixteenth Century*, edited by A. Wear, R. K. French, and I. M. Lonie, 155–174. Cambridge: Cambridge University Press, 1985.

Lopez Piñero, Jose M. and Maria Luz Terrada Ferrandis. "La Obra de Juan Tomas Porcell, 1565, y Los Origines de la Anatomia Patologica Moderna." *Medicina & Historia* 34 (1967): 4–15.

Lunsingh Scheurleer, Th. H. "Un Ampithéâtre d'Anatomie Moralisée." In *Leiden University in the Seventeenth Century: An Exchange of Learning*, edited by Th. H. Lunsingh Scheurleer and G. H. M. Posthumus Meyjes, 217–77. Leiden: University of Leiden Press / E. J. Brill, 1975.

Lunsingh Scheurleer, Th. H. and G. H. M. Posthumus Meyjes, eds. *Leiden University in the Seventeenth Century: And Exchange of Learning*. Leiden: Universitaire Pers Leiden/E. J. Brill, 1975.

Lüthy, Christoph. "An Aristotelian Watchdog as Avant-Garde Physicist: Julius Caesar Scaliger." *The Monist* 84, no. 4 (2001): 542–61.

Lüthy, Christoph. *David Gorlaeus (1591–1612): An Enigmatic Figure in the History of Philosophy and Science*. History of Science and Scholarship in the Netherlands, 13. Amsterdam: Amsterdam University Press, 2012.

Lüthy, Christoph. "The Fourfold Democritus on the Stage of Early Modern Science." *Isis* 91, no. 3 (2000): 443–79.

Luyendijk-Elshout, A. M. "Der Einfluss der italienischen Universitäten auf die medizinische Facultät Leiden." In *Die Renaissance im Blick der Nationen Europas*, edited by Georg Kauffmann, 339–353. Wiesbaden: Harrasowitz, 1991.

Maclean, Ian. "Foucault's Renaissance Episteme Reassessed: An Aristotelian Counterblast." *Journal of the History of Ideas* 59, no. 1 (1998): 149–66.

Maclean, Ian. *Logic, Signs and Nature in the Renaissance*. Cambridge: University of Cambridge Press, 2002.

Maehle, Andreas-Holger. *Drugs on Trial: Experimental Pharmacology and Therapeutic Innovation in the Eighteenth Century*. Leiden: Brill, 1999.

Margócsy, Dániel. *Commercial Visions: Science, Trade, and Visual Culture in the Dutch Golden Age*. Chicago: University of Chicago Press, 2014.

Marr, Alexander, Raphaële Garrod, José Ramón Marcaida, and Richard J. Oosterhoof, eds. *Logodaedalus: Word Histories of Ingenuity in Early Modern Europe*. Pittsburgh: University of Pittsburgh Press, 2018.

Martin, Craig. "With Aristotelians Like These, Who Needs Anti-Aristotelians? Chymical Corpuscular Matter Theory in Niccolò Cabeo's Meteorology." *Early Science and Medicine* 11, no. 2 (January 1, 2006): 135–61.

Mattern, Susan P. *The Prince of Medicine: Galen and the Roman Empire*. Oxford: Oxford University Press, 2013.

Maulitz, Russell. "Pathology." In *The Cambridge History of Science: Volume 6: The Modern Biological and Earth Sciences*, edited by John V. Pickstone and Peter J. Bowler, 6:367–82. The Cambridge History of Science. Cambridge: Cambridge University Press, 2009.

Maulitz, Russell. "The Pathological Tradition." In *Companion Encyclopedia of the History of Medicine*, edited by W. F. Bynum and Roy Porter, 2 vols., vol. 1, 169–191. London and New York: Routledge, 1993.

McVaugh, Michael R. "Determining a Drug's Properties: Medieval Experimental Protocols." In "Testing Drugs and Trying Cures," edited by E. Leong and A. Rankin, *Bulletin of the History of Medicine* (2017): 183–209.

McVaugh, Michael. "Losing Ground: The Disappearance of Attraction from the Kidneys." In *Blood, Sweat and Tears: The Changing Concepts of Physiology From Antiquity into Early Modern Europe*, edited by Manfred Horstmanshoff, Helen King, and Claus Zittel, 103–137. Leiden/Boston: Brill, 2012.

McVaugh, Michael R. "Quantified Medical Theory and Practice at Fourteenth-Century Montpellier." *Bulletin of the History of Medicine*. (1969): 397–413.

McVaugh, Michael R. "The *Experimenta* of Arnau of Vilanova." *Journal of Medieval and Renaissance Studies*. (1971): 107–118.

Meinecke, Bruno. "Consumption (Tuberculosis) in Classical Antiquity." *Annals of Medical History*, 9 (1927): 379–402.

Mikkeli, Heikki. "The Status of the Mechanical Arts in the Aristotelian Classifications of Knowledge in the Early Sixteenth Century." In *Sapientiam Amemus: Humanismus und Aristotelismus in der Reanissance*, edited by Paul Richard Blum, 109–126. Munich: Fink, 1999.

Moes, Robert J., and C. D. O'Malley. "Realdo Colombo: 'On Those Things Rarely Found in Anatomy' An Annotated Translation From the 'De Re Anatomica' (1559)." *Bulletin of the History of Medicine* 34, no. 6 (1960): 508–28.

Molhuysen, P. C., ed. *Bronnen Tot de Geschiedenis Der Leidsche Universiteit*. 7 vols. Rijks Geschiedkundige Publicatiën, nos. 20, 29, 38, 45, 48, 53, and 56. The Hague: Martinus Nijhoff, 1913–1923.

Molhuysen, P. C. and P. J. Blok, eds. *Nieuw Nederlandsch Biographisch Woordenboek.* Leiden: A. W. Sijthoff's Uitgevers-Mattschappij, 1911.

Moran, Bruce T. *Andreas Libavius and the Transformation of Alchemy: Separating Chemical Cultures with Polemical Fire.* Science History Publications/Watson Pub. International, 2007.

Moran, Bruce T. *Chemical Pharmacy Enters the University: Johannes Hartmann and the Didactic Care of Chymiatria in the Early Seventeenth Century.* Madison, Wisconsin: American Institute of the History of Pharmacy, 1991.

Murphy, Hannah. *A New Order of Medicine: The Rise of Physicians in Reformation Nuremberg.* Pittsburgh: University of Pittsburgh Press, 2019.

Nance, Brian K. "Determining the Patient's Temperament: An Excursion into Seventeenth-Century Medical Semeiology." *Bulletin of the History of Medicine* 67, no. 3 (1993): 417–38.

Nasser, M., A. Tibi, and E. Savage-Smith. "Ibn Sina's *Canon of Medicine*: 11th century rules for assessing the effects of drugs." The James Lind Library (www.jameslindlibrary.org). Accessed Monday 23 February 2009.

Nauert, Charles G. "Humanists, Scientists, and Pliny: Changing Approaches to a Classical Author." *The American Historical Review* 84, no. 1 (1979): 72–85.

Newman, William R. *Atoms and Alchemy: Chymistry and the Experimental Origins of the Scientific Revolution.* Chicago: The University of Chicago Press, 2006.

Newman, William R. "Elective Affinity before Geoffroy: Daniel Sennert's Atomistic Explanation of Vinous and Acetous Fermentation." In *Matter and Form in Early Modern Science and Philosophy*, edited by Gideon Manning, 99–124. Leiden: Brill, 2012.

Newman, William R. "From Alchemy to 'Chymistry.'" In *The Cambridge History of Science. Early Modern Science*, edited by Katharine Park and Lorraine Daston, 3:497–517. The Cambridge History of Science. Cambridge: Cambridge University Press, 2006.

Newman, William R. "The Place of Alchemy in the Current Literature on Experiment." In *Experimental Essays—Versuche zum Experiment*, edited by Michael Heidelberger and Friedrich Steinle, 9–33. Baden-Baden: Nomos, 1998.

Newson, Linda A. *Making Medicines in Early Colonial Lima, Peru: Apothecaries, Science and Society.* Leiden: Brill, 2017.

Nicolson, Malcolm. "The Art of Diagnosis: Medicine and the Five Senses." In *Companion Encyclopedia of the History of Medicine*, edited by W. F. Bynum and Roy Porter, 2 vols., vol. 2, 801–825. London and New York: Routledge, 1993.

Niebyl, Peter H. "The Non-Naturals." *Bulletin of the History of Medicine* 45, no. 5 (1971): 486–92.

Nutton, Vivian. "Galen on Theriac: Problems of Authenticity." In *Galen on Pharmacology: Philosophy, History, and Medicine*, edited by Armelle Debru, 133–151. Leiden: Brill, 1997.

Nutton, Vivian. "Greek Science in the Sixteenth-Century Renaissance." In *Renaissance and Revolution: Humanists, Scholars, Craftsmen and Natural Philosophers in Early Modern Europe*, edited by J. V. Field and Frank A. J. L. James, 15–28. Cambridge: Cambridge University Press, 1993.

Nutton, Vivian, ed. *Principles of Anatomy According to the Opinion of Galen by Johann Guinter and Andreas Vesalius*. London and New York: Routledge, 2017.

Nutton, Vivian. "The Reception of Fracastoro's Theory of Contagion: The Seed That Fell among Thorns?" *Osiris* 6 (1990): 196–234.

Nutton, Vivian. "The Rise of Medical Humanism: Ferrara, 1464–1555." *Renaissance Studies* 11, no. 1 (1997): 2–19.

Nutton, Vivian. "The Seeds of Disease: An Explanation of Contagion and Infection from the Greeks to the Renaissance." *Medical History* 27, no. 1 (January 1983): 1–34.

Ogilvie, Brian. *The Science of Describing: Natural History in Renaissance Europe*. Chicago, 2006.

O'Malley, Charles Donald. *Andreas Vesalius of Brussels: 1514–1564*. Berkeley: Los Angeles: Univ. of California Press, 1964.

Otterspeer, Willem. *Groepsportret Met Dame I. Het Bolwerk van de Vrijheid. De Leidse Universiteit 1575–1672*. Amsterdam: Bert Bakker, 2000.

Otterspeer, Willem. *Groepsportret met Dame II. De vesting van de macht. De Leidse Universiteit 1673–1775*. Amsterdam: Bert Bakker, 2002.

Otterspeer, Willem. *The Bastion of Liberty*. Leiden: Leiden University Press, 2008.

Ottoson, Per-Gunnar. *Scholastic Medicine and Philosophy: A Study of Commentaries on Galen's* Tegni (*ca. 1300–1450*). Naples: Bibliopolis, 1984.

Pagel, Walter. "Harvey and Glisson on Irritability with a Note on Van Helmont." *Bulletin of the History of Medicine* 41, no. 6 (1967): 497–514.

Palmer, Richard. "Medical Botany in Northern Italy in the Renaissance." *Journal of the Royal Society of Medicine* 78 (1985): 149–57.

Palmer, Richard. "Pharmacy in the Republic of Venice in the Sixteenth Century." iIn *The Medical Renaissance of the Sixteenth Century*, edited by A. Wear, R. K. French, and I. M. Lonie, 100–117. Cambridge: Cambridge University Press, 1985.

Park, Katharine. *Secrets of Women: Gender, Generation, and the Origins of Human Dissection*. New York: Zone Books, 2010.

Park, Katharine. "The Criminal and the Saintly Body: Autopsy and Dissection in Renaissance Italy." *Renaissance Quarterly* 47, no. 1 (1994): 1–33.

Parke, Emily C. "Flies from Meat and Wasps from Trees: Reevaluating Francesco Redi's Spontaneous Generation Experiments." *Studies in History and Philosophy of Biological and Biomedical Sciences*, 2014, 34–42.

Pasnau, Robert. "Form, Substance, and Mechanism." *The Philosophical Review* 113, no. 1 (2004): 31–88.

Pattison, Mark. *Isaac Casaubon, 1559–1614*. London: Longmans, Green and Co., 1875.

Perler, Dominik. "Faculties in Medieval Philosophy." In *The Faculties: A History*, edited by Dominik Perler, 97–139. Oxford and New York: Oxford University Press, 2015.

Petit, Caroline. "Hippocrates in the Pseudo-Galenic *Introduction*: Or, How was Medicine Taught in Roman Times?" In *Hippocrates and Medical Education*, edited by Manfred Horstmanshoff, in collaboration with Cornelis Van Tilburg, 343–357. Leiden: Brill, 2010.

Pinault, J. R. "How Hippocrates Cured the Plague." *Journal of the History of Medicine and Allied Sciences* 41, no. 1 (January 1986): 52–75.

Pomata, Gianna. "A Word of the Empirics: The Ancient Concept of Observation and Its Recovery in Early Modern Medicine." *Annals of Science* 68, no. 1 (January 1, 2011): 1–25.

Pomata, Gianna. "Observation Rising: Birth of an Epistemic Genre, 1500–1650." In *Histories of Scientific Observation*, edited by Lorraine Daston and Elizabeth Lunbeck, 45–80. University of Chicago Press, 2011.

Pomata. Gianna. "*Praxis Historialis*: The Uses of *Historia* in Early Modern Medicine." In *Historia: Empiricism and Erudition in Early Modern Europe*, edited by Gianna Pomata and Nancy Siraisi. Cambridge, MA: The MIT Press, 2005.

Pomata, Gianna. "Sharing Cases: The *Observationes* in Early Modern Medicine." *Early Science and Medicine* 15, no. 3 (2010): 193–236.

Pomata, Gianna and Nancy Siraisi, eds. *Historia: Empiricism and Erudition in Early Modern Europe*. Cambridge, MA: The MIT Press, 2005

Powers, John C. *Inventing Chemistry: Herman Boerhaave and the Pedagogical Reform of the Chemical Arts*. Chicago: University of Chicago Press, 2012.

Principe, Lawrence M. *The Aspiring Adept: Robert Boyle and His Alchemical Quest*. Princeton: Princeton University Press, 1998.

Principe, Lawrence M. "The Changing Visions of Chymistry at Seventeenth-Century Jena: The Two Brendels, Rolfinck, Wedel, and Others." *Ambix* 68, no. 2–3 (August 2021): 180–97.

Prögler, Daniela. *English Students at Leiden University, 1575–1650: "advancing Your Abilities in Learning and Bettering Your Understanding of the World and State Affairs"*. Farnham: Ashgate, 2013.

Pugliano, Valentina. "Pharmacy, Testing, and the Language of Truth in Renaissance Italy." *Bulletin of the History of Medicine* 91, no. 2 (2017): 233–73.

Ragland, Evan R. "Chymistry and Taste: Franciscus Dele Boë Sylvius as a Chymical Physician Between Galenism and Cartesianism." *Ambix* 59, no. 1 (March 2012).

Ragland. Evan R. "Experimental Clinical Medicine and Drug Action in Mid-Seventeenth-Century Leiden." *Bulletin of the History of Medicine* 91, no. 2 (2017): 331–361.

Ragland, Evan R. "'Making Trials' in Sixteenth- and Early Seventeenth-Century European Academic Medicine." *Isis* 108, no. 3 (2017): 503–28.

Ragland, Evan R. "Mechanism, the Senses, and Reason: Franciscus Sylvius and Leiden Debates Over Anatomical Knowledge After Harvey and Descartes." In *Early Modern*

Medicine and Natural Philosophy, edited by Peter Distelzweig, Benjamin Goldberg, and Evan R. Ragland, 173–205. Dordrecht: Springer, 2016.

Ragland, Evan R. "Reading Galileo in Conversation with Other Scholars." *Early Science and Medicine* 23, no. 3 (August 25, 2018): 265–77.

Ragland, Evan R. "The Contested *Ingenia* of Early Modern Anatomy." In *Ingenuity in the Making: Matter and Technique in Early Modern Europe*, edited by Richard J. Oosterhoff, José Ramón Marcaida, and Alexander Marr, 112–130. Pittsburgh: University of Pittsburgh Press, 2021.

Randall, J. H. *The School of Padua and the Emergence of Modern Science*. Padua: Editrice Antenore, 1961.

Rankin, Alisha. "Of Antidote and Anecdote: Poison Trials in Sixteenth-Century Europe." *Bulletin of the History of Medicine*, 91, no. 2 (2017): 274–302.

Rankin, Alisha. *Panaceia's Daughters: Noblewomen as Healers in Early Modern Germany*. Chicago: Univ. Chicago Press, 2013.

Rankin, Alisha. *The Poison Trials: Wonder Drugs, Experiment, and the Battle for Authority in Renaissance Science*. University of Chicago Press, 2021.

Raphael, Renée. *Reading Galileo: Scribal Technologies and the Two New Sciences*. Baltimore: Johns Hopkins University Press, 2017.

Reeds, Karen. *Botany in Medieval and Renaissance Universities*. New York: Garland, 1991.

Rey, Roselyne. "Diagnostic différentiel et espèces nosologiques: le cas de la phtisie pulmonaire de Morgagni à Bayle." In *Maladies, médicines et sociéties: approches historiques pour le présent, Actes du Vie colloque d'histoire au présent*, edited by François-Olivier Touati, 185–200. Paris: L'Harmattan, 1993.

Riese, Walther. *The Conception of Disease: Its History, Its Versions and Its Nature*. New York: Philosophical Library, 1953.

Rinaldi, Massimo. "Organising Pathological Knowledge: Théophile Bonet's Sepulchretum and the Making of a Tradition." In *Pathology in Practice*, edited by Silvia De Renzi, Marco Bresadola, and Maria Conforti, 39–55. Abingdon and New York: Routledge, 2018.

Roberts, Benjamin B. *Sex and Drugs before Rock 'n' Roll: Youth Culture and Masculinity during Holland's Golden Age*. Amsterdam University Press, 2012.

Robichaud, Denis J.-J. "Ficino on Force, Magic, and Prayers: Neoplatonic and Hermetic Influences in Ficino's Three Books on Life." *Renaissance Quarterly*, no. 70 (2017): 44–87.

Robison, Kira. *Healers in the Making: Students, Physicians, and Medical Education in Medieval Bologna (1250–1550)*. Leiden and Boston: Brill, 2021.

Rossi, Paolo. *Francis Bacon: From Magic to Science*. Chicago: Univ. Chicago Press, 1968.

Ruestow, Edward G. *Physics at Seventeenth and Eighteenth-Century Leiden: Philosophy and the New Science in the University*. The Hague: Martinus Nijhoff, 1973.

Sabra, A. I. *The Optics of Ibn Al-Haytham, Books I–III: On Direct Vision*. 2 vols. London: Warburg Institute, 1989.

Santing, Catrien. "Spreken vanuit het graf. De stoffelijke resten van Willem van Oranje in hun politiek-culturele betekenis." *Bijdragen en Mededelingen betreffende de Geschiedenis der Nederlanden* (2003): 181–207.

Savoia, Paolo. "Skills, Knowledge, and Status: The Career of an Early Modern Italian Surgeon." *Bulletin of the History of Medicine* 93, no. 1 (2019): 27–54.

Sawday, Jonathan. *The Body Emblazoned: Dissection and the Human Body in Renaissance Culture*. London; New York: Routledge, 1994.

Scarborough, John, and Vivian Nutton. "The Preface of Dioscorides' Materia Medica: Introduction, Translation, and Commentary." *Transactions and Studies of the College of Physicians of Philadelphia* IV (1982): 187–227.

Schickore, Jutta. *About Method: Experimenters, Snake Venom, and the History of Writing Scientifically*. Chicago and London: University of Chicago Press, 2017.

Schiefsky, Mark J. *Hippocrates 'On Ancient Medicine': Translated with Introduction and Commentary*. Brill: Leiden, 2005.

Schlegelmilch, Ulrich. "Andreas Hiltebrands Protokoll eines Disputationscollegiums zur Physiologie und Pathologie (Leiden 1604)." In *Frühneuzeitliche Disputationen: Polyvalente Produktionsapparate gelerhten Wissens*, edited by Marion Gindhart, Hanspeter Marti, and Robert Seidel, 49–88. Köln, Weimar, Vienna: Böhlau, 2016.

Schmitt, Charles B. "Aristotle Among the Physicians." In *The Medical Renaissance of the Sixteenth Century*, edited by A. Wear, R. K. French, and I. M. Lonie, 1–16. Cambridge: Cambridge University Press, 1985.

Schmitt, Charles B. "Experience and Experiment: A Comparison of Zabarella's View with Galileo's in *De Motu*." *Studies in the Renaissance* 16 (1969): 80–138.

Schouten, J. *Johannes Walaeus: Zijn Betekenis Voor de Verbreiding van de Leer van de Bloedsomloop*. Assen: Van Gorcum, 1972.

Schullian, Dorothy M. "Coiter, Volcher." In *Complete Dictionary of Scientific Biography*, 342–343. Vol. 3. Detroit, MI. Charles Scribner's Sons (2008): 342–343.

Shackelford, Jole. *A Philosophical Path for Paracelsian Medicine: The Ideas, Intellectual Context, and Influence of Petrus Sevirinus (1540/2–1602)*. Copenhagen: Museum Tusculanum Press, 2004.

Shackelford, Jole. "Documenting the Factual and the Artifactual: Ole Worm and Public Knowledge." *Endeavour* 23 (1999): 65–71.

Shank, Michael H. "From Galen's Ureters to Harvey's Veins." *Journal of the History of Biology* 18, no. 3 (1985): 331–35.

Shapin, Steven. *A Social History of Truth: Civility and Science in Seventeenth-Century England*. Chicago: University of Chicago Press, 1994.

Shapin, Steven, and Simon Schaffer. *Leviathan and the Air-Pump: Hobbes, Boyle, and the Experimental Life*. Princeton: Princeton University Press, 1985.

Shotwell, R. Allen. "Animals, Pictures, and Skeletons: Andreas Vesalius's Reinvention of the Public Anatomy Lesson." *Journal of the History of Medicine and Allied Sciences* 71 (2015): 1–18.

Shotwell, R. Allen. "The Great Pox and the Surgeon's Role in the Sixteenth Century." *Journal of the History of Medicine and Allied Sciences*, 72 (2016): 21–33.

Shotwell, R. Allen. "The Revival of Vivisection in the Sixteenth Century." *Journal of the History of Biology* 46, no. 2 (2013): 171–97.

Singer, P. N. "Galen." *The Stanford Encyclopedia of Philosophy*. Winter 2021 Edition. Edward N. Zalta, ed. https://plato.stanford.edu/archives/win2021/entries/galen/.

Singer, P. N., editor and translator. *Galen: Selected Works*. Oxford and New York: Oxford University Press, 1997.

Singer, P. N. "Levels of Explanation in Galen." *The Classical Quarterly* 47, no. 2 (1997): 525–42.

Siraisi, Nancy. *Avicenna in Renaissance Italy: The Canon and Medical Teaching in Italian Universities after 1500*. Princeton: Princeton University Press, 1987.

Siraisi, Nancy. "Disease and symptom as problematic concepts in Renaissance medicine." In *Res et Verba in der Renaissance*, edited by Eckhard Kessler and Ian Maclean, 217–240. Wiesbaden: Harrasowitz Verlag, 2002.

Siraisi, Nancy. "Giovanni Argenterio and Sixteenth-Century Medical Innovation: Between Princely Patronage and Academic Controversy." *Osiris* 6 (1990): 161–80.

Siraisi, Nancy. "Historia, actio, utilitas: Fabrici e le scienz della vita nel Cinquecento." In *Il Teatro dei Corpi: Le Pitture Colorate D'Anatomia di Girolamo Fabrici D'Acquapendente*, edited by Maurizio Rippa Bonati and Jose Pardo-Tomas, 63–73. Milan: Mediamed Edizioni Scientifiche Srl., 2004.

Siraisi, Nancy. "Medicine, 1450–1620, and the History of Science." *Isis* 103, no. 3 (2012): 491–514.

Siraisi, Nancy. *Medicine and the Italian Universities, 1250–1600*. Leiden: Brill, 2001.

Siraisi, Nancy. *Medieval and Early Renaissance Medicine: An Introduction to Knowledge and Practice*. Chicago: University of Chicago Press, 2009.

Siraisi, Nancy. *Taddeo Alderotti and his Pupils: Two Generations of Italian Medical Learning*. Princeton, N.J.: Princeton University Press, 1981.

Siraisi, Nancy. *The Clock and the Mirror: Girolamo Cardano and Renaissance Medicine*. Princeton: Princeton University Press, 1997.

Siraisi, Nancy. "Vesalius and Human Diversity in De Humani Corporis Fabrica." *Journal of the Warburg and Courtauld Institutes* 57 (1994): 60–88.

Skaarup, Bjørn Okholm. *Anatomy and Anatomists in Early Modern Spain*. Farnham, Surrey and Burlington, VT: Ashgate, 2015.

Smith, Pamela H. *The Body of the Artisan: Art and Experience in the Scientific Revolution*. Chicago: The University of Chicago Press, 2004.

Spronsen, J. W. "The Beginning of Chemistry." In *Leiden University in the Seventeenth Century: An Exchange of Learning*, edited by Th. H. Lunsingh Scheurleer and G. H. M. Posthumus Meyjes, 328–349. Leiden: University of Leiden Press / E. J. Brill, 1975.

Stanglin, Keith D. *Arminius on the Assurance of Salvation: The Context, Roots, and Shape of the Leiden Debate, 1603–1609*. Leiden: Brill, 2007.

Steinle, Friedrich, Cesare Pastorino, and Evan R. Ragland. "Experiment in Renaissance Science." *Encyclopedia of Renaissance Philosophy*, edited by Marco Sgarbi. Springer, 2019.

Stolberg, Michael. "A Woman Down to Her Bones: The Anatomy of Sexual Difference in the Sixteenth and Early Seventeenth Centuries." *Isis* 94, no. 2 (2003): 274–99.

Stolberg, Michael. "Bedside Teaching and the Acquisition of Practical Skills in Mid-Sixteenth-Century Padua." *Journal of the History of Medicine and Allied Sciences* (2014): 633–64.

Stolberg, Michael. "Empiricism in Sixteenth-Century Medical Practice: The Notebooks of Georg Handsch." *Early Science and Medicine*, 18m no. 6 (2013), 487–516.

Stolberg, Michael. *Experiencing Illness and the Sick Body in Early Modern Europe*. Basingstoke: Palgrave Macmillan, 2014.

Stolberg, Michael. "Learning from the Common Folks. Academic Physicians and Medical Lay Culture in the Sixteenth Century." *Social History of Medicine* 27, no. 4 (2014): 649–67.

Stolberg, Michael. "Post-Mortems, Anatomical Dissections and Humoral Pathology in the Sixteenth and Early Seventeenth Centuries." In *Pathology in Practice*, edited by Silvia De Renzi, Marco Bresadola, and Maria Conforti, 79–95. Abingdon and New York: Routledge, 2018.

Stolberg, Michael. "Teaching Anatomy in Post-Vesalian Padua: An Analysis of Student Notes." *Journal of Medieval and Early Modern Studies* 48, no. 1 (January 1, 2018): 61–78.

Stolberg, Michael. *Uroscopy in Early Modern Europe*. Translated by Logan Kennedy and Leonhard Unglaub. Farnham, Surrey: Ashgate, 2015.

Stroup, Alice. *A Company of Scientists: Botany, Patronage, and Community at the Seventeenth-Century Parisian Royal Academy of Sciences*. Berkeley: University of California Press, 1990.

Struik, Dirk J. "Ceulen, Ludolph van." In *Complete Dictionary of Scientific Biography*. Vol. 3. Detroit, MI: Charles Scribner's Sons, 2008.

Swan, Claudia. *Art, Science, and Witchcraft in Early Modern Holland: Jacques de Gheyn, 1565–1629*. Cambridge: Cambridge University Press, 2005.

Teigen, Philip M. "Taste and Quality in 15th- and 16th- Century Galenic Pharmacology." *Pharmacy in History* 29, no. 2 (1987): 60–68.

Temkin, Owsei. *Galenism: Rise and Decline of a Medical Philosophy*. Ithaca: Cornell University Press, 1973.

Temkin, Owsei. "The Classical Roots of Glisson's Doctrine of Irritation." *Bulletin of the History of Medicine* 38, no. 4 (1964): 297–328.

Temkin, Owsei. "The Scientific Approach to Disease: Specific Entity and Individual Sickness." In *The Double Face of Janus and Other Essays in the History of Medicine*, 41–455. Baltimore: Johns Hopkins University Press, 1977.

Thorndike, Lynn. *A History of Magic and Experimental Science*, 8 vols. New York: Columbia Univ. Press, 1923–1958.

Tieleman, Teun. "Galen on the Seat of the Intellect: Anatomical Experiment and Philosophical Tradition." In *Science and Mathematics in Ancient Greek Culture*, edited by C. J.Tuplin and T. E. Rihil, 257–273. Oxford: Oxford University Press, 2002.

Tjon Sie Fat, Leslie. "Clusius' Garden: A Reconstruction." In *The Authentic Garden: A Symposium on Gardens*, edited by Leslie Tjon Sie fat and Erik de Jong, 3–12. Leiden: Clusius Foundation, 1991.

Touwaide, Alain. "Therapeutic Strategies: Drugs." In *Western Medical Thought from Antiquity to the Middle Ages*, edited by Mirko D. Grmek, translated by Antony Shugaar, 259–72, 266. Cambridge, MA: Harvard University Press, 1998.

Tracy, Theodore, S.J. "Heart and Soul in Aristotle." In *Essays in Ancient Greek Philosophy*, edited by John Anton and Anthony Preus, 321–339. Albany: SUNY Press, 1983.

Van Berkel, Klaas. *Citaten uit het boek der natuur*. Amsterdam: Bert Bakker, 1998.

Van Berkel, Klaas. *Isaac Beeckman on Matter and Motion*. Baltimore: Johns Hopkins, 2013.

Van Berkel, Klaas. "The Dutch Republic: Laboratory of the Scientific Revolution." *BMGN-Low Countries Historical Review* 125 (2010): 81–105.

Van Berkel, Klaas, Albert van Helden, and Lodewijk Palm, eds. *A History of Science in the Netherlands: Survey, Themes and Reference*. Leiden: Brill, 1999.

Van Bunge, Wiep. *From Stevin to Spinoza: An Essay on Philosophy in the Seventeenth-Century Dutch Republic*. Leiden: Brill, 2001.

Van der Eijk, Philip. *Medicine and Philosophy in Classical Antiquity: Doctors and Philosophers on Nature, Soul, Health, and Disease*. Cambridge: Cambridge University Press, 2005.

Van Gemert, Lia. "Johan van Beverwijck Als 'Instituut.'" *De Zeventiende Eeuw* 8 (1992): 99–106.

Van Lieburg, Marius. "The Early Reception of Harvey's Theory on Bloodcirculation in the Netherlands," *Histoire des sciences médicales*, no. 17 (1982): 102–105

Van Maanen, R. C. J. "De Leidse bevolkingsaantallen in de 16de en 17de eeuw. Enkele kanttekeningen," *Leids Jaarboekje voor geschiedenis en oudheidkunde van Leiden en omstreken*, 101 (2009): 41–70.

Van Miert, Dirk. *Humanism in an Age of Science: The Amsterdam Athenaeum in the Golden Age, 1632–1704*. Leiden: Brill, 2009.

Ventura, Iolanda. "Galenic Pharmacology in the Middle Ages: Galen's *On the Capacities of Simple Drugs* and its Reception between the Sixth and Fourteenth Century." In *Brill's Companion to the Reception of Galen*, edited by Petros Bouras-Vallianatos and Barbara Zipser, 393–433. Leiden: Brill, 2019.

Verbeek, Theo. *Descartes and the Dutch: Early Reactions to Cartesian Philosophy, 1637–1650*. Carbondale: Southern Illinois University Press, 1991.

Vermij, Rienk. *The Calvinist Copernicans: The New Astronomy and the Dutch Republic*. Amsterdam: Koninklijke Nederlandse Akademie van Wetenschappen, 2002.

Vogt, Sabine. "Drugs and Pharmacology." In *The Cambridge Companion to Galen*, edited by R. J. Hankinson, 304–22. Cambridge Companions to Philosophy. Cambridge: Cambridge University Press, 2008.

Vollgraff, J. A. "Snellius' Notes on the Reflection and Refraction of Rays." *Osiris* 1 (1936): 718–725.

Von Staden, Heinrich. "Experiment and Experience in Hellenistic Medicine." *Bulletin of the Institute of Classical Studies* 22 (1975): 178–199.

Von Staden, Heinrich. *Herophilus: The Art of Medicine in Early Alexandria: Edition, Translation and Essays*. Cambridge University Press, 1989.

Von Staden, Heinrich. "Teleology and Mechanism: Aristotelian Biology and Early Hellenistic Medicine." In *Aristotelische Biologie: Intentionen, Methoden, Ergebnisse*, edited by Wolfgang Kullman and Sabine Föllinger, 183–208. Stuttgart: Franz Steiner, 1997.

Von Staden, Heinrich. "The Discovery of the Body: Human Dissection and Its Cultural Contexts in Ancient Greece." *The Yale Journal of Biology and Medicine* 65 (1992): 223–41.

Wall, Cecil. *A History of of the Worshipful Society of Apothecaries of London, vol. 1: 1617–1815*, edited by H. C. Cameron and E. A. Underwood. Oxford: Oxford University Press, 1963.

Wear, Andrew. "Explorations in Renaissance Writings on the Practice of Medicine." In *The Medical Renaissance of the Sixteenth Century*, edited by A. Wear, R. K. French, and I. M. Lonie, 118–45. Cambridge: Cambridge University Press, 1985.

Wear, Andrew. *Knowledge and Practice in English Medicine, 1550–1680*. Cambridge: Cambridge University Press, 2000.

Wesdorp, I.C.E. "The Physician Dr. Nicolaes Tulp." In *Nicolaes Tulp: The Life and Work of an Amsterdam Physician and Magistrate in the 17th Century*, edited by S.A.C. Dudok van Heel et al. Second Edition. Amsterdam: Six Art Promotion Bv., 1998.

Wiesenfeldt, Gerhardt. *Leerer Raum in Minervas Haus. Experimentelle Naturlehre an Der Universität Leiden, 1675–1715*. Amsterdam: Royal Netherlands Academy of Arts and Sciences, 2004.

Wilson, Adrian. "On the History of Disease-Concepts: The Case of Pleurisy." *History of Science* 38 (2000): 271–319.

Wilson, Margaret D. "History of Philosophy in Philosophy Today; and the Case of the Sensible Qualities." *The Philosophical Review* 101, no. 1 (1992): 191–243.

Wightman, William P. D. "'Quid Sit Methodus?' 'Method' in Sixteenth Century Medical Teaching and 'Discovery.'" *Journal of the History of Medicine and Allied Sciences* 19, no. 4 (1964): 360–76.

Winterbottom, Anne E. "Of the China Root: A Case Study of the Early Modern Circulation of Materia Medica." *Social History of Medicine* 28 (2014): 22–44.

Zanello, Marc *et al.*, "The Death of Henry II, King of France (1519–1559). From Myth to Medical and Historical Fact." *Acta Neurochirurgica* (2014)

Zilsel, Edgar. "The Sociological Roots of Science." *American Journal of Sociology* 47 (1942): 544–562.

Index

Page numbers in italics refer to figures.